Digital Radiography

An Introduction

Euclid Seeram, RT(R), BSc, MSc, FCAMRT

Medical Imaging Degree Studies

British Columbia Institute of Technology

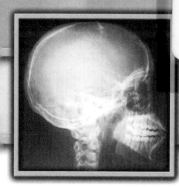
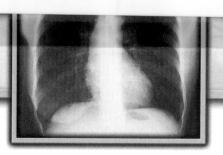
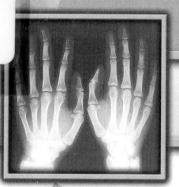

DELMAR
CENGAGE Learning

Australia • Brazil • Japan • Korea • Mexico • Singapore • Spain • United Kingdom • United States

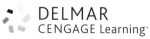

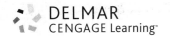

DELMAR
CENGAGE Learning

Digital Radiography: An Introduction

Euclid Seeram

Vice President, Career and Professional Editorial: Dave Garza

Director of Learning Solutions: Matthew Kane

Senior Acquisitions Editor: Sherry Dickinson

Managing Editor: Marah Bellegarde

Product Manager: Natalie Pashoukos

Editorial Assistant: Anthony Souza

Vice President, Career and Professional Marketing: Jennifer Ann Baker

Marketing Director: Wendy Mapstone

Senior Marketing Manager: Michelle McTighe

Marketing Coordinator: Erica Ropitzky

Production Director: Carolyn Miller

Production Manager: Andrew Crouth

Senior Content Project Manager: Kenneth McGrath

Senior Art Director: David Arsenault

> For product information and technology assistance, contact us at
> **Cengage Learning Customer & Sales Support, 1-800-354-9706**
> For permission to use material from this text or product,
> submit all requests online at **www.cengage.com/permissions**
> Further permissions questions can be emailed to
> **permissionrequest@cengage.com**

Library of Congress Control Number: 2009937308

ISBN-13: 978-1-4018-8999-9

ISBN-10: 1-4018-8999-9

Delmar
Executive Woods
5 Maxwell Drive
Clifton Park, NY 12065
USA

Cengage Learning is a leading provider of customized learning solutions with office locations around the globe, including Singapore, the United Kingdom, Australia, Mexico, Brazil, and Japan. Locate your local office at **www.cengage.com/global**

Cengage Learning products are represented in Canada by Nelson Education, Ltd.

To learn more about Delmar, visit **www.cengage.com/delmar**

Purchase any of our products at your local bookstore or at our preferred online store **www.CengageBrain.com**

Notice to the Reader

Printed in the United States of America
1 2 3 4 5 XX 11 10 09

This book is dedicated with love and sincere appreciation to my lovely wife Trish, the cutest Chaplain I know, and to our son Dave and daughter-in-law Priscilla, two wise and caring young people.

CONTENTS

Digital radiography, as expected, has taken over from screen-film radiography in the medical imaging world. It is the most common imaging examination in medicine and still at the forefront of patient diagnosis in the highly technological imaging world of computed tomography, magnetic resonance imaging, diagnostic ultrasound, positron emission tomography and other complex imaging modalities. Digital radiographs need complex image processing to enable clinicians to fully visualize image detail. These digital images must be able to be stored, are often transmitted from location to location and the digital imaging technologies must meet quality standards to fulfill the diagnostic requirements for the patient's benefit.

There is a real need for radiologic technologists/radiographers and radiologists to understand the physical principles and technical details of digital radiography imaging systems. Such systems include computed radiography, flat-panel digital systems, digital fluoroscopy and digital mammography. This text provides an insight and an understanding of these imaging modalities. It goes further to put the acquisition of these images in context of the digital environment through an explanation of the basic digital image processing, image storage and transmission and explains the process of quality control in digital radiography.

The name Euclid Seeram has become synonymous with radiography education. Euclid has decades of experience in the teaching of medical imaging sciences and particularly in CT. During this time he has gained world-wide respect as an educator. In this text Euclid has sought and gained input from other experienced people in the field of digital radiography such as **Charles E Willis, PhD., DABR,** Associate Professor, Department of Imaging Physics, The University of Texas MD Anderson Cancer Center, Houston, Texas; and **Barry Burns, MS., RT(R)., DABR,** Professor, Division of Radiologic Science, School of Medicine, University of North Carolina, Chapel Hill, North Carolina. Their experience and knowledge have added to the depth and quality of treatment of the digital radiography topics.

Euclid has the gift of being able to explain difficult concepts in a way that students can grasp. This has been seen in his other texts such as his well-known text *Computed Tomography—Physical Principles, Clinical Applications & Quality Control.* This book continues in this tradition and makes complex concepts easier to understand.

Students will appreciate the detail, ease of explanation and depth and breadth of the treatment of the topics in digital radiography.

Furthermore Euclid has demonstrated a continual quest for knowledge in the medical imaging sciences field via his numerous lifelong education pursuits. Having completed courses in digital radiography from several notable experts in the field as well as a course on medical imaging informatics from Stanford University, Euclid is willing to share this knowledge with the imaging community. These efforts continue to make him a successful author and educator.

For those studying in the field of medical imaging or for those just wishing to gain a high level appreciation of digital radiography, we highly recommend this book.

Another great text by a great educator.

Rob Davidson, PhD, MAppSc (MI), BBus, FIR
Associate Professor
Head, Discipline of Medical Radiations
RMIT University
Melbourne, Australia

and

Stewart C. Bushong, Sc.D., FAAPM, FACR
Professor of Radiologic Science
One Baylor Plaza
Houston, Texas

The motivation for writing this book stems from the continued technical evolution of digital radiographic imaging systems; picture archiving and communication systems (PACS) and the growth of what is popularly referred to as medical imaging informatics; and more importantly, the lack of textbooks on this subject for radiologic technologists.

The continued evolution of these digital radiographic imaging systems is marked by the refinement of current physical principles, the introduction of new technologies and the development of engineering tools to make these imaging devices perform at optimum levels to meet the needs of various clinical imaging requirements. Notable technical developments for example include the introduction of digital mammography systems and the continued evolution of digital image processing, both pre-processing and post-processing software for digital radiography, and quality control tools and procedures for digital radiography imaging systems.

Purpose

The purpose of this textbook is four-fold as follows:

1. To provide comprehensive coverage of the physical principles of digital radiography imaging systems and associated technologies, such as PACS and medical imaging informatics

2. To lay the theoretical foundations necessary for the effective use of digital radiography in clinical practice

3. To enhance communication among radiology personnel such as technologists, radiologists, medical physicists, biomedical engineers, and between radiology personnel and vendors

4. To meet the educational requirements of various radiologic technology professional organizations including the American Society of Radiologic Technologists, the American Registry for Radiologic Technologists, the Canadian Association of Medical Radiation Technologists, the College of Radiographers in the United Kingdom, as well as those in Africa, Asia, Australia, and continental Europe.

Content and Organization

The content and organization of the book are based on the following structure:

- Brief historical developments of digital radiography imaging systems
- Digital image processing fundamentals
- Physical principles and technological aspects of digital radiography imaging modalities
- Effective use of technologies that are integral components of digital imaging systems, such as for example, PACS, medical imaging informatics and Quality Control procedures

CHAPTER 1 presents an overview of the technologies that constitute the subject matter of this book including a discussion of the limitations of film-based radiography and the major structural components of digital radiography imaging systems as well as brief description of the image acquisition detectors, PACS, and medical imaging informatics.

CHAPTER 2 provides a detailed description of the topic of digital image processing, a topic that is of particular importance in today's digital clinical imaging practice.

CHAPTER 3 deals with the basic physics and technology of Computed Radiography (CR) and describes specifically, the physics of photostimulable luminescence, CR technical components, image processing, exposure control in CR, image quality descriptors for CR, and presents an overview of artefacts. Finally the chapter concludes with a brief introduction of selected quality control tests for CR, using quality criteria for assessment.

CHAPTER 4 addresses the effective use of computed radiography imaging equipment in clinical practice. It addresses the causes of sub-optimal images, selection of technical factors, and other considerations.

CHAPTER 5 is devoted to flat-panel digital radiography imaging systems and includes a description of the different types of flat-panel digital imaging systems, design characteristics, operating principles, image processing and imaging performance characteristics such as spatial resolution, modulation transfer function, dynamic range, detective quantum efficiency, image lag and image artifacts.

CHAPTER 6 provides a description of the technical aspects and image processing for digital fluoroscopy systems, based on image intensifiers and flat-panel digital detectors, as well as the fundamental physical principles of digital subtraction angiography.

CHAPTER 7 describes the essential technological aspects of digital mammography. Topics include types of detectors, digital image processing, and various applications such as digital tomosynthesis, and computer-aided detection and diagnosis for example.

CHAPTER 8 deals with the major components and core technologies of PACS in detail followed by an outline of the bare essentials of information systems and communication standards for digital radiology, including DICOM (Digital Imaging and Communications in Medicine), HL-7 (Health Level-7), and the technical framework of IHE (Integrating the Health Care Enterprise).

CHAPTER 9 outlines the major components of medical imaging informatics, an evolving field for the digital radiography community. Examples of these components include health information systems, the electronic health record, systems integration, information technology (IT) security fundamentals, and the skills and certification of a PACS technologist.

CHAPTER 10, presents a detailed description of the elements of quality control (QC) in digital radiography. Topics described include components of QC, a definition of "Quality," understanding processes and errors in digital radiography, responsibilities for digital radiography QC, and an overview of digital mammography QC.

Features

Each chapter begins with Objectives and a list of Key Terms to help the reader identify important concepts they need to learn. Illustrations and photographs throughout the book reinforce and enhance learning and retention of material. Chapters conclude with review questions, which provide readers with an opportunity to check their learning progress. Definitions for the key terms and concepts can be found in the glossary at the end of the book.

Use and Scope

The purpose of this comprehensive text is to meet the wide and varied requirements of its users, students and educators alike. Therefore this book can meet many different educational and program needs. *Digital Radiography-An Introduction* can be used as the primary text for introductory digital imaging courses at the diploma, associate, and baccalaureate degree levels. Additionally, it can be used as a resource for continuing education programs; it functions as a reference text for other technical professionals working in radiology. Finally it provides the required overview of the physical principles and technological considerations, and may be viewed as providing the needed prerequisites for graduate-level (Master's Degree) courses in Digital Radiography.

The content is intended to meet the educational requirements of various radiologic technology professional associations including the American Society of Radiologic Technologists, the American Registry for Radiologic Technologists, the Canadian Association of Medical Radiation Technologists, the College of Radiographers in the United Kingdom, as well as those in Africa, Asia, Australia, and continental Europe.

Digital Radiography has become an integral part of the education of radiologic technologists and related professionals who play a significant role in the care and management of patients undergoing both routine and other sophisticated imaging procedures.

Enjoy the pages that follow and remember that with your knowledge and skills in digital radiography, your patients will benefit from your wisdom.

Euclid Seeram, RT(R), BSc, MSc, FCAMRT
British Columbia, Canada

ACKNOWLEDGMENTS

The single most important and satisfying task in writing a book of this nature is to acknowledge the help and encouragement of those individuals who perceive the value of its contribution to the medical imaging sciences literature. It is indeed a pleasure to express sincere thanks to several individuals whose time and efforts have contributed tremendously to this book.

First and foremost, I must thank my two contributors who gave their time and expertise to write Chapters 4 and 10 in this book. I am indebted to Dr Charles Willis, PhD, Department of Imaging Physics, University of Texas MD Anderson Cancer Center, Houston, Texas; and to Barry Burns, MS, Division of Radiologic Science, School of Medicine, University of North Carolina, Chapel Hill, North Carolina. Furthermore I am grateful to my good friend and colleague Anthony Chan, MEng, MSc, PEng, CEng, CCE, at the British Columbia Institute of Technology (BCIT) and Canadian award-winning Biomedical Engineer who provided good explanations of the engineering aspects of making digital detectors and other technical aspects of PACS, such as DICOM and HL-7. In addition, I must also thank Bruno Jaggi, DiplT, BASc, MASc, PEng, an expert Biomedical Engineer at BCIT whose course and regular discussions on digital image processing provided me with the theoretical background for a better understanding image post processing operations.

The content of this book is built around the works and expertise of several noted medical physicists, radiologists, computer scientists, and biomedical engineers who have done the original research. In reality, they are the tacit authors of this text, and I am truly grateful to all of them. In this regard, I owe a good deal of thanks to Dr Anthony Siebert, PhD of the University of California at Davis, and Dr Charles Willis, PhD, The University of Texas, MD Anderson Cancer Center; two expert physicists in Digital Radiography and from whom I have learned the physics and technical aspects of digital radiography through their seminars and workshops that I have attended. Furthermore I am also grateful to several other physicists from whom I have learned much about digital imaging physics through their published writings. These include Dr Perry Sprawls, PhD (Emory University); Dr Kerry Krugh, PhD (Medical Physicist, The Toledo Hospital, Toledo, Ohio); Dr John Yorkston, PhD (Senior Research Scientist, Clinical Applications Research, Carestream Health Inc. Rochester, NY); Dr Martin Spahn, PhD (Siemens AG, Medical Solutions); Dr Ehsan Samei, PhD (Medical Physicist and Associate Professor at Duke University); Dr Beth Schueler, PhD (Medical Physicist, Mayo Clinic); and Jeff Shepard, MS (Senior Medical Physicist, MD Anderson Cancer Center). One more medical physicist to whom I owe thanks is Dr John Aldrich, PhD, Vancouver General Hospital, University of British Columbia, whose seminars on digital radiography and other topics, have taught me quite a bit. Thanks John.

Additionally, I must acknowledge the efforts of all the individuals from Digital Radiography vendors who have assisted me generously with technical details and photographs of their systems for use in the book. In particular, I am grateful to Lew Potts of Fuji Medical Systems; David Robitalle of Konica-Minolta; Dr Ralph Schaetzing, PhD of Agfa Healthcare (Belgium); and Richard Weisfield, PhD from dpiX, LLC, Palo Alto, (USA). Thanks so much for this assistance. These vendors are acknowledged in the respective figure legends.

In this book I have used several illustrations and quotes from original papers published in the professional literature and I am indeed thankful to all the publishers and the authors (such as A Seibert, PhD; Charles Willis, PhD; Ehsan Samei, PhD; Yorkson, PhD, for example) who have done the original work, and have provided me with permission to reproduce them in this textbook. I have purposefully used several quotes so as not to detract from the authors' original meaning. I personally believe that these quotes and illustrations have added significantly to the clarity of the explanations. In this regard, I am appreciative of the Radiological Society of North America (RSNA) for use of materials from *Radiographics* and *Radiology*; Springer Science and Business Media, for materials from *European Radiology*; the American Association of Physicists in Medicine (AAPM), for materials from *Medical Physics*; Wiley-Blackwell Publishers Inc., for materials from *Australian Radiology*, and the British Institute of Radiology for materials from the *British Journal of Radiology*. Furthermore, *Radiologic Technology* (Journal of the American Society of Radiologic Technologists) and the *Indian Journal of Radiology and Imaging* were helpful with other information and I am grateful to the editors. There are several Radiologists who graciously gave of the permission as well and I would like to list some of their names here; Dr J Park, MD and Dr M Korner, MD; and Dr E Siegel, MD; and Dr B Reiner, MD.

Additionally, I must acknowledge the work of the several reviewers of this book (listed on a separate page) who offered constructive comments to help improve the quality of the chapters. Their efforts are very much appreciated.

The people at Delmar, Cengage Learning deserve special thanks for their hard work, encouragement and support of this project. They are Natalie Pashoukos, product manager, who did significant prior work on the chapters as they were submitted, and who also provided me with the encouragement that kept me on track in meeting deadlines. Additionally, Sherry Dickinson, senior acquisitions editor, provided support to bring this work to fruition. I must also thank the individuals in the production department at Cengage Learning for doing a wonderful job on the manuscript to bring it to its final form. In particular, I am grateful to Sathyabama Kumaran, Project Manager (PreMedia Global) in Chennai, India, and her production team, who have worked exceptionally hard during the production of this book, especially in the copyediting and page-proof stages.

Finally, my family deserves special mention for their love, support, and encouragement while I worked into the evenings on the manuscript. I appreciate the efforts of my lovely wife, Trish, a warm, caring and overall special person in my life; our son David, a brilliant young editor and publisher of his own online digital photography magazine called *PhotographyBB* (available at Photographybb.com) that has a world-wide audience, and our beautiful daughter-in-law, Priscilla, a smart, remarkable and caring young woman, and who is also responsible for the design of *PhotographyBB* magazine. Thanks for everything, especially for thinking that I am the greatest husband and Dad. I would also like to acknowledge here the love, support, and encouragement of both my mother, Betty and my father, Samuel, who passed away five years ago (thanks for having me and thanks for the memories Dad); my father-in-law Edward Penner, and my mother-in-law, Joan (who earned the title "the most well-read person I know" from me, and who passed away six years ago). I love all of you.

Last but not least, I must thank my students who have diligently completed my courses on digital imaging modalities, PACS and digital image processing in Radiology, at both the diploma and degree levels. Thanks for all the challenging questions.

Keep on learning and enjoy the pages that follow.

Euclid Seeram, RT(R), BSc, MSc, FCAMRT
British Columbia, CANADA.

Charles E. Willis, PhD, DABR
Associate Professor
Department of Imaging Physics
The University of Texas MD Anderson Cancer Center
Houston, Texas

Barry Burns, MS, RT(R), DABR
Professor,
Division of Radiologic Science
School of Medicine,
University of North Carolina,
Chapel Hill, North Carolina

REVIEWERS

Arlene M. Adler, MEd, RT(R), FAERS
Director/Professor
Department of Radiologic Sciences
Indiana University Northwest
Gary, IN

Rex Ameigh, MSLM, BSRT(R)
Director/Associate Professor
Department of Allied Health Science/Radiologic
 Technology Program
Austin Peay State University
Clarksville, TN

Jeffrey C. Fannin, MSRS, RT(R)(CT)(ARRT), RDMS
Assistant Professor
Department of Imaging Sciences
Morehead State University
Morehead, KY

Jeff Killion, PhD, RT(R)(QM)
Assistant Professor
Department of Radiologic Science
Midwestern State University
Wichita Falls, TX

Cynthia L. Liotta, MS, RT(R)(CT)
Program Director/Assistant Professor
Department of Radiologic Sciences
Gannon University
Erie, PA

Pamela Moseley, MPH, RT(R)
Directory of Radiology Informatics
Rochester General Hospital
Rochester, NY

Regina C. Panettieri, MPA, RT(R)(CT)
Assistant Professor
Department of Nursing and Allied Health
 (Radiologic Technology)
Bronx Community College
Bronx, NY

Anita R. Phillips, BS, MEd, (ARRT)
Program Director
Department of Radiography
Cape Fear Community College
Wilmington, NC

Andrew Shappell, MEd, RT(R)(MR)(CT)(QM)
Assistant Professor/Clinical Coordinator
Department of Radiographic Imaging
Rhodes State College
Lima, OH

Robert J. Slothus, MS, RT(R)
Director/Associate Professor
Department of Medical Radiography
The Pennsylvania College of Technology
Williamsport, PA

Kelli Bahr Summers, BS, RT(R)
Program Director
Department of Radiologic Technology
Mountain State University
Beckley, WV

CHAPTER 1

Digital Radiography: An Overview

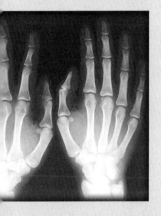

OBJECTIVES

Upon completion of this chapter, the student should be able to:

1. Define the term digital radiography.

2. Describe the essential steps in the production of a radiograph.

3. Explain the major elements of the film characteristic curve.

4. State the fundamental limitations of film-based radiography.

5. Describe the major technical components of a digital radiography imaging system.

6. State the meaning of the term *integrating the health care enterprise*.

7. Explain briefly the essential characteristics of four digital radiography imaging modalities.

8. Define the term picture archiving and communication systems (PACS) and identify its major components.

9. Identify the primary considerations of quality assurance in digital radiography.

10. State what is meant by the term medical imaging informatics, and identify the potential skill set of the technologist as informaticist.

KEY TERMS

Bits

Chemical processing

Computed radiography (CR)

Data acquisition

Digital fluoroscopy

Digital mammography

Digital radiography

Direct conversion

Film characteristic curve

Film speed

Filmless imaging

Film-screen mammography

Film-screen radiography

Flat-Panel Digital Radiography

Hospital information systems (HIS)

Image communications

Image and information management

Indirect conversion

Integrating the health care enterprise (IHE)

Medical imaging informatics (MII)

Optical density (OD)

Picture archiving and communication systems (PACS)

Quality assurance (QA)/quality control (QC)

Radiology information system (RIS)

Introduction

Film-screen radiography has been the workhorse of radiology ever since the discovery of X-ray by W. C. Roentgen in 1895. Today film-screen radiography has entered into the domain of digital imaging, or **filmless imaging** as it is sometimes referred to. It is the goal of radiology departments to eliminate film-based imaging systems and introduce new technologies for the purpose of improving diagnostic interpretation and digital image management and to reduce the radiation dose to patients. These technologies include not only digital image acquisition modalities but also digital image processing and display, storage, and image communication, or image transmission. Specifically, digital image acquisition modalities include computed radiography (CR), digital radiography (DR), digital mammography, digital fluoroscopy for routine gastrointestinal fluoroscopy and vascular imaging, computed tomography (CT), magnetic resonance imaging (MRI), nuclear medicine, and diagnostic medical sonography (Brennan, McEntee, Stowe, & Seeram, in press).

The purpose of this chapter is to present a broad overview of the elements of digital radiography imaging systems and to lay the overall framework and foundations for the rest of this book.

This chapter and hence the book will not describe inherent digital imaging modalities such as CT and MRI. Additionally, the other imaging modalities, such as nuclear medicine and diagnostic medical sonography, will not be covered in this book.

 ## Digital Radiography: A Definition

The term **digital radiography** as used in this book refers to projection radiography, whereby computers process data collected from patients using special electronic detectors that have replaced the X-ray film cassette. In this regard, digital radiography has also been referred to as filmless radiography. The detectors measure and convert X-ray attenuation data from the patient into electronic (analog) signals that are subsequently converted into digital data for processing by a computer (Korner et al., 2007; Seibert, 2007; Verma & Indrajit, 2008). The result of this processing is a digital image that must be converted so that it can be viewed

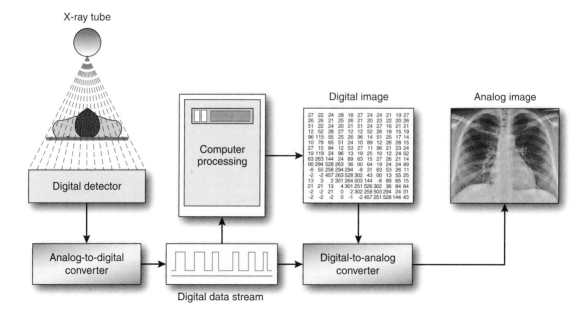

FIGURE 1-1. The major system components and the essential steps in the production of a digital image.
Source: *Delmar, Cengage Learning*

on a computer monitor. The displayed image can then be manipulated using a variety of digital image processing techniques to enhance the interpretation of diagnostic radiology images (Seeram & Seeram, 2008). Digital radiography also includes image and information management systems, image storage, and image and data communications. The major system components and the essential steps to digital image production are illustrated in Figure 1-1.

Film–Based Radiography: A Brief Review

Basic Steps in the Production of a Radiograph

The production of a film-based radiographic image involves several steps, as illustrated in Figure 1-2. X-rays pass through the patient and fall upon the film to form a latent image. The latent image is then rendered visible using chemical processing and subsequently displayed on a lightview box for viewing and interpretation by a radiologist. The film image appears with varying degrees of blackening as a result of the amount of exposure transmitted by different parts of the anatomy. More exposure produces more blackening and less exposure produces less blackening, as

is clearly illustrated in Figure 1-3. This blackening is referred to as the film density and the difference in densities in the image is referred to as the film contrast. The film, therefore, converts the radiation transmitted by the various types of tissues (tissue contrast) into film contrast.

An image displayed on a lightview box transmits light into the eyes of the radiologist, who interprets the image. This transmitted light can be measured using a densitometer and is referred to as the optical density (OD), defined as the log of the ratio of the intensity of the light falling upon the film from the lightview box (original intensity = I_0) to the intensity of the transmitted light (I_t) through the film. This is given by the algebraic expression

$$OD = \log I_0/I_t$$

The OD is used to describe the degree of film blackening as a result of radiation exposure, and it can be measured by a densitometer.

The Film Characteristic Curve

The film contrast can be described by what is popularly known as the film characteristic curve or the Hurter-Driffield (H and D) curve. The curve is a plot of the OD to the radiation exposure (or, more accurately, the logarithm of the relative exposure) used in the imaging process. The purpose

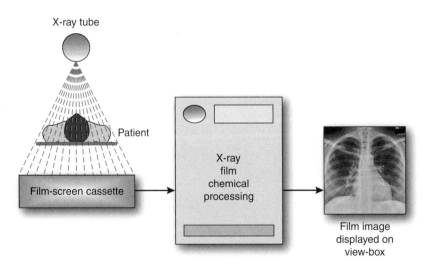

FIGURE 1-2. The basic steps in the production of a film–based radiographic image.
Source: *Delmar, Cengage Learning*

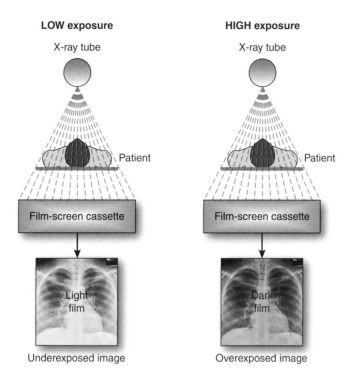

LOW exposure

X-ray tube

Patient

Film-screen cassette

Light
film

Underexposed image

HIGH exposure

X-ray tube

Patient

Film-screen cassette

Dark
film

Overexposed image

FIGURE 1-3. The visual image quality feedback in film–based radiography as a result of low and high exposures.
Source: *Delmar, Cengage Learning*

of the curve is to indicate the degree of contrast or different densities that a film can display using a range of exposures. An idealized characteristic curve for film-screen radiography is shown in Figure 1-4; it has three main segments: the toe, the slope (straight-line portion), and the shoulder. While the toe and shoulder indicate underexposure and overexposure respectively, the slope represents the useful portion of the curve and reflects acceptable exposure, or the range of useful densities. This simply means that if an exposure falls at the toe region (OD = 0.12–0.20), the image will be light and generally useless. If the exposure falls in the shoulder region of the curve (OD = about 3.2), the image will be black and serve no useful purpose in providing a diagnosis. If the exposure falls within the slope of the curve (OD = 0.3–2.2), the image contrast (density) will be acceptable, and this region of the curve contains the useful range of exposures. A final note about the characteristic curve is the base plus fog density, which ranges in general from 0.1 to 0.2 OD and represents the

film density when no exposure is used, as shown in Figure 1-4.

There are four other factors that can be described using the characteristic curve: the film speed, average gradient, film gamma, and film latitude. Only film speed and film latitude will be reviewed here. The interested reader should refer to any standard radiography physics text for a further description of the other terms.

The **film speed** refers to the sensitivity of the film to radiation. It is inversely proportional to the exposure (E) and can be expressed algebraically as

$$Film\ speed = 1/E$$

This means that films with high speeds (fast films) require less exposure than films with low speeds (slow films). Conversely, the film latitude describes the range of exposures that would produce useful densities (contrast). While wide exposure latitude films can respond to a wide range of exposures, films with narrow exposure latitude can respond

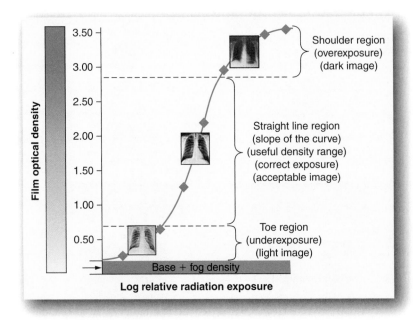

FIGURE 1-4. The idealized characteristic curve (H and D curve) for film–screen radiography.
Source: *Delmar, Cengage Learning*

only to a small range of exposures. In the latter situation, the technologist has to be very precise in the selection of the exposure technique factors for the anatomical part under investigation. This is mainly because the film emulsion has a nonlinear response to chemical processing (Bushong, 2009; Seibert & Boone, 2005).

Limitations of Film-Screen Radiography

Film-based radiography has been the workhorse of radiology ever since the discovery of X-rays in 1895, and despite its successful use for over 100 years and the present use in many departments, one of the major problems with the radiographic imaging process is poor image quality if the initial radiation exposure has not been accurately determined. For example, if the radiation exposure is too high, the film is overexposed and the processed image appears too dark and the radiologist cannot make a diagnosis from such an image. Alternatively, if the radiation exposure is too low, the processed image appears too light and not useful to the radiologist, as shown in Figure 1-4. In both of these situations, the

images lack the proper image density and contrast, and would have to be repeated to provide an acceptable image quality needed to make a diagnosis. Additionally, the patient would be subjected to increased radiation exposures due to the repeated exposures.

There are other problems associated with film-based radiography. For example:

1. As a radiation detector, film-screen cannot show differences in tissue contrast less than 10%. This means that film-based imaging is limited in its contrast resolution. For example, while the contrast resolution (mm at 0.5% difference) for film-screen radiography is 10, it is 20 for nuclear medicine, 10 for ultrasound, 4 for CT, and 1 for MRI (Bushong, 2009). The spatial resolution (line pairs/mm) for radiography, however, is the highest of all the other imaging modalities, and can range from 5–15 line pairs/mm (Bushong, 2009). This is the main reason why radiography has been so popular through the years.

2. As a display medium, the optical range and contrast for film are fixed and limited. Film can only display once, using the optical range and contrast determined by the exposure technique factors that produced the image. In order to change the image display (optical range and contrast), another set of exposure technique factors would have to be used, thus increasing the dose to the patient from repeated exposures.

3. As an archive medium, film is usually stored in envelopes and housed in a large room. It thus requires manual handling for archiving and retrieval by an individual.

These problems, however, can be overcome by a digital radiography imaging system.

A Digital Radiographic Imaging System: Major Components

The major technical components of a digital radiography system are illustrated in Figure 1-5 and include the data acquisition, computer data processing, image display and post processing, image storage, image and data communications, and image and information management. Each of these will now be described briefly.

Data Acquisition

Data acquisition refers to the collection of X-rays transmitted through the patient. It is the first step in the production of the image. For digital radiography, special electronic (digital) detectors are used that replace the X-ray film cassette used in film-based radiography. These detectors are of several types and utilize various technologies to convert X-rays to electrical (analog) signals. For example, while one type of detector will first convert X-rays into light, followed immediately by the conversion of the light into electrical signals, another type of digital detector will avoid the light-electricity conversion process and convert X-rays directly into electrical signals. The analog signals must then be converted into digital data for processing by a computer. The conversion of analog signals into digital data is the function of the analog-to-digital converter (ADC).

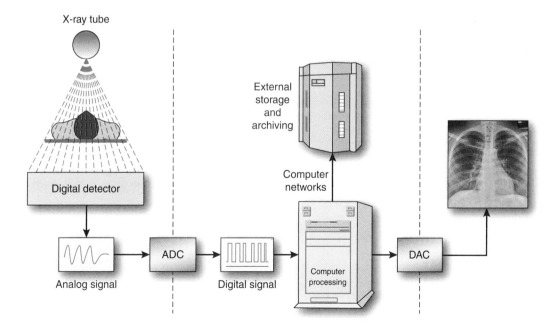

FIGURE 1-5. The major technical components of a digital radiography system.
Source: *Delmar, Cengage Learning*

Computer Data Processing

The ADC sends digital data for processing by a computer. The computer uses special software to create or build up digital images using the binary number system. While humans use the decimal number system (which operates with base 10, that is, 10 different numbers; 0,1,2,3,4,5,6,7,8,9), computers use the binary number system (which operates with base 2, that is, 0 or 1). These two digits are referred to as binary digits, or **bits**. Bits are not continuous; rather, they are discrete units. Computers operate by processing and transforming these discrete units (binary numbers) into other discrete units. To process the name Euclid, for example, it would first have to be converted into digital data (binary representation), which would appear as 01000101 01010101 01000011 01001100 01001001 01000100.

Image Display and Post Processing

The output of computer processing, that is, the digital image, must first be converted into an analog signal before it can be displayed on a monitor for viewing by the observer. Such conversion is the function of the digital-to-analog converter (DAC). The image displayed for initial viewing can be processed using a set of operations and techniques, referred to as post-processing techniques, to transform the input image into an output image that suits the needs of the observer (radiologist) in order to enhance diagnosis. For example, these operations can be used to reduce the image noise, enhance image sharpness, to simply change the image contrast, or to stitch several images together to form one image. The effect of one common and popular digital image-processing tool, referred to as gray-scale mapping, can be seen in Figure 1-6.

Image Storage

The vast amount of images generated for the wide range of digital radiology examinations must be stored not only for retrospective analysis but also for medico-legal purposes. Today, various kinds of storage devices and systems are used for this purpose, for example, magnetic tapes, disks, and laser optical disks for long-term storage. In a PACS environment, for example, a storage system such as a RAID (redundant array of independent disks) is not uncommon. It is important to note that those images that are stored in a short-term archival system are deleted after a period of time defined by the institution.

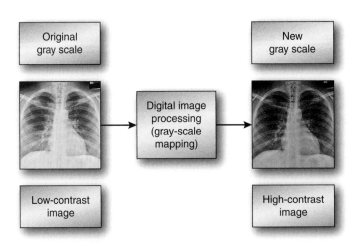

FIGURE 1-6. The digital image-processing tool of gray-scale mapping can change the picture quality to suit the needs of the viewer.
Source: *Delmar, Cengage Learning*

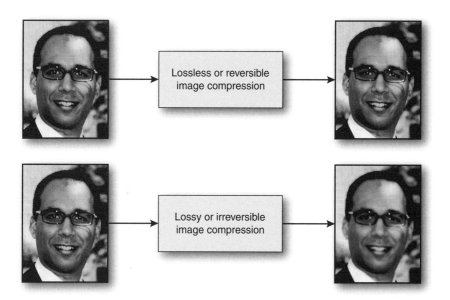

FIGURE 1-7. The effects of two image–compression methods on picture quality.
Source: *Courtesy of David Seeram*

Image and Data Communications

Image and data communications are concerned with the use of computer communication networks to transmit images from the acquisition phase to the display/viewing and storage phase. If the image transmission is within the hospital (Intranet), local area networks (LANs) are used. If, however, the images have to be sent outside the hospital to remote locations (Internet), networks such as wide area networks (WANs) must be used.

Recently, picture archiving and communication systems (PACS) are being used for storing/archiving and communicating images in the digital radiology department. In addition, information systems, such as radiology information systems (RIS) and hospital information systems (HIS) are now being integrated with the PACS via computer networks, using communications standards such as DICOM (Digital Imaging and Communications in Medicine) and HL-7 (Health Level-7), for effective management of patient information.

An important element of image and data communications is that of image compression (Seeram & Seeram, 2008). The purpose of image compression is to reduce storage space (and hence costs) and decrease the image transmission time. Two popular compression methods for use in digital radiology are lossless, or reversible, compression, and lossy, or irreversible, compression. While in the former, there is no loss of information when the image is decompressed, the latter will result in some loss of information. The effects of these two compression methods on visual image quality are illustrated in Figure 1-7, which shows a photograph of the author's son, David, a warm, caring, and overall brilliant young man.

Image and Information Management

Image and information management refers to the use of PACS and information systems such as RIS and HIS to manage the vast number of images and text data produced in a digital radiology department with databases and file management software. While the RIS and HIS handle essentially textual information, specifically dealing with business operations for the entire hospital, the PACS handle images generated by the various digital imaging modalities (to be described later).

Integrating the Health Care Enterprise

Another important aspect of digital image acquisition and PACS-RIS-HIS integration is integrating the health care enterprise (IHE), a model for ensuring that the standards for communication such as DICOM and HL-7 work effectively to facilitate integration. The concept of IHE had its origins in 1998, when two major organizations, the Radiological Society of North America (RSNA) and the Healthcare Information and Management Systems Society (HIMSS), developed what they refer to as a Technical Framework that is based on three essential elements: a data model, an actor, and an integration profile. These will be discussed in more detail in a later chapter.

Digital Radiography Modalities

Digital radiography includes several imaging modalities coupled to the PACS-RIS-HIS image and information systems and based on the technologies mentioned above. The imaging modalities include computed radiography (CR), flat-panel digital radiography (DR), digital mammography (DM), and digital fluoroscopy (DF) and the laser film digitizer. Imaging modalities and the PACS-RIS-HIS systems must be fully integrated for overall effective and efficient operations.

This section will provide an overall orientation by describing how these modalities work in the most fundamental way. Each of them will be described in detail in later chapters.

Computed Radiography

Computed radiography (CR) makes use of photostimulable or storage phosphors to produce digital images using existing X-ray imaging equipment. A computer is used to process data collected by radiographic means to produce digital images of the patient.

In 1983, Fuji Medical Systems introduced a CR imaging system for use in clinical practice. Other companies such as Agfa, Kodak, Konica, and Cannon, to mention only a few, now manufacture CR imaging systems.

In CR, a photostimulable phosphor such as barium-fluoro-halide is coated on an imaging plate (IP) that is housed in a cassette (similar in appearance to a film-screen cassette) to protect it from damage and exposure to foreign materials. The IP then is considered the digital detector in CR. (Korner et al., 2007; Seibert, 2007; Verma & Indrajit, 2008).

The basic steps in the production of a CR image are shown in Figure 1-8 and include the following:

1. The IP is exposed to X-rays, which causes electrons in the phosphor to move to another energy level, where they remain trapped, creating a latent image.

2. The plate is then taken to the CR reader/processor (digital image processor) where it is scanned by a laser beam, which causes the trapped electrons to return to their original orbit, and in the process, light is emitted.

3. This light is collected by a light guide and sent to a photomultiplier tube (PMT). The electrical signal output from the PMT is subsequently converted into digital data.

4. A digital processor processes the digital data to produce a CR image that can be viewed on a monitor.

5. The IP is exposed to a bright light to erase it (the residual latent image is removed).

6. The IP can now be used again.

One of the significant differences between CR and film-screen radiography is that the exposure latitude of CR is about 10^4 times wider than that of the widest range of film-screen systems. This difference and others, as well as similarities, will be described further in the chapter on CR.

A major drawback of CR systems is their limited ability to image detail (spatial resolution). While the spatial resolution of a CR is about 3–5 line pairs/mm, it is about 10–15 line pairs/mm for film-screen radiographic imaging systems. However, the contrast resolution for CR systems can be manipulated, which makes it superior to the fixed film-screen systems in this respect.

One important objective descriptor of digital image quality is the detective quantum efficiency (DQE). The DQE is a measure of how efficiently a

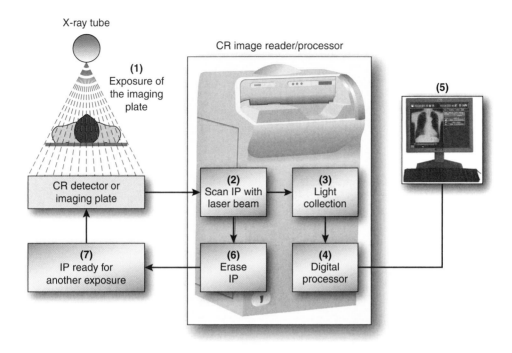

FIGURE 1-8. The fundamental steps in the production of a CR image. See text for explanation of the numbers 1–7.
Source: *Delmar, Cengage Learning*

digital detector can convert the X-rays collected from the patient into a useful image (Verma & Indrajit, 2008). The DQE for CR is much better than for film-screen systems. This means that CR can convert X-rays from the patient into useful data, over a wider exposure range, compared with film-screen detectors. CR will be described in more detail in Chapter 3.

Flat-Panel Digital Radiography

Flat-Panel Digital Radiography systems have been developed to overcome the shortcomings of CR systems. As the name implies, the digital detector is designed as a flat-panel and it is totally different in design structure and function to the CR detector image panel. Currently, there are two categories of flat-panel digital radiography imaging systems, based on the type of detector used (Korner et al., 2007; Lanca & Silva, 2009; Seibert, 2007; Spahn, 2005; Verma and Indrajit, 2008), popularly referred to as: (1) Indirect conversion digital radiography systems (2) Direct conversion digital radiography systems.

The basic components of these detectors and the steps in the production of an image for indirect and direct conversion systems are illustrated in Figures 1-9A and 1-9B, respectively.

In Figure 1-9A, X-rays are first converted into light using a phosphor such as cesium iodide. The emitted light from the phosphor falls upon a matrix array of electronic elements to create and store electrical charges in direct proportion to the X-ray exposure. The charges produce electrical signals, which are subsequently digitized and processed by a computer to produce an image.

Direct conversion digital radiography systems use detectors that convert X-rays directly into electrical signals. As shown in Figure 1-9B, X-rays fall upon a photoconductor (selenium, for example) that is coupled to a matrix array of electronic elements to produce electrical signals. These signals are digitized and processed by a computer to produce an image.

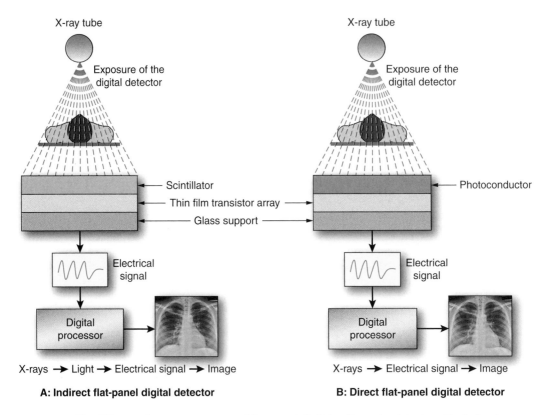

FIGURE 1-9. The difference between two types of flat-panel digital radiography detectors, the indirect flat-panel system (A) and the direct flat-panel system (B).
Source: *Delmar, Cengage Learning*

The second type of indirect conversion detector is shown in Figure 1-10. This type uses an array of charge-coupled devices (CCDs) instead of an array of electronic elements as identified in the first type (Figure 1-9A). The CCDs are coupled to a scintillator phosphor, cesium iodide (as shown). X-rays fall upon the phosphor to produce light, which then falls upon the CCD array, which in turn converts the light into electrical signals that are then digitized and processed by a computer to produce an image.

It is important to note that after all electrical charges are read out, the flat-panel digital detector can be erased and is ready to be used again. In addition, flat-panel detectors offer several advantages, including a high DQE and spatial resolution comparable to CR systems. Furthermore, the digital detectors used in CR and flat-panel digital radiography have a characteristic response to radiation exposure

(shown in Figure 1-11) that is fundamentally different to the film characteristic curve. The digital detector output signal is linear with the input radiation exposure. This linear response produces wider exposure latitudes compared to the film characteristic curve, which has limited exposure latitudes (defined by their slopes). Herein lies a significant advantage of the digital detector. The wide exposure latitude of the digital detector will produce acceptable images even when the input exposure is low or high. As mentioned earlier, in film-screen radiography, a low exposure will produce a light image and a high exposure will produce a dark image, neither of which are useful for patient diagnosis and therefore both would have to be repeated, thus increasing the radiation dose to the patient. These will be discussed in more detail in the respective chapters on CR (Chapter 3) and flat-panel digital radiography (Chapter 5).

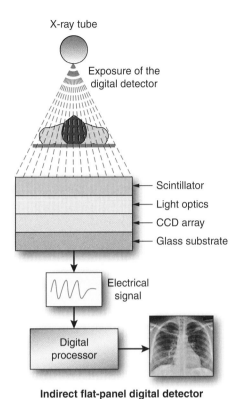

FIGURE 1-10. An indirect flat-panel digital detector using a CCD array to produce digital images of a patient.
Source: *Delmar, Cengage Learning*

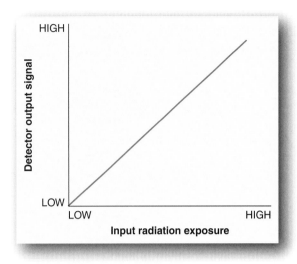

FIGURE 1-11. A digital detector provides a linear response to radiation exposure. This graph shows that a digital detector has a wide exposure latitude compared to a film-screen image receptor.
Source: *Delmar, Cengage Learning*

Digital Mammography

Mammography is radiography of the breast and is often referred to as soft-tissue imaging. **Film–screen mammography** requires a great deal of special technical considerations in order to detect breast cancer. Film-screen mammography suffers from all of the limitations of film-screen radiography described earlier. Digital mammography overcomes these limitations and offers several benefits as well. One such major benefit is that digital mammography allows the observer to use digital image-processing tools to enhance diagnostic interpretation of the image.

Digital mammography systems currently utilize CR detectors and flat-panel digital detectors, including direct and indirect conversion detectors, as well as CCD arrays to image the breast. Additionally,

digital mammography uses computer-aided diagnosis (CAD) software to help radiologists enhance their detection of microcalcifications and malignant lesions and also provides the so-called "second reader" approach (Mashesh, 2004; Pisano & Yaffe, 2005). Other applications of digital mammography include telemammography, digital tomosynthesis, dual energy subtraction, breast angiography. Digital mammography and its associated applications will be described in Chapter 7.

Digital Fluoroscopy

The application of digital image processing to fluoroscopy is referred to as **digital fluoroscopy** (Bushong, 2009). One of the major goals of digital fluoroscopy is to improve the perception of contrast resolution, compared to conventional fluoroscopy, by using digital image-processing software. Other advantages of digital fluoroscopy are gray-scale processing, temporal frame averaging, and edge enhancement, to mention only a few.

While radiography produces static images, fluoroscopy produces dynamic images acquired in real time to allow for the study of motion of organ

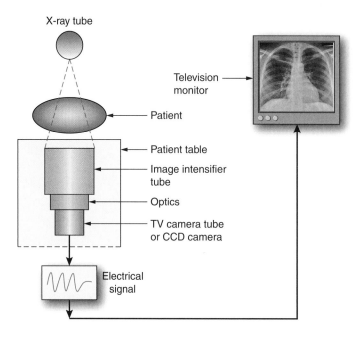

X-ray tube

Television monitor

Patient

Patient table

Image intensifier tube

Optics

TV camera tube or CCD camera

Electrical signal

FIGURE 1-12. The major technical components of a conventional fluoroscopic imaging system.
Source: *Delmar, Cengage Learning*

systems and hollow internal structures, such as the gastrointestinal tract, as well as the blood circulatory system.

A conventional fluoroscopy imaging system is shown in Figure 1-12; it consists of a fluoroscopic X-ray tube, an image intensifier tube (the radiation detector), associated optics, a television (TV) or CCD camera tube, and a television monitor for image display and viewing.

A digital fluoroscopy system, in contrast, is shown in Figure 1-13; it consists of all of the imaging components found in a conventional fluoroscopic imaging system with a few differences. In digital fluoroscopy, the output signal (an electrical signal) from the TV/CCD video system is digitized by the ADC and sent to a computer for image processing. The detector in digital fluoroscopy is also the image intensifier tube, since it captures the radiation passing through the patient. Recently, flat-panel digital detectors are also being used in some digital fluoroscopy systems.

The application of digital fluoroscopy to angiography is referred to as digital subtraction angiography (DSA), in which pre-contrast and post-contrast images can be digitally subtracted in real time. The goal of such operations is to improve the observer's perception of low-contrast vessels by subtracting or removing the tissues that interfere with visualization of vascular structures. Two such subtraction methods include temporal subtraction, in which images are subtracted in time, and energy subtraction, in which images are subtracted using different kilovoltages. Digital fluoroscopy will be described in detail in Chapter 6.

Picture Archiving and Communication Systems

The digital radiography modalities described above all produce digital images that must be displayed for interpretation, stored and archived for medico-legal purposes and retrospective analysis, and transmitted to remote locations to accommodate the needs of users such as surgeons in the operating room, emergency physicians, and other users either within or outside an institution. To perform this task efficiently and effectively requires

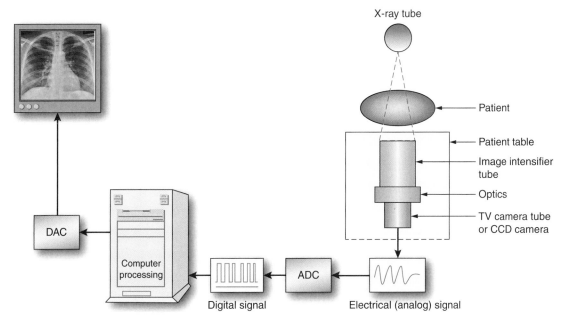

FIGURE 1-13. The major technical components of a digital fluoroscopic imaging system. Note that a computer is used to process digital data from the analog-to-digital converter.
Source: *Delmar, Cengage Learning*

the use of PACS. PACS have therefore become the backbone of digital radiology departments. The term image management and communication systems (IMACS) has also been used to describe the various functions performed by this technology; however, the more common and popular term used today is PACS.

Definition of PACS

There are several definitions of PACS in the literature; however, one that is simple and meaningful and will be used in this book is provided by Samei et al. (2004), who define PACS as:

"a comprehensive computer system that is responsible for the electronic storage and distribution of medical images in the medical enterprise. The system is highly integrated with digital acquisition and display devices and is often related closely to other medical information systems, such as the Radiology Information System (RIS) or Hospital Information System (HIS)."

Major System Components

The major components of PACS are shown in Figure 1-14 and include image acquisition devices, a PACS computer, devices called interfaces, and display workstations, all of which are connected and linked to the HIS and RIS through digital communication networks.

The PACS computer is the heart of the system and is a "high-end" computer or server. Images and patient data (demographics, for example) are sent from the digital image acquisition modalities and the HIS and the RIS to the PACS computer, which has a database server as well as an archive system. Common forms of archiving in a PACS environment include laser optical disks, a redundant array of independent disks (RAID), and magnetic tapes.

Display workstations, or softcopy workstations as they are often referred to, serve to display images on a monitor for the purpose of image interpretation. In addition, these workstations are of various types depending on the degree of use by the observer. Although radiologists must have high-resolution diagnostic workstations that

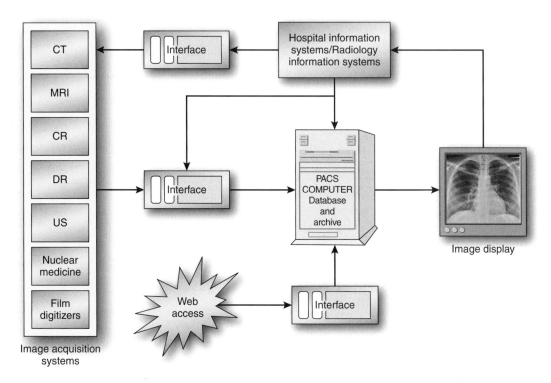

FIGURE 1-14. A typical PACS system showing the major technical components required from acquisition of the image to the display of the image for viewing and interpretation. In this system, users can access images stored in the PACS using Web technology.
Source: *Delmar, Cengage Learning*

allow them to interpret images and provide a diagnosis of the patient's medical condition, technologists often use review workstations for general assessment of image quality before the images are sent to the PACS. A major feature of workstations is that they allow users to perform digital post processing of images for the purpose of enhancing diagnosis. For example, images can be compressed to reduce storage space and decrease image transmission times.

In order for the PACS to work efficiently and effectively, certain requirements must be met. One such requirement is the use of industry health care standards for data and image communications. Two standards that are currently used in a PACS environment are the DICOM and HL-7 standards (Indrajit, 2007; Indrajit & Verma, 2007). While DICOM is concerned primarily with images from the digital image acquisition modalities, HL-7 is concerned mainly with textual information from the HIS and RIS.

Since the PACS contains confidential patient data and information, it is essential that they be secured; hence data security is of central importance in a digital hospital as well as in a PACS environment.

The interfaces shown in Figure 1-14 serve to facilitate easy communications between the image acquisition modalities and the HIS/RIS with the PACS computer, and they also allow individuals to use the World Wide Web to access the PACS computer.

PACS will be described in more detail in Chapter 8.

Quality Assurance in Digital Radiography

Quality assurance (QA) and quality control (QC) procedures are effective strategies to ensure continuous quality improvement of a product. In radiology, QA/QC policies and procedures and related activities are all intended to:

- Ensure that patients are exposed to minimum radiation using the ALARA (as low as reasonably achievable) philosophy.
- Produce optimum image quality for diagnosis.
- Reduce the costs of radiology operations.

For digital radiography systems, QA and QC are beginning to evolve, and special tools are now available to test the performance of digital imaging equipment, as well as the components of PACS. For example, QC tests for CR systems, dark noise, exposure index calibration, and so on, are now becoming commonplace, and already, technologists are performing these tests on a routine basis (AAPM, 2006).

The fundamentals of QC for digital radiography imaging systems will be described in Chapter 10.

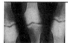 ## Medical Imaging Informatics

Digital imaging departments and the digital hospital now operate in the information technology (IT) domain. Digital image acquisition technologies; digital image processing; digital image display, storage, and archiving; and digital image communications all utilize IT concepts. IT is a growing field, and it is becoming increasingly popular in all aspects of society. It involves the use of computer technology coupled with communications technology to solve problems in society, including medical imaging and health care.

What Is Medical Imaging Informatics?

The application of information technology to medical imaging is referred to as medical imaging informatics (MII). Medical imaging plays a significant role in health care, since images can be used for diagnosis, assessment and planning (e.g., assessing the extent of a tumor and helping to prepare an approach to management), guidance of procedures, communication, education, training, and research. These functions require the use of IT.

IT involves such topics as information systems, standards for communicating both text and image data, computer communication networks, Web technology, image and text handling, privacy, security, and confidentiality issues, and last but not least, digital image processing.

The Technologist as Informaticist

The total digital medical imaging department will require that technologists have additional skills related to IT. Already these departments have what is referred to as a PACS administrator (a technologist in some departments or an IT person in others) whose function is solely dedicated to ensuring the integrity of the PACS. To be effective and efficient in this role, technologists must not only educate themselves in all aspects of IT but also continue to learn more about the digital world of radiology, including digital image processing (Seeram & Seeram, 2008). This will lead to a new role function for the technologist as informaticist (Seeram, 2004).

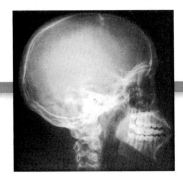

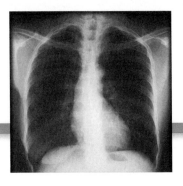

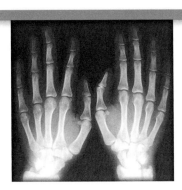

REVIEW QUESTIONS

1. Define the term "digital radiography" as used in this book.

2. Describe the basic steps in the production of a radiograph and briefly describe each of them,

3. Explain the main features of the film characteristic curve (the H and D curve).

4. What are three limitations of film-screen radiography?

5. What are the main technical elements of a digital radiography imaging system?

6. Briefly explain what is meant by the term "integrating the health care enterprise."

7. Describe four digital radiographic imaging modalities and the fundamental characteristics of each.

8. What is a PACS and its associated technical components?

9. What are the reasons for quality assurance/quality control in digital radiography?

10. What is meant by the term "medical imaging informatics"? List the potential skill set for a technologist informaticist.

REFERENCES

American Association of Physicists in Medicine (AAPM) Report No 93 (2006). *Acceptance Testing and Quality Control of Photostimulable Storage Phosphor Imaging Systems.* College Park, MD: Amercian Association of Physicists in Medicine.

Bushong, S. (2009). *Radiologic Science for Technologists* (9th Edition). Philadelphia: Elsevier Mosby.

Indrajit, I. K. (2007). Digital imaging and communication in medicine: A basic review. *Indian Journal of Radiology and Imaging, 17,* 5–7.

Korner, M., Weber C. H., Wirth, S., Klaus-Jürgen Pfeifer; Maximilian F. Reiser; and Marcus Treitl (2007). Advances in digital radiography: Physical principles and system overview. *Radiographics, 27,* 675–686.

Lanca, L., & Silva, A. (2009). Digital radiography detectors: A technical overview Part 1. *Radiography, 15,* 58–62.

Mahesh, M. (2004). Digital mammography: An overview. *Radiographics, 24,* 1747–1760.

Nagy, P. G. (2008). Using informatics to improve the quality of radiology. *Applied Radiology,* Suppl. December, 14–17.

Pisano, E. D., & Yafee, M. J. (2005). Digital mammography. *Radiology, 234,* 353–362.

Samei, E., Seibert, J. A., Andriole, K., Aldo Badano; Jay Crawford; Bruce Reiner; Michael J. Flynn; and Paul Chang (2004). General guidelines for purchasing and acceptance testing of PACS equipment. *Radiographics, 24,* 313–334.

Seeram, E. (2004). Digital image processing. *Radiologic Technology, 75*(6), 435–455.

Seeram, E., & Seeram, D. (2008). Image postprocessing in digital radiology: A primer for technologists. *Journal of Medical Imaging and Radiation Sciences, 39,* 23–44.

Seibert, J. A. (2007). Digital radiography: CR vs DR? Time to reconsider the options, the definitions, and current capabilities. *Applied Radiology, 2,* 4–7.

Seibert, J. A., & Boone, J. M. (2005). X-Ray imaging physics for nuclear medicine technologists Part 2: X-Ray interactions and image formation. *Journal of Nuclear Medicine, 33,* 3–18.

Spahn, M. (2005). Flat-panel detectors and their clinical applications. *European Journal of Radiology, 15,* 1943–1947.

Verma, B. S., & Indrajit, I. K. (2007). DICOM, HL7 and IHE: A basic primer on Healthcare Standards for Radiologists. *Indian Journal of Radiology and Imaging 17,* 66–68.

Verma, B. S., & Indrajit, I. K. (2008). Advent of digital radiography: Part 1. *Indian Journal of Radiology and Imaging, 18,* 113–116.

CHAPTER 2

Digital Image Processing Concepts

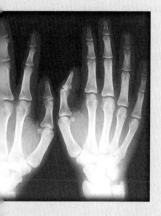

OBJECTIVES

Upon completion of this chapter, the student should be able to:

1. Define the term digital image processing.

2. Outline briefly the evolution of digital image processing.

3. State how images are formed and how they are represented.

4. Identify and describe briefly five classes of digital image processing operations.

5. Describe four characteristics (matrix size, pixel, voxel, bit depth) of a digital image and how they affect the appearance of the image.

6. Explain the three steps in digitizing an image.

7. Identify four digital image processing operations and explain the principles of each of them.

8. Describe the features of a histogram.

9. Explain what is meant by a look-up table in digital image processing.

10. Define the terms windowing, window width (WW), and window level (WL).

11. Describe the effect of the WW and the WL on the image gray-scale appearance.

12. Describe the difference between spatial location filtering and spatial frequency filtering.

13. State the effect of three spatial frequency filtering techniques (low-pass and high-pass filtering, and unsharp masking) on the visual appearance of an image.

14. State the effect of geometric operations on an image.

KEY TERMS

Analog image
Analog-to-digital converter (ADC)
Bit depth
Convolution
Density resolution
Digital image
Digital image processing
Field-of-view (FOV)
Fourier transform (FT)
Geometric operation
Global processing operation
Gray-scale processing
Histogram
Image analysis
Image compression
Image enhancement
Image restoration
Image synthesis

Inverse Fourier transform
Local processing operation
Low-pass filtering
Matrix
Pixels
Pixel size
Quantization
Sampling
Scanning
Spatial frequency domain
Spatial location domain
Spatial resolution
Unsharp masking
Voxel
Window level (WL)
Window width (WW)
Windowing

Introduction

In Chapter 1, digital radiography was defined as projection radiography whereby a computer is used to process data acquired from the patient to generate digital images. These images are subsequently displayed for viewing and interpretation by an observer. In radiology, the image-viewing task of the technologist is to assess the overall image quality (image density, contrast, detail, noise, distortion, artifacts, and accurate positioning of the anatomy) and the viewing task of the radiologist is mainly detection of pathology. This task is dependent on the quality of the image submitted by the technologist, who can manipulate the images through the use of digital image processing techniques in order to enhance the diagnostic ability of the radiologist.

The purpose of this chapter is to outline the essential elements of digital image processing as it relates to digital radiography. First, a definition of digital image processing will be given, followed by a brief description of the history and application areas of digital image processing. Second, image representation and the basic concepts of digital image processing will be discussed.

 ## Definition of Digital Image Processing

Digital Image Processing simply means the processing of images using a computer. The data collected from the patient during imaging is first converted into digital data (numerical representation of the patient) for input into a computer (input image), and the result of computer processing is a digital image (output image). These numerical images can be changed in several ways, to suit the viewing needs of the radiologist, in an effort to improve and enhance diagnostic interpretation and management of the vast amount of images acquired from patients.

Digital image processing has become commonplace in digital radiology departments and is now part of the routine skills of technologists and radiologists.

 ## Brief History

NASA

The history of digital image processing dates back several decades to the United States National Aeronautics and Space Administration (NASA) space program. The Jet Propulsion Laboratory, California Institute of Technology in Pasadena also made notable developments in this field. NASA used digital image processing to manipulate images beamed back to Earth from the Ranger spacecraft, for example, to improve visualization of the surface of the moon. Later benefits from the space program's research were applied to other fields such as photography, biology, forensics, defense, remote sensing, and medicine, including medical imaging.

Medical Imaging

All digital radiography imaging modalities including CR, flat-panel digital radiography, digital mammography, and digital fluoroscopy, utilize digital image processing as a central feature of their operations. Additionally, other digital imaging modalities such as CT, MRI, diagnostic ultrasound, and nuclear medicine incorporate digital image processing as an essential tool to manipulate and enhance digital images. For this reason, it is important that technologists and radiologists alike become well versed in the nature, scope, and principles of digital image processing. This chapter offers one small step in that direction.

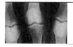 ## Image Formation and Representation

One of the first steps in becoming aware of and versatile with digital image processing is to understand the general nature of images. In this regard, Castleman (1994), an image processing expert, uses set theory to classify images based on their form and the method used to produce them. He conceptualizes images as a subset of all objects, and that image set contains subsets within it, such as visible and invisible images, optical images, and mathematical images. Visible images include photographs,

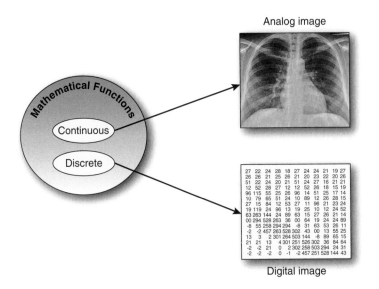

FIGURE 2-1. **Mathematical images include both continuous and discrete functions.**
Source: *Delmar, Cengage Learning*

drawings, and paintings, and invisible images include temperature, pressure, and elevation maps. Optical images include holograms, for example, and mathematical images include continuous and discrete functions, as is illustrated in Figure 2-1.

Mathematical images are important in the world of digital imaging. For example, the classical sine wave is a continuous function that can be converted into a discrete function, both of which will generate two categories of images, namely, analog and digital images (Figure 2-1).

Analog Images

If the image of the chest in Figure 2-1 is scanned from left to right using a light source (positioned in front of the image) and a photomultiplier tube (PMT-positioned behind the image) to detect the transmitted light, the light intensity will change continuously with respect to dark and bright spots on the image. The PMT would generate an output signal in which its intensity varies continuously depending on the location of the light on the image. This signal is called an analog signal, and it represents the image scanned by the light source and the PMT. Such an image is called an analog image, because it is generated from a continuous function. It is important to note that in radiology, images displayed on analog monitors for viewing and interpretation are **analog images**.

Digital Images

In digital radiography, a **digital image** is a numerical representation of the patient, as is illustrated in Figure 2-2. The following points are noteworthy:

1. The output from a digital radiography detector is an analog (electrical) signal.

2. This signal is sent to an **analog-to-digital converter (ADC)**.

3. The ADC changes the continuous analog signal into discrete digital data. This is an important step in generating a digital image, simply because a computer requires discrete data (0s and 1s) for operation.

4. The result of computer processing is a digital image. Since radiologists and technologists do not view numerical representations (digital images), these must be converted into a form suitable for human viewing. Hence, the digital image is converted into a visible physical image, an analog image.

In summary, digital image processing is defined by as "subjecting numerical representations of objects to a series of operations in order to obtain a desired result" (Castleman, 1996). This chapter will subsequently outline the essential elements of several operations.

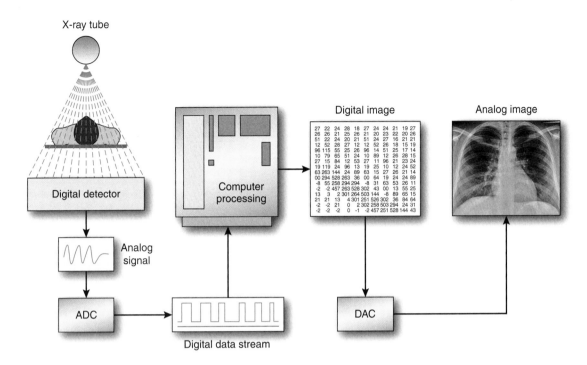

FIGURE 2-2. A digital image is a numerical representation of the patient. A computer is used to process the data from the digital detector to produce a digital image.
Source: *Delmar, Cengage Learning*

Image Domains

The images obtained in radiology can be represented in two domains, based on how they are acquired. These include (1) the spatial location domain, and (2) the spatial frequency domain.

As mentioned earlier, the digital image is a numerical image arranged in such a manner that the location of each number in the image can be identified using an X-Y coordinate system. Each pixel can be located using the X-Y coordinate system. The X-axis describes the horizontal location of the pixel (the column where the pixel is located) and the Y-axis describes the vertical location of the pixel (the row where the pixel is located) as illustrated in Figure 2-3. For example, the first pixel in the upper left corner of the image is always identified as 0,0. The spatial location 5, 3 in Figure 2-3 will describe a pixel that is located 5 pixels to the right of the left hand side of the image and 3 lines down from the top of the image. As noted by Baxes (1994) "often, the X location is referred to as the pixel number and the Y location

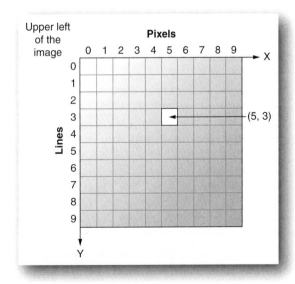

FIGURE 2-3. A right-handed coordinate system for locating any pixel that makes up a digital image. In this case, the arrows and associated numbering show the exact location of two pixels.
Source: *Delmar, Cengage Learning*

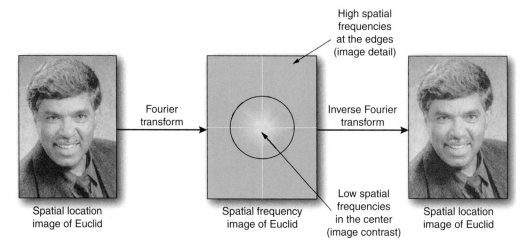

High spatial
frequencies
at the edges
(image detail)

Fourier
transform

Inverse Fourier
transform

Low spatial
frequencies
in the center
(image contrast)

Spatial location
image of Euclid

Spatial frequency
image of Euclid

Spatial location
image of Euclid

FIGURE 2-4. An image of Euclid in the spatial location domain (left) can be transformed using the Fourier transform into an image in the spatial frequency domain (right).
Source: *Delmar, Cengage Learning*

as the line number". Such an image is said to be in the spatial location domain.

Images can also be acquired in the spatial frequency domain. For example, MRI acquires data from the patient in the frequency domain. The term frequency refers to the number of cycles per unit length, that is, the number of times a signal changes per unit length. While small structures within an object (patient) produce high frequencies that represent the detail in the image, large structures produce low frequencies and represent contrast information in the image.

In digital radiography, digital image processing can transform one image domain into another image domain. For example, an image of Euclid in the spatial location domain, can be transformed into a spatial frequency domain image, as illustrated in Figure 2-4. The Fourier Transform (FT) is used to perform this task. The FT is mathematically rigorous and will not be covered in this text. The FT converts a function in the time domain (say signal intensity versus time) to a function in frequency domain (say, signal intensity versus frequency). The inverse Fourier Transform denoted by FT^{-1} is used to transform an image in the frequency domain back to the spatial location domain for viewing by radiologists and technologists. Physicists and engineers on the other hand, would probably prefer to view images in the frequency domain.

One of the primary goals for doing this is to facilitate image processing that can enhance or suppress certain features of the image. For example, the image can be enhanced for sharpness, in which case the low frequencies are suppressed, or it can be smoothed to enable better visualization of homogeneous structures by suppressing high frequencies via digital image processing in the frequency domain.

 ## Classes of Digital Image Processing Operations

The operations used in digital image processing to transform an input image into an output image to suit the needs of the human observer are several. Baxes (1994) identifies at least five fundamental classes of operations: image enhancement, image restoration, image analysis, image compression, and image synthesis. Although it is not within the scope of this text to describe all of these in any great detail, it is noteworthy to mention the purpose of each of them and state their particular operations. For a more complete and thorough description, the interested reader should refer to the work of Baxes (1994).

- *Image enhancement:* The purpose of this class of processing is to generate an image that is more pleasing to the observer. Certain characteristics such as contours and shapes can be enhanced to improve the overall quality of the image. The operations include contrast enhancement, edge enhancement, spatial and frequency filtering, image combining, and noise reduction.

- **Image restoration**: The purpose of image restoration is to improve the quality of images that have distortions or degradations. Image restoration is commonplace in spacecraft imagery. Images sent to Earth from various camera systems on spacecrafts suffer distortions/degradations that must be corrected for proper viewing. Blurred images, for example, can be filtered to make them sharper.

- *Image analysis:* This class of digital image processing allows measurements and statistics to be performed, as well as image segmentation, feature extraction, and classification of objects. Baxes (1994) indicates that "the process of analyzing objects in an image begins with image segmentation operations, such as image enhancement or restoration operations. These operations are used to isolate and highlight the objects of interest. Then the features of the objects are extracted resulting in object outlines or other object measures. These measures describe and characterize the objects

in the image. Finally, the object measures are used to classify the objects into specific categories." Segmentation operations are used in 3D medical imaging (Seeram, 2009).

- **Image compression**: The purpose of image compression of digital images is to reduce the size of the image in order to decrease transmission time and reduce storage space (Seeram, 2005, 2006). In general, there are two forms of image compression, lossy and lossless compression. In lossless compression there is no loss of any information in the image (detail is not compromised) when the image is decompressed. In lossy compression, there is some loss of image details when the image is decompressed. The latter has specific uses, especially in situations when it is not necessary to have exact details of the original image (Seeram & Seeram, 2008). A more recent form of compression that has been receiving attention in digital diagnostic imaging is that of wavelet (special waveforms) compression. The main advantage of this form of compression is that there is no loss in either spatial and frequency information. Image compression will be described further in Chapter 8.

- *Image synthesis:* These processing operations "create images from other images or non-image

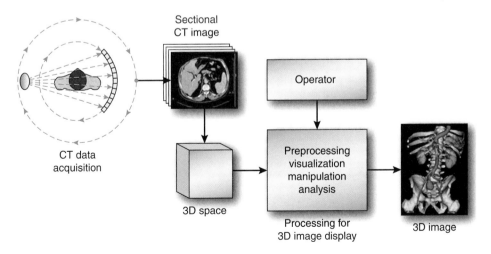

FIGURE 2-5. 3D imaging is an example of image synthesis. Note that a new image—the 3D image—is created from a set of transverse sectional images collected from the imaging modality.
Source: *3D image is provided by the courtesy of Philips Medical Systems, Andover, Mass*

data. These operations are used when a desired image is either physically impossible or impractical to acquire, or does not exist in a physical form at all" (Baxes, 1994). Examples of operations are image reconstruction techniques, which are the basis for the production of CT and MR images, and 3D visualization techniques, which are based on computer graphics technology (Seeram, 2009). This is illustrated in Figure 2-5.

Image synthesis will not be described further in this book.

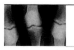

Characteristics of the Digital Image

A digital image can be described with respect to several characteristics or fundamental parameters, including the matrix, pixels, voxels, and the bit depth (Brennan, McEntee, Stowe, & Seeram, in press; Castleman, 1996; Indrajit & Verma, 2007; Pooley, et al., 2001; Seeram, 2004, 2008; Seeram & Seeram, 2009; Seibert, 1995).

Matrix

Apart from being a numerical image, there are other elements of a digital image that are important to our understanding of digital image processing. A digital image is made up of a 2D array of numbers called a matrix. The matrix consists of columns (M) and rows (N) that define small square regions called picture elements, or pixels. The dimension of the image can be described by M, N and the size of the image is given by the relationship

$$M \times N \times k \text{ bits}$$

When $M = N$, the image is square. Generally, diagnostic digital images are rectangular in shape. When imaging a patient using a digital imaging modality, the operator selects the matrix size for the examination, sometimes referred to as the **field-of-view (FOV)**. In this case, one dimension of the matrix size is used to represent the FOV and is the dimension of the anatomy to be imaged. Typical matrix sizes are shown in Table 1-1. It is important to note that as images become larger, they require more processing time and more storage space, as well more time to be transmitted to remote locations. In this regard, image compression is needed to facilitate storage and transmission requirements.

Pixels

The pixels that make up the matrix are generally square. Each pixel contains a number (discrete value) that represents a brightness level, which reflects the tissue characteristics being imaged. For example, while in radiography and CT, these numbers are related to the atomic number and mass density of the tissues, in MRI, they represent other characteristics of tissues such as proton density and relaxation times.

The **pixel size** can be calculated using the relationship:

$$\text{Pixel Size} = \text{FOV}/\text{Matrix Size}$$

TABLE 1-1. Typical matrix sizes used in digital medical imaging, at the time of writing this book.

Digital Imaging Modality	Matrix Size and Typical Bit Depth
Nuclear Medicine	128 x 128 x 12
Magnetic Resonance Imaging	256 x 256 x 16
Computed Tomography	512 x 512 x 16
Digital Subtraction Angiography	1024 x 1024 x 10
Computed Radiography	3520 x 4280 x 12
Digital Radiography (Flat-Panel Imagers)	3000 x 3000 x 12–16
Digital Mammography	4096 x 4096 x 12

For digital imaging modalities, the larger the matrix size, the smaller the pixel size (for the same FOV) and the better the spatial resolution. The effect of the matrix size on picture clarity can be seen in Figure 2-6.

Voxels

Pixels in a digital image represent the information contained in a volume of tissue in the patient. Such volume is referred to as a **voxel** (**vo**lume **el**ement). Tissue voxel information is converted into numerical values and expressed in the pixels, and these numbers are assigned brightness levels, as illustrated in Figure 2-7.

Bit Depth

In the relationship, M x N x k bits, the term "k bits" implies that every pixel in the digital image matrix M x N is represented by k binary digits. The number of bits per pixel is the bit depth. Since the binary number system uses the base 2, k bits = 2^k.

Therefore, each pixel will have 2^k gray levels. For example, in a digital image with a bit depth of 2, each pixel will have 2^2 (4) gray levels (density). Similarly, a bit depth of 8 implies that each pixel will have 2^8 (256) gray levels or shades of gray. The effect of bit depth is clearly seen in Figure 2-8. Table 1-1 also provides the typical bit depth for diagnostic digital images.

Appearance of Digital Images

The characteristics of a digital image, that is, the matrix size, the pixel size, and the bit depth, can affect the appearance of the digital image, particularly its spatial resolution and its contrast resolution.

The matrix size has an effect on the detail, or spatial resolution, of the image. The larger the matrix size (for the same FOV), the smaller the pixel size, hence the better the appearance of detail (Figure 2-6). Additionally, as the FOV decreases without a change in matrix size, the size of the pixel decreases as well (recall the relationship pixel size = FOV/matrix size), thus improving detail. The operator selects a larger matrix size when imaging larger body parts, such as the chest, in order to show small details in the anatomy.

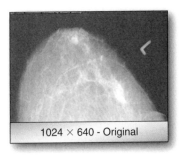

1024 × 640 - Original

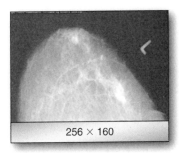

256 × 160

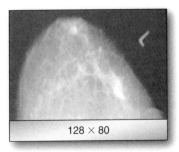

128 × 80

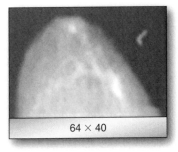

64 × 40

FIGURE 2-6. The effect of matrix size on picture quality. As the matrix size increases for the same FOV, picture quality improves; that is, the image becomes sharper. Source: *Images are the courtesy of Bruno Jaggi, PEng–Biomedical Engineer–British Columbia Institute of Technology*

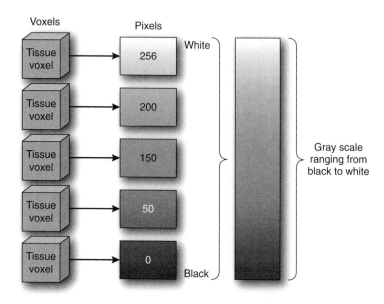

FIGURE 2-7. The tissues contained in voxels are converted into numerical values that are represented in the pixels. These values are converted into a gray scale, where the lower numbers are represented as black and the higher numbers are represented as white.
Source: *Delmar, Cengage Learning*

The bit depth has an effect on the number of shades of gray, hence the density resolution of the image. This is clearly apparent in Figure 2-8.

Steps in Digitizing an Image

In order to understand filmless imaging technology in the radiology department, it is first essential to understand the fundamental steps to digitizing images, because similar steps apply to any digital imaging modality.

There are three steps to digitizing an image, as shown in Figure 2-9: scanning, sampling, and quantization. Each of these will now be described briefly.

In scanning, the image is first divided into an array of pixels. The second step, sampling, simply involves measuring the brightness level of each of the pixels using special devices such as a photomultiplier tube (PMT). The signal from the PMT is an analog signal (voltage waveform) that must be converted into a digital image for processing by a computer. The third step in digitizing an image is quantization. This is a process whereby the brightness levels obtained from sampling are assigned an integer (zero or a negative or positive number) called a gray level. The image is now made up of a range of gray levels. The total number of gray levels is called the gray scale.

The ADC (Figure 2-2) plays an important role in the process of converting an analog signal into digital data for input into a computer. The ADC consists of several components that will divide up the analog signal into equal parts. For example, a 2-bit ADC will convert the analog signal into 4 (2^2) equal parts, resulting in 4 gray levels. An 8-bit ADC will divide up the analog signal into 256 (2^8) parts, resulting in 256 gray levels. The image digitization steps are shown in Figure 2-9.

Digital imaging modalities have 12 to 32-bit ADCs. The greater the bits, the more accurately the signals from the detectors can be digitized for a faithful reproduction of the original signal. This means that image quality is better with higher-bit ADCs compared to lower-bit ADCs.

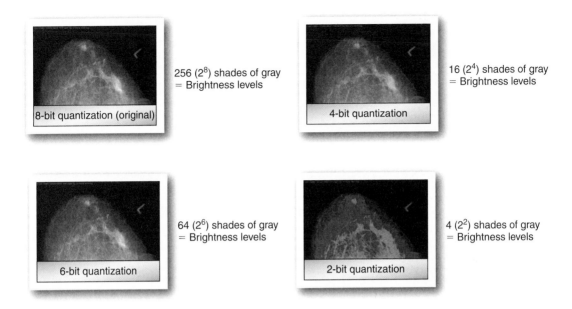

FIGURE 2-8. The effect of bit depth on the shades of gray in an image (density resolution). The higher the bit depth the greater the shades of gray.
Source: *Images courtesy of Bruno Jaggi, PEng–Biomedical Engineer–British Columbia Institute of Technology*

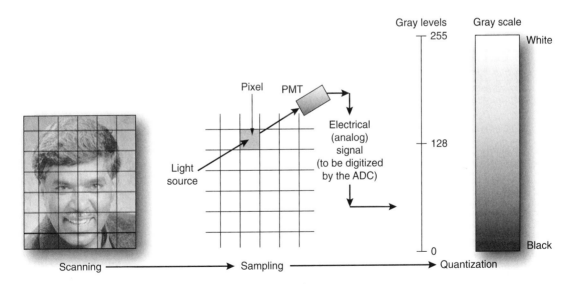

FIGURE 2-9. The essential steps in digitizing an image.
Source: Seeram E. (2004). Digital Image Processing. *Radiologic Technology*, vol 75, No 6, 435–452. (*Reproduced by permission of the ASRT*)

TABLE 2-2. Common digital image processing operations used in diagnostic digital imaging technologies.

Digital Imaging Modality	Common Image Processing Operations
Computed Tomography	Image Reformatting, Windowing, Region of Interest (ROI), Magnification, Surface and Volume Rendering, Profile, Histogram, Collage, Image Synthesis
Magnetic Resonance Imaging	Windowing, Region of Interest (ROI), Magnification, Surface and Volume Rendering, Profile, Histogram, Collage, Image Synthesis
Digital Subtracting Angiography/ Digital Fluoroscopy	Analytic Processing, Subtraction of Images out of a Sequence, Gray-Scale Processing, Temporal Frame Averaging, Edge Enhancement, Pixel Shifting
Computed Radiography/ Digital Radiography	Partitioned Pattern Recognition, Exposure Field Recognition, Histogram Analysis, Normalization of Raw Image Data, Gray-Scale Processing (Windowing), Spatial Filtering, Dynamic Range Control, Energy Subtraction, etc

Source Seeram E: Digital Image Processing. *Radiologic Technology* 2004, vol 75, No 6: 435–452. (*Reproduced by permission of the ASRT*)

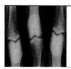

Digital Image Processing Operations: General Concepts

Another important concept in digital image processing is processing itself. Both past and current day processing technologies include a wide range of image processing algorithms for use in digital radiology (Baxes, 1994; Huang, 2004; Seeram, 2009; Seeram & Seeram, 2008). These include point processing operations such as gray-scale processing (windowing, image subtraction, and temporal averaging); local processing operations (such as spatial filtering, edge enhancement, and smoothing); and global operations such as the FT. It is not within the scope of this chapter to describe the details of these processing algorithms; however, a conceptual overview of these operations for single images (as opposed to multiple images) will be presented since a number of them are used in digital radiology, several examples of which are shown in Table 2-2.

Image processing operations are intended to change the intensity values of the pixels in the input image and display the resulting changes in the output image with the goal of changing the characteristics of the image to suit the needs of the observer in order to enhance diagnosis. This chapter will outline the elements of those operations that are specifically intended to change and optimize image contrast, improve image detail by sharpening the image, and decrease the noise present in the image.

Point Processing Operations

A point processing operation is simple and the most frequently used in digital diagnostic imaging. The basic framework for this operation is illustrated in Figure 2-10. The value of the one (point) input image pixel is mapped onto the corresponding output image pixel; that is, the output image pixel value at the same location as on the input image matrix depends on the value of the input image pixel. The operation (algorithm) allows the entire input image matrix to be scanned pixel by pixel, using a "pixel point process" (Baxes, 1994), until the entire image is transformed.

One common point processing operation is referred to as gray-level mapping or gray-scale processing. Other terms that are used to describe gray-level mapping are "contrast stretching," "contrast enhancement," "histogram modification," "histogram stretching," or simply "windowing." Windowing is the most commonly used image processing operation in digital diagnostic imaging, including computed radiography, digital radiography using flat-panel detectors, CT, and MRI.

Image contrast and brightness transformations can be done using a variety of processing techniques, and it is noteworthy here to describe the fundamental concepts of at least two common methods used in digital radiology, the look-up-table (LUT) method and the windowing method. Before describing each

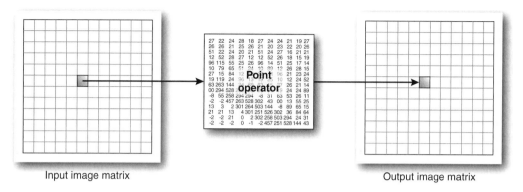

FIGURE 2-10. The point-processing digital operator.
Source: *Delmar, Cengage Learning*

of these, the concept of a histogram must be understood.

Histogram

A **histogram** is a graph of the number of pixels in the entire image or part of the image having the same gray levels (density values) plotted as a function of the gray levels, as shown in Figure 2-11. Changing the histogram of the image can alter its brightness and contrast. If the histogram is modified or changed, the brightness and contrast of the image will change as well. This operation is called histogram modification or histogram stretching. A wide histogram implies more contrast and a narrow histogram will show less contrast. If the values of the histogram are concentrated in the lower end of the range of values, the image appears dark; conversely, the image appears bright at the higher end of the range.

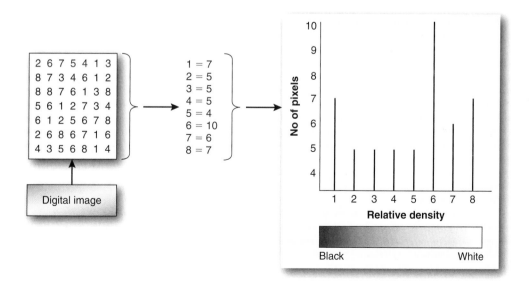

FIGURE 2-11. A digital image can be converted into a histogram in which the number of pixels is plotted as a function of the relative density. Adjusting the histogram will change the density of the image.
Source: *Delmar, Cengage Learning*

Look-up Table

To illustrate the concept of a look-up table (LUT), two excellent examples from Sprawls (2004) will be given here, a numerical example and a graphical example. First, consider Figure 2-12, which shows a low-contrast numerical image with a contrast difference, (that is, the object relative to the background) of 10 (40-30) where 40 represents the background contrast and 30 represents the object contrast. The LUT is then used to change the low-contrast numerical image to a high-contrast image by assigning numbers to the input values 40

and 30 that will subsequently change them into 90 and 10, respectively. The contrast difference for the new output image (on the right) is now 80 (90-10) and therefore this image appears as a high-contrast image. During digital image processing, the LUT determines the numbers assigned to the input pixel values that change them into output pixel values, resulting in a change in contrast and brightness of the image (Seeram, 2009; Seeram & Seeram, 2008).

Conversely, consider Figure 2-13A, which shows a plot of the input image pixel values as a function

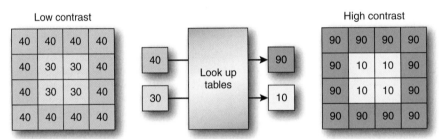

Contrast is changed by changing pixel values.

FIGURE 2-12. Image manipulation allows the operator to change a low-contrast image into a high-contrast image using a look-up table.
Source: *Courtesy of Dr Perry Sprawls, PhD*

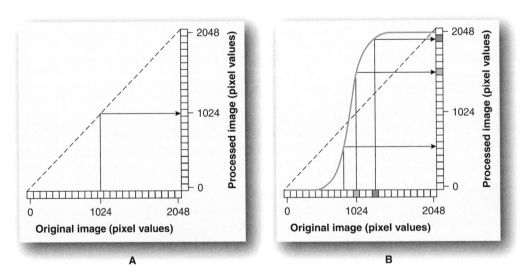

FIGURE 2-13. The pixel values in the input image plotted as a function of the pixel values in the output image result in a straight line (A); however, a LUT curve is also possible (B). The latter is the characteristic H and D curve for film.
Source: *Courtesy of Dr Perry Sprawls, PhD*

of the output image pixel values. In this case the values are the same. For example, the value 1024 for the input image matches the value 1024 for the output image. The resulting graph is a straight line. Are LUT curves possible? The answer is yes, as is clearly apparent in Figure 2-13B. This is the classic characteristic curve (H and D) for film. Finally, in Figure 2-14, three LUT curves are shown: a latitude curve, a high-contrast curve, and an invert curve. Recall that the slope of the characteristic curve

influences the contrast of the image. A steep slope results in a high-contrast image while a small slope (less than 45°) will result in decreased contrast.

Digital radiographic imaging systems (such as CR for example) utilize a wide range of LUTs stored in the system for the different types of clinical examinations (chest, spine, pelvis, extremities, for example). The operator should therefore select the appropriate LUT to match the part being imaged. An important point to note here is that since digital radiographic detectors have wide exposure latitude and a linear response, the image displayed without processing may appear as a low-contrast image. A processing example for a chest image using the LUT is shown in Figure 2-15.

Windowing

The digital image processing technique known as windowing is also intended to change the contrast and brightness of an image. A digital image is made up of numbers, and by definition the range of the numbers is the window width (WW) and the center of the range is defined as the window level (WL). The range of the pixel values (gray levels) and displayed image contrast range are shown in Figure 2-16. The WW controls image contrast and the WL controls the brightness of the image. In an image, the displayed gray levels will range from −1/2WW+WL to +1/2WW+WL (Seeram, 2009). The numbers above the maximum are assigned 255, and those numbers below the minimum will be assigned 0. The displayed WW and WL values

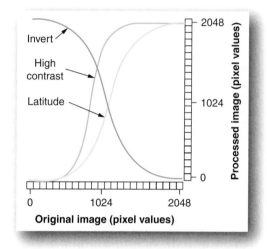

FIGURE 2-14. Other LUT curves are possible when the input pixel values are plotted as a function of the output pixel values, such as the three curves shown.
Source: *Courtesy of Dr Perry Sprawls, PhD*

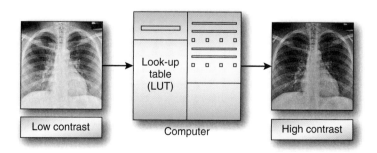

FIGURE 2-15. The effect on a chest image of using an LUT to convert a low-contrast image into a high-contrast image.
Source: *Delmar, Cengage Learning*

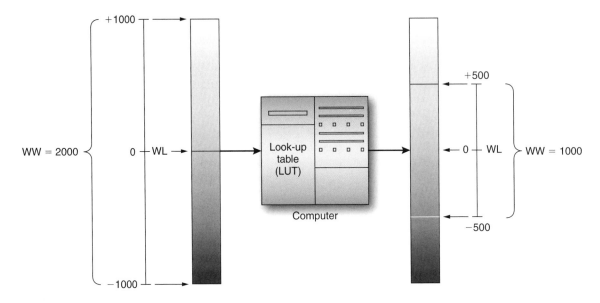

FIGURE 2-16. A graphical illustration of the effect of using an LUT to change a wide range of pixel values (WW = 2000/WL = 0) into a narrow range of pixel values (WW = 1000/WL = 0).
Source: *Delmar, Cengage Learning*

are always shown on the image. Narrow WW provides higher image contrast (short-scale contrast) and a wide WW will show an image with less contrast. This effect is shown in Figure 2-17. Conversely, when the WL is increased, the image becomes darker since more of the lower numbers will be displayed (Figure 2-18).

It is interesting to note that image subtraction and temporal averaging are also classified as point processing operations. These are used routinely in digital subtraction angiography. Essentially, in image subtraction, the pixel values from post-contrast images are subtracted from pixel values from the first pre-contrast image (mask) to show contrast-filled blood vessels with the other structures removed in order to enhance the diagnostic impressions of the radiologist. Temporal averaging refers to subtraction of images in time. In particular, temporal averaging involves averaging a set of images to reduce image noise. The greater the number of images averaged, the lesser the image noise. The interested reader should refer to Pooley et al. (2001) and Seibert (1995) for further details of these two techniques.

Local Processing Operations

A local processing operation is one in which the output image pixel value is obtained from a small area of pixels around the corresponding input pixel, as illustrated in Figure 2-19. Because a small area of pixels, or group of pixels, is used, these operations are also referred to as area or group processes. A notable example is that of spatial frequency filtering.

As described earlier in this text, an image in the spatial location domain can be transformed into an image in the spatial frequency domain. The spatial frequency domain image would be made of high spatial frequencies that represent detail and low spatial frequencies that represent contrast information. The idea of using spatial frequency filtering (processing) is to use the high and low frequencies to change the characteristics of the image to suit the needs of the observer in order to enhance diagnosis. For example, spatial frequency processing can sharpen, smooth, and blur images, as well as reduce the noise in the image and extract certain features of interest from it.

Spatial frequency filtering can be done in the frequency domain or it can be done in the spatial

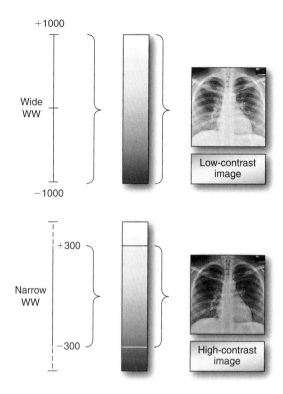

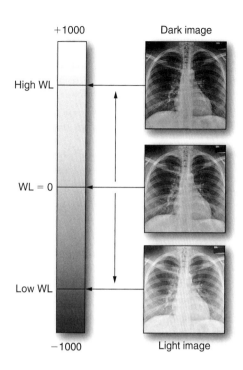

FIGURE 2-17. The effect of changing the window width (WW) on the contrast of a chest image. A narrow WW results in an image of higher contrast, while the window level (WL) remains fixed.
Source: Seeram E. (2004). Digital Image Processing. *Radiologic Technology*, vol 75, No 6, 435–452. (*Reproduced by permission of the ASRT*)

FIGURE 2-18. The effect of changing the window level (WL) on image brightness. As the WL decreases (low WL), the image increases in brightness for a fixed WW.
Source: Seeram E. (2004). Digital Image Processing. *Radiologic Technology*, vol 75, No 6, 435–452. (*Reproduced by permission of the ASRT*)

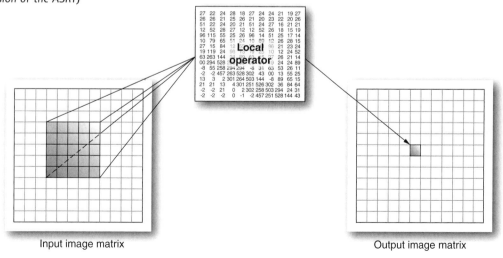

Input image matrix

Output image matrix

FIGURE 2-19. A local processing digital operator uses a defined region of pixels in the input image to change one pixel value in the output image.
Source: *Delmar, Cengage Learning*

location domain. While the former uses the FT, the latter makes use of the pixel values themselves.

Spatial Location Filtering–Convolution

A common example of filtering in the spatial location domain is convolution (Figure 2-20). The algorithm for convolution can be described as:

"the value of the output pixel depends on a group of pixels in the input image that surround the input pixel of interest: in this case P5. The new value for P5 in the output image is calculated by obtaining its weighted average and that of its surrounding pixels. The average is computed using a group of pixels called a convolution kernel, in which each pixel in the kernel is a weighting factor, or a convolution coefficient. In general the size of the kernel is a 3 x 3 matrix. Depending on the type of processing, different types of convolution kernels can be used, in which case the weighting factor is different." (Seeram, 2009).

In the act of processing, the kernel scans across the entire image, pixel by pixel. Every pixel in the input image, the pixels surrounding it, and the kernel are used to calculate the corresponding output pixel value. It can be seen from Figure 2-20, that

each calculation requires 9 multiplications and 9 summations. This arithmetic can be time-consuming, so special hardware (array processors) is used to speed up these calculations.

Spatial Frequency Filtering: High–Pass Filtering

The high-pass filtering process, also known as edge enhancement or sharpness, is intended to sharpen an input image in the spatial domain that appears blurred. The algorithm is such that first the spatial location image is converted into spatial frequencies using the FT, followed by the use of a high-pass filter that suppresses the low spatial frequencies to produce a sharper output image (Seeram & Seeram, 2008). This process is shown in Figure 2-21. The high-pass filter kernel is also shown.

Spatial Frequency Filtering: Low–Pass Filtering

A low-pass filtering process makes use of a low-pass filter to operate on the input image with the goal of smoothing. The output image will appear blurred. Smoothing is intended to reduce noise and the displayed brightness levels of pixels; however, image detail is compromised. This is illustrated in Figure 2-22. The low-pass filter kernel is also shown.

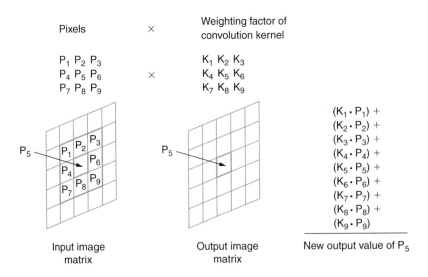

FIGURE 2-20. An example of the convolution technique. See text for further explanation.
Source: Seeram E. (2004). Digital Image Processing. *Radiologic Technology*, vol 75, No 6, 435–452. *(Reproduced by permission of the ASRT)*

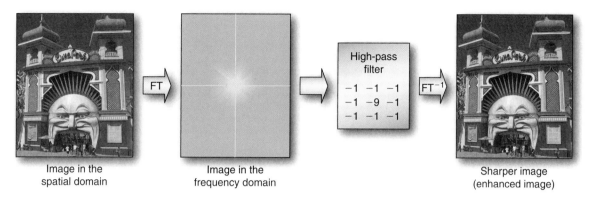

FIGURE 2-21. The effect of using a high-pass digital filter on the quality of the output image. Note that in order to use this filter, the input image is first changed from a spatial location image into a spatial frequency image. The filter operates on the frequencies to sharpen the output image.
Source: *Delmar, Cengage Learning*

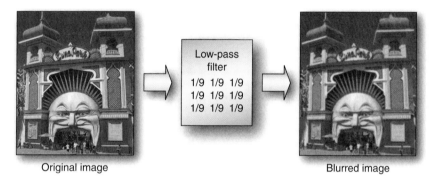

FIGURE 2-22. The effect of a low-pass filter on the quality of the output image. In this case, the output image is blurred.
Source: *Delmar, Cengage Learning*

Spatial Frequency Processing: Unsharp (blurred) Masking

The digital image processing technique of unsharp (blurred) masking uses the blurred image produced from the low-pass filtering process and subtracts it from the original image to produce a sharp image, as illustrated in Figure 2-23, where it can be seen that the output image appears sharper.

Global Processing Operations

The term "global" implies that all the pixels in the entire input image are used to change the value of a pixel in the output image. The conceptual framework for global processing operations is shown in Figure 2-24. One popular global operation is to use the FT in filtering images in the frequency domain rather than in the spatial location domain (Baxes, 1994). These techniques can process images for edge enhancement, image sharpening, and image restoration. It is not within the scope of this text to describe the details of global processing operations.

Geometric Operations

Another class of image processing operations that are sometimes used in digital radiology is that of geometric operations. These techniques allow the

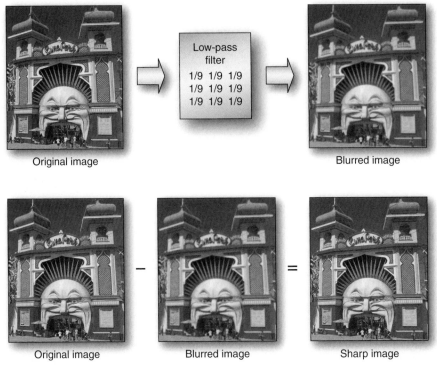

FIGURE 2-23. The digital processing technique of unsharp masking can be used to sharpen the output image.
Source: *Delmar, Cengage Learning*

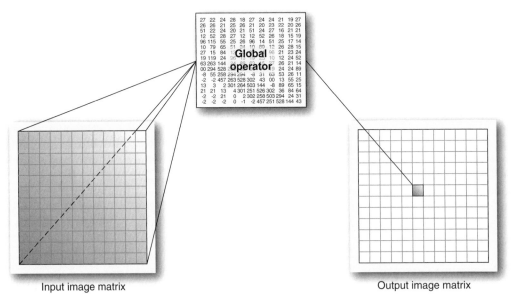

FIGURE 2-24. A global processing digital operator uses all of the pixels in the input image to change one pixel value in the output image.
Source: *Delmar, Cengage Learning*

user to change the position or orientation of pixels in the image rather that the brightness of the pixels. Geometric operations result in the scaling, sizing, rotation, and translation of images, once again, to enhance diagnosis.

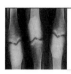

Image Post-Processing: An Essential Tool for Technologists

Digital image post-processing is a range of techniques that allow the user to change the appearance of a digital image displayed on a monitor for viewing and interpretation. These techniques, for example, allow both the gray scale and the sharpness of the image to be manipulated to enhance diagnostic interpretation. Image post-processing is now a routine activity in digital medical imaging, and it is also an essential tool in the PACS environment. Already, technologists and radiologists are actively involved in using the tools of image processing, such as the digital image processing operations and techniques outlined in this chapter. Education programs for both technologists and radiologists are also beginning to incorporate digital image processing as part of their curriculum. Such activities will serve to improve communications between radiologists, medical imaging physicists, and biomedical engineers, as well as with equipment vendors. A course on image post-processing for medical imaging technology programs may include topics such as the nature of digital images; image processing operations and their applications in digital radiology, to include specific post-processing operations in CR, DR, CT, MRI, digital subtraction angiography, digital fluoroscopy, and 3D Imaging; and image compression fundamentals. Finally, programs may use the commercially available image processing software Adobe Photoshop® for laboratory exercises that students can engage in to strengthen and enhance their understanding of image post-processing (Seeram & Seeram, 2008).

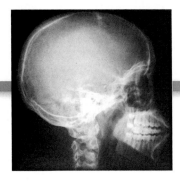

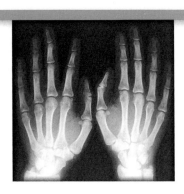

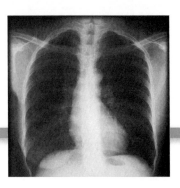

REVIEW QUESTIONS

1. State the meaning of the term "digital image processing."
2. Briefly trace the evolution of digital imaging processing.
3. What is the difference between an analog image and a digital image?
4. Explain the difference between the spatial location domain and the spatial frequency domain.
5. List five classes of digital image processing operations and explain the goal of each of them.
6. Describe the major features of each of the following characteristics of a digital image:
   a. Matrix
   b. Pixel
   c. Voxel
   d. Bit depth
7. What is the relationship between pixel size, FOV, and matrix size?
8. What physical characteristic of tissues does the pixel number represent?
9. How many shades can be seen in an image with a bit depth of 10?
10. What is the main controlling factor for the spatial resolution of a digital image?
11. Explain the effect on the appearance of the digital image as the bit depth is reduced.
12. Describe the three steps in digitizing an image.
13. State the goal of each of the four digital image processing operations: point processing, local processing, global processing, and geometric processing operations.
14. What information is contained in an image histogram?

15. State the meaning of the terms "windowing," "window width," and "window level."
16. Explain the influence of the WW and WL on image gray-scale appearance
17. What is the difference between spatial location filtering and spatial frequency filtering of an image?
18 Explain the effects of using a high-pass filter and a low-pass filter on an image.
19. What is the visual effect of an unsharp (masking) digital image processing technique on an image?
20. What is the purpose of a geometric digital image processing operation?

REFERENCES

Baxes, G. A. (1994). *Digital Image Processing: Principles and Applications*. New York: John Wiley & Sons, Inc.

Brennan, P., McEntee, M., & Seeram, E. *Digital Diagnostic Imaging*. Oxford: Blackwell Publishers. In press.

Castleman, K. R. (1996). *Digital Image Processing*. Englewood Cliffs: NJ, Prentice Hall.

Huang, H. K. (2004). *PACS and Imaging Informatics*. New York: John Wiley & Sons, Inc.

Indrajit, I. K., & Verma, B. S. (2007). Digital imaging in radiology practice: An introduction to few fundamental concepts. *Indian Journal of Radiology and Imaging, 17*, 230–236.

Pooley, R. A., McKinney, J. M., & David A. Miller (2001). Digital fluoroscopy. *Radiographics, 21*, 521–534.

Seeram, E. (2005). Digital image compression. *Radiologic Technology, 76*(6), 449–459.

Seeram, E. (2006). Using irreversible compression in digital radiology: A preliminary study of the opinions of radiologists. *Progress in Biomedical Optics and Imaging* (pp. 276–284). Proceedings of SPIE: San Diego, CA.

Seeram, E. (2009). *Computed Tomography: Physical Principles, Clinical Applications, and Quality Control* (3rd ed.). Philadelphia: WB Saunders Co.

Seeram, E. & Seeram, D. (2008). Image postprocessing in digital radiology: A primer for technologists. *Journal of Medical Imaging and Radiation Sciences, 39*(1), 23–44.

Seibert, A. J. (1995). Digital image processing basics. *RSNA Categorical Course in Physics*, 121–142.

Sprawls, P. (2008). Personal communications. Emory University.

CHAPTER 3

Computed Radiography: Physics and Technology

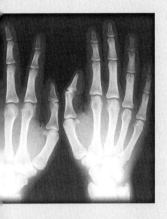

OBJECTIVES

On completion of this Chapter, you should be able to:

1. List terms synonymous with computed radiography (CR).

2. Trace the history of CR.

3. Identify and describe four primary steps involved in the CR imaging process.

4. Explain the fundamental physics of the formation of CR images.

5. Describe the structure of the CR imaging plate.

6. Describe how the CR reader works.

7. Outline the pre-processing and post-processing operations used in CR imaging.

8. Describe the response of the CR imaging plate to radiation exposure.

9. Outline the use of exposure indicators in CR.

10. Identify and describe briefly four image quality descriptors for CR.

11. Define the term "artifact."

12. Identify several sources of artifacts in CR and the remedy for each of them.

13. Identify the basic elements of a quality control program for CR.

KEY TERMS

Acceptance testing (AT)
Artifact
Cassette-based systems
Cassette-less systems
Contrast enhancement
CR reader
CR workstation
Detective quantum
    efficiency (DQE)
Dose creep
Dual-sided reading
Edge enhancement
Erasure of the IP
Exposure field recognition
Exposure index (EI)
Exposure indicator
Fading
High resolution IP
Image acquisition
Imaging cycle

Imaging plate (IP)
Image processing
Laser scanning
Latent image
Measured histogram
Noise
Photodetector
Photostimulable
    luminescence (PSL)
Photostimulable phosphors
    (PSP)
Post-processing
Pre-processing operations
QC test
Quality control tool
Scanning technologies
Sensitivity number (S)
Spatial frequency processing
Standard resolution IP
Stored (known) histogram

Introduction

The basic principles of computed radiography (CR) were introduced in Chapter 1. In review, CR is a digital radiographic imaging modality in which a digital detector is used to capture X-rays transmitted through the patient. CR is based on the phenomenon of photostimulable luminescence that is exhibited by photostimulable phosphors. The CR digital detector is made of a photostimulable phosphor, which, when struck by X-rays, creates a latent image. The latent image is rendered visible when the detector is scanned by a laser beam to produce light (photostimulable luminescence) that is subsequently converted into electrical signals. These signals are digitized and processed by a computer that produces the CR image using special digital image processing algorithms.

The purpose of this chapter is to describe in detail the CR imaging system in terms of the basic physics of the CR detector and the technology needed to produce a CR image. In addition, the chapter will outline the essential elements of image processing, exposure control, image quality, and image artifacts in CR.

Terms Synonymous with CR

In the medical imaging literature, several other terms have been used to refer to CR. These include photostimulable luminescence (PSL), storage phosphor radiography (SPR), digital luminescence radiography (DLR), photostimulable storage phosphor (PSP) radiography, and digital storage phosphor (DSP) radiography. The term that has become commonplace, however, is computed radiography (CR) and, therefore, it will be used throughout this book.

A Brief History of CR

The history of CR is linked to photostimulable phosphors (PSP) and the phenomenon of photostimulable luminescence (PSL), and it can be traced back to the 1600s to the discovery of the Bolognese stone (glowing stone) in Italy. Later, in the 1800s,

Becquerel worked on the notion of de-excitation of atoms by optical means. This was followed by several notable developments, as shown in Figure 3-1.

It was in 1983 that commercialization of CR imaging systems for use in diagnostic radiology began, when Fuji introduced their FCR-101 unit. This was followed by other manufacturers, most notably Kodak and Agfa, whose systems became popular as well (Andriole, 1996, 2002; Lanca & Silva, 2009).

Today there are at least four manufacturers actively engaged in CR research, technology development, and marketing. They are Fuji, Kodak, Agfa Gavaert (Belgium), and Konica. The interested reader may visit their respective Web sites for their most recent developments in hardware and software.

The CR Imaging System

The CR imaging system components are shown in Figure 3-2. It is clearly apparent that the imaging process consists of four primary steps: image acquisition, image plate scanning and erasure, image processing, and image display. In addition to these, there are secondary steps that must be considered, as well as what the American Association of Physicists in Medicine (AAPM) refers to as "implementation issues." These issues address the practical use of CR and include technical concerns such as the use of grids, radiation exposure, technique selection, and so forth. These characteristics will be described in Chapter 4.

Image Acquisition

As illustrated in Figure 3-2, image acquisition refers to X-ray exposure of the phosphor plate storage, or imaging plate (IP) as it is popularly referred to. It is at this point that the technologist must pay careful attention to technical details, such as positioning, centering of the X-ray beam, selection of the appropriate IP, grid selection, and correct radiographic exposure technique factors (kVp, mAs).

Image acquisition also refers to the mechanism of X-ray interaction with the phosphor to produce

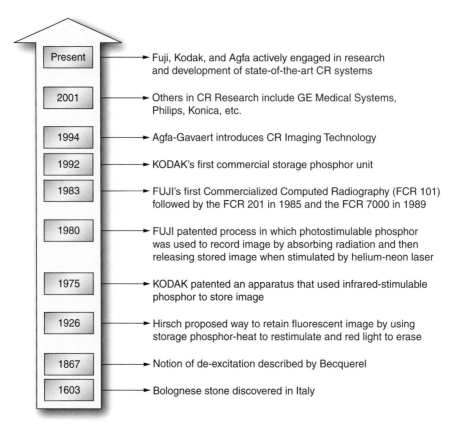

FIGURE 3-1. Notable developments in the history of CR based on photostimulable lumi-nescence. As can be seen, three manufacturers, most notably Agfa, Fuji, and Kodak, have been actively engaged in CR research and development.
Source: *Delmar, Cengage Learning*

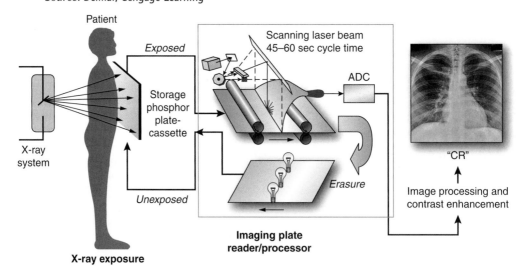

FIGURE 3-2. The CR imaging system components.
Source: Samei, E., Seibert, J. A., Andriole, K, et al. (2004). PACS Equipment Overview. *Radiographics* 24, 313–334. (*Reproduced by permission of the Radiological Society of North America*)

a latent image and subsequent scanning of the IP by a laser beam to produce photostimulable luminescence (PSL). The scanning of the IP takes place in the imaging plate reader/processor (Figure 3-2). This readout process essentially consists of laser scanning, detection, conversion of the PSL, and digitization of the signal by the analog-to-digital converter (ADC), as shown in Figure 3-2. These elements will be described in detail later in the chapter.

Image Processing

Image processing in CR refers to the use of several digital operations for pre-processing and post-processing of the CR image data. Pre-processing deals with shading corrections, pattern recognition, and exposure field recognition. Post-processing of the CR image data refers to contrast enhancement (image grayscale processing) and edge enhancement, a technique that is based on spatial frequency processing (Chapter 2). Additionally, energy subtraction imaging can be done in CR using a special algorithm to create separate images of bone and soft tissue. Image processing will be elaborated on in the section on image processing in this chapter.

Image Display, Storage, and Communications

After images have been processed, they are displayed for viewing and interpretation on a picture archiving and communication systems (PACS) environment, the technologist determines and assesses the overall image quality of the image and subsequently sends the image to the PACS. Once in the PACS, images are retrieved for interpretation by a radiologist.

In CR, images are displayed on a computer workstation. These workstations have either a cathode-ray tube (CRT) display monitor or an active-matrix liquid crystal display (LCD) device. The workstation allows the technologist to do any post-processing on images before they are communicated to the PACS for storage. Image storage and archiving in a CR-PACS environment include the use of magnetic tapes and disks, magneto-optical disks, optical disks, and digital videodisks (DVDs).

Finally, communication of the CR image to the PACS is accomplished via computer networks and other suitable technologies.

Basic Physics of CR Image Formation

The CR imaging process, that is, the image acquisition in particular, consists of a three-step cycle of image formation, as illustrated in Figure 3-3. The imaging plate (IP) consists of a photostimulable storage phosphor (PSP) layered on a base to provide support. Photostimulable phosphors have the property of creating and storing a latent image when exposed to X-rays. To render the latent image visible, the PSP must be scanned by a laser beam of a specific wavelength. Laser scanning produces a luminescence (light) that is proportional to the stored latent image (Schaetzing, 2003). This luminescence is referred to as photostimulated luminescence (PSL).

After laser scanning, the PSP IP is erased by exposing it to a high intensity light beam to get rid of any residual latent image. This step is important so that the IP can be used again and again for several X-ray exposures. In this section, the basic physics of photostimulable storage phosphor X-ray exposure and photostimulated luminescence will be described.

Nature of PSPs

As can be seen in Figure 3-3, the IP contains the PSP. The phosphors used in radiology must have certain physical characteristics to be useful in CR imaging. For example, phosphors should have good X-ray absorption efficiency and must be capable of being stimulated by a helium-neon (He Ne) laser. Additionally, the luminescence light must be compatible with the photomultiplier tube (PMT) phosphor (for proper detection and capture) and the time for luminescence must be shorter than 1 μsec (Fuji, 2002). Finally, these phosphors should be able to store the latent image for a number of hours without compromising the signal from the IP (Seibert, 2004).

The phosphors that meet the above requirements and are used by several manufacturers are, in general, Barium Fluoro Halide: Europium (BaFX: Eu^{2+}). The halide (X) can be chlorine (Cl), bromine (Br), or iodine (I), or a mixture of them (Neitzel, 2005). The phosphor is usually doped with Eu^{2+}, which

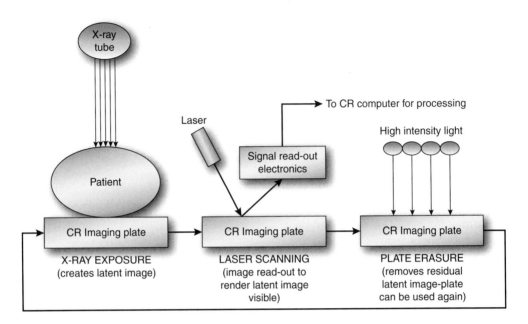

FIGURE 3-3. The CR image acquisition process is a cycle consisting of three steps: X-ray exposure of the IP, laser scanning of the exposed IP, and erasure of the IP for subsequent re-use.
Source: *Delmar, Cengage Learning*

acts as an activator to improve the efficiency of PSL. Another phosphor used in CR is BaFBr/I: Eu^{2+} (Seibert, 2004) and recently cesium bromide (CsBr: Eu2+) is being considered as a PSP for CR imaging (Neitzel, 2005). As mentioned above, good X-ray absorption efficiency is one of the requirements of a PSP for CR imaging. Such efficiency depends on not only the kVp (X-ray energy) used but also the thickness of the phosphor used in the IP. In Figure 3-4, the X-ray absorption efficiency of BaFBr PSP is shown and compared with the X-ray absorption efficiencies of the rare earth phosphor gadolinium oxysulfide (Gd_2O_2S) and cesium iodide (CsI). Figure 3-4 shows that between 35 keV and about 50 keV, BaFBr attenuates (absorbs) X-rays much better than Gd_2O_2S rare earth screens because of the lower k-edge absorption of barium. Note, however, that at energies lower than 35 keV and greater than 50 keV, Gd_2O_2S attenuates much better than BaFBr (Seibert, 2004).

Latent Image Formation and PSL

X-ray exposure of the PSP IP creates a latent image, and laser scanning of the exposed IP produces PSL. The information captured from the PSL is used to create the CR image. The physics of latent image creation and the mechanism of PSL are complex and beyond the scope of this book; however, the basic physics of image formation will be highlighted here. The interested reader should refer to the review article by Rowlands (2002) for a detailed description of the physics of CR.

The mechanics of how PSPs are thought to work is shown in Figure 3-5. When X-rays fall upon the PSP IP, the europium atoms are ionized by the radiation and the electrons move from the valence band (ground state) to the conduction band (higher energy). Electrons in the conduction band are free to travel to a so-called "F-center." The *F* comes from the German word *farbe*, meaning color (Fuji, 2002). The number of trapped electrons is proportional to the absorbed radiation. It is at the point in the process that the electrons are spatially distributed to create the latent image (Seibert, 2004). In addition to this mechanism, X-ray exposure of the IP causes it to fluoresce (emit light when it is exposed to X-rays) for a very brief duration.

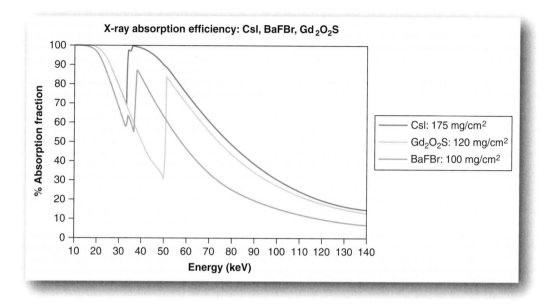

X-ray absorption efficiency: CsI, BaFBr, Gd₂O₂S

FIGURE 3-4. X-Ray absorption efficiency as a function of X-ray energy for BaFBr, Gd_2O_2S, and CsI phosphors. The mg/cm^2 is the typical thickness of the phosphor.
Source: Seibert, J. A. (2004). Computed radiography technology 2004. In L. W. Goldman & M. V. Yester (Eds.), *Specifications, Performance, and Quality Assurance of radiographic and Fluoroscopic Systems in the Digital Era.* College Park, Maryland: American Association of Physicists in Medicine [AAPM]. *(Reproduced by permission)*

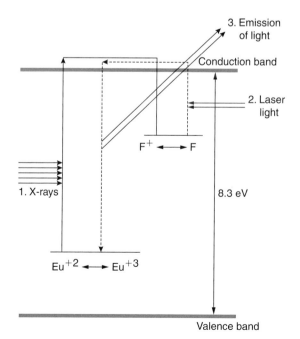

FIGURE 3-5. The mechanism of latent image creation and photostimulable luminescence (PSL).
Source: *Delmar, Cengage Learning*

To render the latent image visible, the PSP IP is taken to the CR reader/processor to be scanned by a laser beam. This process is referred to as photostimulated excitation (Fuji, 2002). While in the CR reader, the PSP IP is scanned systematically (to be described later in the chapter). The laser light used must be capable of being absorbed by the F-centers. This absorption causes the trapped electrons to move up to the conduction band, where they are free to return to the valence band, thus causing the Eu^{3+} to return to the Eu^{2+} state. This transition of the electrons from a higher energy state to a lower energy state (ground state) results in an emission of bluish-purple light (~415 nm wavelength). This is referred to as photostimulable luminescence (PSL) in the IP (AAPM, 2006; Bushong, 2009). This PSL is very different from the fluorescence described earlier.

The lasers used today for PSL in CR units are semiconductor lasers that produce light with a 680 nm wavelength compared to He Ne lasers that produce light with a 633 nm wavelength used in earlier CR units.

The PSL from the IP is collected by a special light-collection device and sent to a photomultiplier tube that produces an electrical signal. This signal is subsequently digitized by the ADC and sent to a computer for processing and CR image creation.

PSL Characteristics

There are several characteristics of PSL that are important in CR imaging. These include the light spectra related to the PSP IP and fading (Fuji, 2002). The light spectra of the PSP include the storage phosphor stimulation and the PSL emission spectra shown in Figure 3-6. The critical point to note is that the stimulation spectra are different from the PSL emission spectra. This is important to CR imaging since it is the PSL emission being captured by the PMT that creates the CR image.

Fading is a term that refers to the time it takes for the latent image to disappear. The latent image can last for several hours; however, it is important to read the exposed IP in a reasonable time so as not to compromise the PSL signal. For example, the PSL decreases by about 25% if the time between exposure and image reading is 8 hours or more (Fuji, 2002).

CR Technology

The CR imaging system is shown in Figure 3-2. The components of significance in this illustration are the imaging plate (IP) and the imaging plate reader/processor. Other components, such as image display and image processing, will be described later in the chapter.

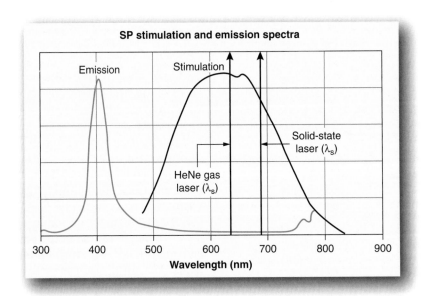

FIGURE 3-6. The emission and stimulation spectra of the IP in CR. The stimulation spectra of two lasers, a helium–neon gas laser and a solid-state laser diode (photostimulable excitation), are different from the emission (PSL) spectra. This difference is critical in CR imaging.
Source: Schaetzing R (2004). In L. W. Goldman & M. V. Yester (Eds.), *Specifications, Performance, and Quality Assurance of Radiographic and Fluoroscopic Systems in the Digital Era.* College Park, Maryland: American Association of Physicists in Medicine [AAPM]. (Reproduced by permission)

The CR Imaging Plate

The digital detector used in CR imaging is the imaging plate (IP). A cross section of the IP showing the major structural components is shown in Figure 3-7. The IP consists of the PSP layer on a base that provides support. In addition, the IP structure consists of two protective layers, an electroconductive layer and a light-shielding layer. The support holds the other components of the IP together and provides mechanical strength. One of these critical components is the photostimulable phosphor. The phosphor is mixed with an organic binder (a polymer such as polyester, for example) and coated onto the support layer. Two layers coat the phosphor, a front and a back protective layer (Figure 3-7). The front protective layer must be constructed so that it provides durability during multiple uses. This layer must also allow light from the laser and the stimulated light to pass through it. The purpose of the electroconductive layer, shown in Figure 3-7, is to reduce any problems when the IP is transported in the CR reader (CR scanner or processor) and static electricity problems that may degrade image quality. Some IPs have a barcode for easy identification.

Essentially, there are two types of IPs, a standard resolution IP and a high resolution IP. While standard IPs have thick phosphor layers and absorb more radiation, high resolution IPs have thinner phosphor layers and provide sharper images compared to thick phosphors. The sharpness is due to the fact that thinner phosphors reduce the lateral spread of the laser light.

In terms of radiographic speed, thick phosphor IPs have faster speeds than high resolution IPs (slow speeds), similar to the cassettes used in conventional radiography. Of course, the high resolution IPs will be used for extremity imaging and other small parts where detail (sharpness) is critical. The imaging plate size varies depending upon the manufacturer; however, 17" × 17" (43 × 43 cm), 17" × 14" (43 × 35 cm), 14" × 17" (35 × 43 cm), and 14" × 14" (35 × 35 cm) plates are not uncommon. Smaller sizes are also available. CR IPs are housed in cassettes similar to conventional film-screen cassettes, with the IP replacing the film, and there are no intensifying screens. The CR cassette is usually made of aluminum (Fuji) or an aluminum honeycomb panel. While the front of the cassette is radiolucent, the back of the cassette is designed with a lead backing to prevent backscatter radiation from getting to the IP. Backscatter will lead to image artifacts.

The IP Imaging Cycle

One of the advantages of CR is that the IP can be used over and over again for several hundreds of exposures. During imaging, the IP goes through the imaging cycle shown in Figure 3-2. This cycle basically consists of at least three steps: X-ray exposure of the IP, readout of the exposed IP, and erasure of the IP. In the first step, the "ready-to-use" IP is exposed to X-rays using radiographic exposure factors (kVp, mAs) suitable to the needs of the examination. X-ray exposure produces an immediate light emission, but also creates a latent image in the form of energy storage in the phosphor. The energy stored is directly proportional to the intensity of X-rays striking the phosphor. The exposed IP is then readout in the CR reader (CR processor) to render the latent image visible. While in the CR reader, a laser light scans the IP to produce the photostimulated luminescence, as described earlier. The mechanics and electronics of this readout procedure will be described in the next section. Finally, in the third step of the IP imaging cycle, the IP is erased using a high intensity light to

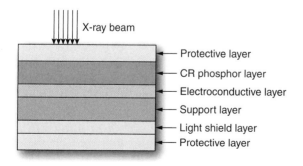

FIGURE 3-7. A cross section of a typical imaging plate (IP) used in CR imaging, showing the major structural components.
Source: *Delmar, Cengage Learning*

remove any residual energy after the IP has been scanned by the laser beam. The erased IP is now ready to be used again.

The CR Reader: Types

The CR reader, or scanner as it is sometimes referred to, is a machine for scanning the exposed IP to render the latent image visible. To do this efficiently and effectively requires a set of technical components engineered precisely to allow the IP to be scanned, erased, and made available for repeated use by the technologist. The purpose of the CR reader is to render the latent image stored on the exposed IP visible. The electrical signal generated as a result of scanning the IP is amplified and subsequently digitized.

There are two types of CR systems: cassette-based systems and cassette-less systems.

Cassette-Based Systems

These systems use individual IPs of different sizes analogous to cassette-based film-screen radiography. As seen in Figure 3-2, an exposed IP has to be physically taken to a CR reader unit for scanning to acquire an image from the IP, followed by erasure of the IP and subsequent transported of the IP in the unit itself for reuse. This means that the IP is in contact with various transport mechanisms that may in time result in plate/phosphor damage.

Cassette-less Systems

These systems evolved to overcome some of the problems with cassette-based systems. One such problem, as mentioned above, is related to the physical task of taking an exposed IP to the CR reader for processing, as well as the mechanical transport of the IP in the reader itself. Cassette-less CR systems incorporate a single fixed IP encased in a special housing that forms a stationary part of the unit. There is also no contact with the IP in the unit when it is read. The single fixed IP can accommodate various exposure sizes ranging from 17" × 17" and 14" × 14" to 10" × 12" and 8" × 10" or 10" × 8". These varying sizes will have varying matrix sizes as well.

Once the fixed stationary IP is exposed, the patent image is acquired using a scanning technology appropriate to the system.

The CR Reader: Scanning Technologies

Acquiring the image from the exposed IP can be accomplished by point-scan (P-S) CR readers, (Figure 3-8A) or more recently by line-scan CR readers (Figure 3-8B).

The major components of a P-S CR reader are shown in Figure 3-8A. These include the laser source, IP transport mechanism, light channeling guide, photodetector, and the analog-to-digital converter (ADC). Each of these will now be described briefly.

First, the IP is removed from the cassette and is placed on the transport mechanism for scanning by a laser beam. The movement of the IP is referred to as the "slow-scan" direction and the laser beam movement across the IP is called the "fast-scan" direction (Seibert, 2004). The laser beam is used to stimulate the trapped electrons (latent image) in the exposed IP. In the past, gas lasers such as a helium-neon (He-Ne) laser were used; however, current CR readers use solid-state laser diodes that emit a red laser beam having wavelengths of about 670–690 nm (Schaetzing, 2003). The laser stimulation of the IP causes it to emit light (by photo-stimulable luminescence (PSL) that is of a much different wavelength than the stimulating laser light.

Second, the emitted light from the IP is optically filtered and collected by the light channeling guide, or light collection optics as it is sometimes referred to. This light (PSL) is then sent to the photodetector (a photomultiplier tube in the case of Figure 3-8A or charge-couple devices (CCDs) as in the case of Figure 3-8B), which converts the PSL into an electrical signal (analog signal) that is first amplified and then digitized by the ADC. It is not within the scope of this book to describe the mechanics of amplification. Amplification is sometimes referred to as "signal conditioning" (Schaetzing, 2003).

Finally, the analog signal from the photodetector is sent to the ADC for digitization, as described in Chapter 2. Digitization involves both sampling the analog signal and quantization. Depending on the amplification, the ADC will produce 8 to16 bits of quantization per pixel, providing discrete gray levels ranging from 2^8 to 2^{16} (Schaetzing, 2003; Seibert, 2004).

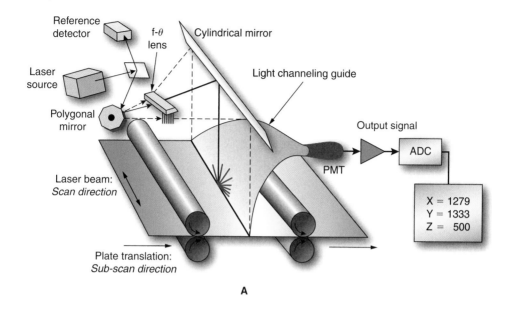

A

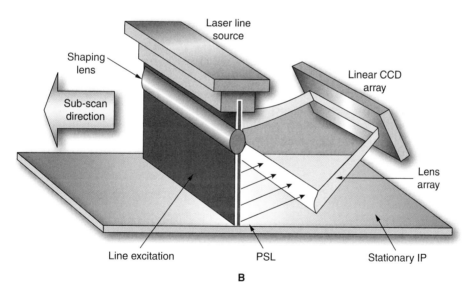

B

FIGURE 3-8. The major technical components of two types of CR Readers. While a Point Scan Reader is illustrated in A, a Line Scan Reader is shown in B.
Source: Seibert, J.A. (2004). Computed radiography technology 2004. In L. W. Goldman & M. V. Yester (Eds.), *Specifications, Performance, and Quality Assurance of radiographic and Fluoroscopic Systems in the Digital Era*. College Park, Maryland: American Association of Physicists in Medicine [AAPM]. (*Reproduced by permission*)

As mentioned earlier, current CR readers employ line-scan principles (Figure 3-8B), as opposed to the point-scan image acquisition (Figure 3-8A) just described. These systems use several linear laser sources, a lens system, and a linear array of CCD photodetectors (Arakawa, Hiroaki, Kuwabara, Suzuki, Suzuki, & Hagiwara, 2004). While the laser beam is collected and shaped by the lens system (shaping lens), to scan the IP line-by-line (instead of point-by-point for point-scan systems), the PSL

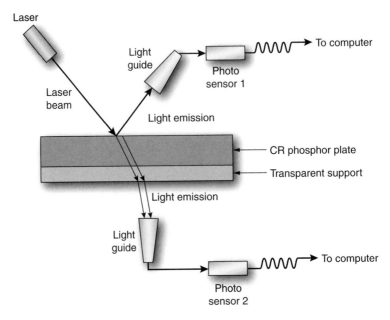

FIGURE 3-9. The mechanism of dual-side reading of the IP in CR imaging.
Source: *Delmar, Cengage Learning*

from the IP is collected by the CCD linear photodetector array. Because of this, the line-scan CR reader is much faster than the point-scan CR reader.

As described above, the IP is scanned on one side to emit the PSL that is used to produce an image. Recently, however, dual-sided reading technology has become available in the more modern CR units. Dual-sided reading of the IP is illustrated in Figure 3-9, in which it can be seen that two sets of photodetectors (dual light collection system) are used to capture PSL from the front and back side of the IP. In this way, more signal is obtained, which improves the signal-to-noise ratio and, hence, improves image quality. Additionally, Schaetzing (2003) reported that a thicker phosphor layer can be used to increase the absorption of X-rays, further improving system efficiency.

After the latent image has been extracted by laser stimulation and collection of the PSL from the IP, the IP must be erased to prepare it for another exposure. Erasure of the IP is done in the CR reader by exposing it to a high intensity light that is brighter than the stimulating laser light, to get rid of any residual signal left on the IP. It is interesting

to note that since the IP is also sensitive to background radiation, as well as scattered radiation from X-ray procedures, it must always be erased before use, especially if the IP has not been used for a period of time.

The CR Workstation

The CR workstation provides the technologist with the opportunity to interact with the entire CR process by facilitating a number of important functions ranging from the input of patient identification or selection of patient data to target exposure and image preview, image processing, quality assurance procedures, image printing, and sending images to the PACS through the Digital Imaging and Communication in Medicine (DICOM) standard.

A typical CR workstation consists of the image processing computer and image display monitor, keyboard, and mouse. In addition, some workstations offer a barcode reader and a magnetic card reader (not shown). While cathode-ray tube (CRT) monitors are used for some CR workstations, liquid crystal display (LCD) monitors have become commonplace. LCD monitors are available in different sizes; however, 21-inch and 20-inch monochrome monitors are not uncommon. A 3-megapixel monitor offers high resolution display of pixels with a bit depth of 8 ($2^8 = 256$). With high resolution monitors, radiologists can perform soft copy reading of CR images.

The keyboard allows the technologist to input relevant information about the CR examination, and the mouse allows the selection of various operations. Some monitors utilize touch-screen technology to enable the technologist to communicate with the software. Finally, the barcode reader enables the registration of the various IPs used.

In general, CR software should be intuitive to provide ease of use of the system. Such software will allow the technologist to perform several functions, including quality assurance tasks and simple and complex image processing operations. Image processing will be described in the next section.

Computer Networking and CR

Once images are acquired and displayed for viewing by the technologist, they must be assessed for image quality and QA before they are sent to the PACS (AAPM, 2006). Additionally, the CR system is interfaced to the hospital information system (HIS) and the radiology information system (RIS). These components, that is, the CR unit (CR reader and workstation), the HIS/RIS, and the PACS should be fully integrated to communicate with each other. While DICOM facilitates the communication of images in the digital radiology environment, the Health Level-7 (HL-7) standard addresses the communication of textual data within the information systems environment. PACS and information systems, as well as computer networking and communications standards such as DICOM and HL-7, will be explored further in Chapter 8.

Digital Image Processing in CR

The overall general concepts of digital image processing were described in Chapter 2. Image processing operations, such as image contrast and brightness control, as well as spatial frequency filtering in which images can be enhanced for sharpness and blurred depending on the viewing needs of the observer, were described in detail.

Image processing in CR can be discussed in terms of pre-processing and post-processing operations, both of which are intended to enhance the visual appearance of the image displayed for viewing on a monitor (soft-copy viewing), in an effort to assist the radiologist in image interpretation (Seeram & Seeram, 2008).

Pre-Processing Operations

There are several pre-processing operations used to identify, correct, and scale the raw image data obtained when the IP is scanned in the CR reader and before the image is displayed for viewing and subject to post-processing (Seibert, 2004, 2006). Pre-processing operations are also referred to as acquisition processing.

Pre-processing operations for digital detectors are several and, more importantly, each manufacturer offers proprietary algorithms for their systems. Therefore, it is not within the scope of this book to describe these algorithms; however, there are a few noteworthy aspects of pre-processing that the technologist must be familiar with and will be reviewed here. According to Seibert (2006), pre-processing in CR is essential to correct the raw digital data collected from the IP and the CR reader that may have imperfections. For example, the IP may have scratches and other marks and the CR reader may have dirt on the light-channeling guide, all of which will lead to image artifacts. In addition, the raw data is scaled to ensure that only the useful anatomic signals are used in the digitization process to improve image quality.

One important pre-processing method in CR is exposure field recognition, also referred to as exposure data recognition (Fuji) and segmentation (Kodak). The basic steps of exposure recognition are shown in Figure 3-10 and include exposure field recognition, histogram analysis, and grayscale rendition. The purpose of exposure recognition is to identify the appropriate raw data values (minimum and maximum values) to be used for image grayscale rendition and to provide an indication of

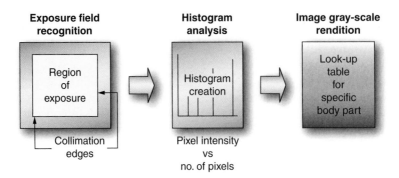

FIGURE 3-10. The basic steps of exposure recognition are exposure field recognition, histogram creation, and grayscale rendition. The histogram in this case is referred to as the scanned or measured histogram to distinguish it from the stored histogram.
Source: *Delmar, Cengage Learning*

the average radiation exposure to the IP CR detector (Flynn, 2003). The latter will be described later in this chapter.

In the first step of exposure field recognition, the collimation edges or boundaries are detected and anatomical structures that should be displayed in the image are identified using specific algorithms, such as the "shift and subtract" method where "the image is subtracted from an identical copy of itself and then shifted onto horizontal and vertical directions by two or more pixels. This produces differential signals at locations of rapid change (e.g., collimator shadows) and identifies the area of interest" (Seibert, 2004). In the second step, a histogram of the information on the IP (including the anatomy and the collimated and opened regions of the image) is created. This is referred to as the measured histogram or scanned histogram, to distinguish it from what is referred to as known or stored histograms, that is, the identical copy of the images of the anatomy under study stored previously in the machine. The CR imaging system will compensate for underexposure or overexposure by matching the measured histogram with the appropriate known histogram using an anatomy-specific template-matching algorithm (Seibert, 2004). This is illustrated in Figure 3-11, where the measured histogram from an overexposure (dotted line) is shifted to match the known histogram (solid line) stored in the machine to produce an acceptable image. This is accomplished by rescaling that

"involves mapping the minimum useful value to a correspondingly small digital value and mapping the maximum useful value to a correspondingly large digital value within the typical output image (10–12 bits)" (Seibert, 2004).

The final step in exposure recognition is grayscale rendition of the image. Grayscale rendition is a procedure that "maps the raw image values for the least penetrated anatomic region to the largest presentation value for display at maximum luminance. The most penetrated anatomic region of interest is mapped to the smallest presentation value for display at minimum luminance. The intermediate raw values are then mapped to presentation values in a monotonically decreasing fashion. This produces a presentation with a black background similar to that of conventional radiographs" (Flynn, 2003). This is illustrated in Figure 3-12. Note that a look-up table (LUT) is used to do this function. Exposure recognition may not always be successful and may fail due to problems with too much scattered radiation, metallic components in the patient such as implants the presence of lead markers, and immobilization devices (Flynn, 2003).

In CR, exposure recognition performs another task and that is to provide an indication as to the amount of radiation falling upon the detector as a result of the exposure technique used by the technologist (Flynn, 2003; Seibert, 2004). This exposure indicator, or exposure index as it is sometimes referred to as, appears on the displayed image and

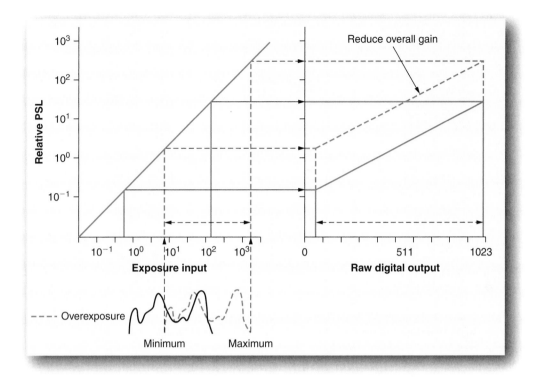

FIGURE 3-11. Digital systems compensate for under or overexposure by automatically adjusting the internal gain of the output conversion stage once the minimum and maximum values are identified; see the overexposure histogram (dotted line). The histogram shifts position but does not change shape. Although not shown, the digital system gain curve can also adjust slope to adjust for variation of the input exposure dynamic range. PSI = photostimulable luminescence
Source: Seibert, J. A. (2003). Digital radiographic image presentation: Preprocessing methods. In E. Samei and M.J. Flynn (Eds.) *Advances in Digital Radiography: RSNA Categorical Course in Diagnostic Radiology Physics* (pp. 63-70). Illinois: RSNA. (*Reproduced by permission*)

serves to provide the technologist with a visual cue as to whether correct or incorrect exposure technique was used. Incorrect exposure techniques are those that result in underexposure or overexposure of the patient. In this regard, the exposure indicator can be used as a quality control tool to facilitate the optimization of radiation protection.

Manufacturers of CR systems report the exposure indicator in different ways, and at present there is no universal standard for reporting exposure indicators. For example, while Fuji Medical Systems (Japan) refers to their exposure indicator as a sensitivity number (S-number), Agfa Medical Systems (New Jersey) uses the log of Median (lgM) value of the histogram and Kodak (New York) uses

the term exposure index (EI). Exposure indicators will be described in more detail later in this chapter.

Post-Processing Operations

Post-processing of the displayed image to suit the viewing needs of the observer, who may want to not only sharpen and reduce the noise in the image but also to enhance the image contrast, logically follows pre-processing. There are several types of post-processing algorithms for use in CR. These in general include contrast enhancement; spatial frequency or edge enhancement; multi-scale, multi-frequency enhancement; and dual-energy and disease-specific processing (Andriole; 2002;

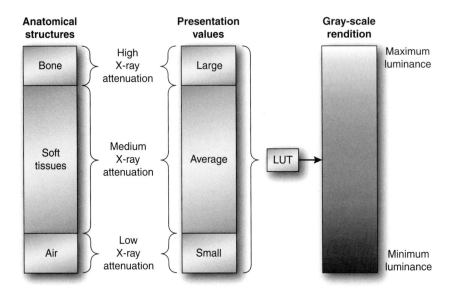

FIGURE 3-12. Grayscale rendition maps the degree of penetration of the anatomical regions to the degree of luminance of the display device. Large and small penetration values are mapped to the maximum luminance and minimum luminance respectively. Source: *Delmar, Cengage Learning*

Davidson, 2005; Flynn 2003; Seeram & Seeram, 2008; Seibert, 2004).

Contrast enhancement is also referred to as contrast scaling, and various manufacturers use different terms to refer to it. For example, while Fuji uses the term gradation processing, Kodak and Agfa use the terms tone scaling and latitude reduction respectively. A more current algorithm is one from Agfa called multi-scale image contrast amplification (MUSICA).

The purpose of contrast enhancement is to optimize the image contrast and density to enhance diagnostic interpretation of the image. Essentially, the pixel values are normalized and rescaled using an LUT. An example of a very common approach for contrast enhancement is the unsharp mask method described in Chapter 2.

Another common post-processing operation is edge enhancement or spatial frequency processing. These algorithms are intended to adjust or control the sharpness or detail of an image by adjusting the frequency components of the image. As described in Chapter 2, an image in the spatial location domain can be transformed into an image in the frequency domain using the Fourier Transform (FT).

The spatial frequency domain image contains both high spatial frequencies (detail information) and low spatial frequencies (contrast information). The effect of frequency processing on an image of the author is shown in Figure 3-13.

More recent algorithms (software) for frequency processing have been introduced by CR vendors, who use their own terminology to describe their software. For example, while Fuji uses the term multi-objective frequency processing (MFP), Agfa and Kodak use the terms multi-scale image contrast amplification (MUSICA) and enhanced visualization processing (EVP). In addition, Philips and Konica have algorithms called unified image quality enhancement (UNIQUE) and hybrid processing, respectively. While UNIQUE is a multi-resolution algorithm, the hybrid algorithm uses distinct frequency components of different anatomical parts on the image to reduce noise and shadowing, resulting in a more natural appearance of the image while maintaining detail. CR manufacturers also offer a wide variety of image processing software for their systems. While it is not realistic to describe them all in this text, a few advanced image-processing options for one manufacturer (Fuji) are highlighted in Table 3-1.

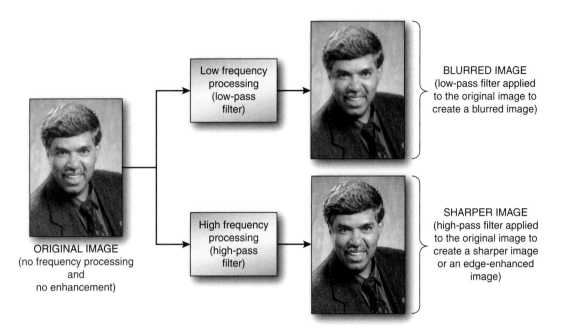

FIGURE 3-13. The visual effects of low- and high-frequency processing (edge enhancement) on a photograph of the author, Euclid Seeram.
Source: *Delmar, Cengage Learning*

TABLE 3-1. Several examples of Fuji's advanced image processing software for their CR imaging systems. (From Fuji's Image Intelligence Brochure, © 2009 FUJIFILM Medical Systems USA, Inc.)

Image Processing Operation	Brief Description
Dynamic Range Control (DRC)	Improves the visualization of areas with different densities in the same image
Energy Subtraction	Using a single exposure of a body part, three different displays such as bone, soft tissue, and the standard exam (chest in this case) to allow visualization and typification of structures that may be obscured by overlying or underlying anatomy
Multi-objective Frequency Processing (MFP)	This is frequency enhancement which adjusts both large and small structures independently within the same image simultaneously
Flexible Noise Control (FNC)	This software separates noise and image signals, enabling selective suppression of noise levels to enhance diagnostic interpretation
Grid Pattern Removal (GPR)	Removes grid patterns from the image to suppress moiré patterns within an image
Image Composition	Separate images are stitched (joined together) to form a single image

It is important that technologists realize that the information content of an image depends primarily on the radiation dose used. During the conduct of an examination, the technologist must strive to use the appropriate exposure technique factors (kVp and mAs) that produce the best possible image quality with the least radiation dose to the patient. This task requires a careful assessment of all the parameters that influence the selection of appropriate exposure technique factors.

The technologist should not depend on the use of inappropriate image processing to improve image quality. As noted by Willis et al (2004), "image processing is not a panacea. Misuses of image processing include compensation for inappropriate radiographic technique, compensating for poor calibration of acquisition and display devices, and surreptitious deletion of non-diagnostic images. Image processing to recover non-diagnostic images to prevent re-exposure should be the last resort, not a routine activity. Routine preprocessing indicates a problem with automatic image processing or technical practice." "The proper use of image processing can produce dramatic improvements in image quality" (Flynn, 2003), and this should be the primary goal of the technologist, who is involved in the use of these image-processing algorithms to enhance digital images for diagnostic interpretation.

Exposure Control in CR

The use of proper exposure technique factors is a vital part of any radiographic examination, since these factors determine the image quality obtained as well as the radiation dose to the patient.

IP Response to Exposure

The response of radiographic film to radiation exposure is well understood as described by the characteristic curve, or the H and D curve as it is often referred to (see Chapter 1). When the exposure is low, the film is underexposed and the image is light and is not acceptable. When the exposure is high, the film is overexposed and the image is dark and is not acceptable. In both cases repeat exposures are required to achieve the proper film density using image receptor exposures that fall within the slope of the characteristic curve. This slope defines the useful range of exposures referred to as the film latitude or dynamic range of the image receptor.

Underexposure of the film results in noisy images while overexposure will result in high doses to the patient.

The above problems are solved by a CR imaging system, since the IP has wider exposure latitude than film, as shown in Figure 3-14. The consequence of this wide dynamic range on the image quality is also clearly shown in Figure 3-14, which illustrates one of the significant advantages of CR. Even if the exposure is too low or too high, the image quality is still acceptable due to the ability of the CR system to perform digital image processing to adjust the image quality to match the image quality that would be produced by the optimum exposure. As seen in Figure 3-14, a low exposure (underexposure) will produce high noise (that can be detected by the radiologist), while a high exposure (overexposure) will produce very good images, compared to the optimum image produced by the optimum exposure (appropriate exposure).

The fundamental problem with high exposures is that of increased radiation dose to the patient. As noted by Seibert (2004), "because of the negative feedback due to underexposures, a predictable and unfortunate use of higher exposures, dose creep, is a typical occurrence. To identify an estimate of the exposure used for a given image, CR manufacturers have devised methods to analyze the digital numbers in the image based upon the calibrated response to known incident exposure." As noted earlier in this chapter, one of the functions of exposure data recognition is to provide an indication of the amount of radiation falling upon the CT IP. This is referred to as the exposure indicator or exposure index (AAPM, 2006) and provides feedback to the operator about the dose that was used to create the image on the detector (Schaefer-Prokop & Neitzel, 2006).

Exposure Indicators

An exposure indicator is a numerical parameter used to monitor the radiation exposure to the IP in CR imaging. The determination of exposure indicators differs among CR vendors. Fuji refers to their exposure indicator as a sensitivity number (S-number); Kodak uses the term exposure index (EI); Agfa uses the term

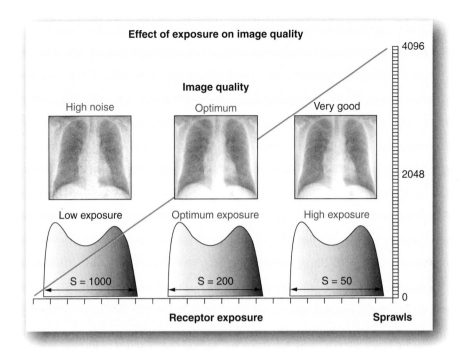

FIGURE 3-14. CR has a wide exposure latitude compared to film–screen radiography. The advantage of this is that CR can produce images that appear visually the same.
Source: *Courtesy of Dr Perry Sprawls-Emory University*

log of the median of the image histogram (LgM-**Log** of **M**edian Values); and Konica uses the term sensitivity value (S-value). Only the first three will be described briefly in this chapter. Exposure indicators used by other vendors will be reviewed in Chapter 10.

Sensitivity Number (S-number) of the Fuji CR System

Fuji's sensitivity number (S) is derived from the following relationship, using a standard resolution IP and under normal processing operations (Seibert, 2004; Goldman, 2004):

$$S = \frac{200}{\text{Exposure to the IP (mR)}}$$

This relationship shows that S is inversely proportional to the exposure; hence a low exposure will result in a high S-number and a high exposure will result in a low S-number. It should be noted that if the exposure to the IP is low, the PMT signal will be weak and must be increased. Conversely, if the

exposure to the IP is high, the PMT signal is strong and must be decreased to produce optimum image quality. Adjusting the PMT's signal in this manner means that the sensitivity of the PMT will be set for the final scan of the IP. Recall that the IP undergoes a first scan to generate a histogram based on the collimation boundaries. This histogram is labeled the scanned histogram to distinguish it from stored histograms (pre-programmed histograms for various body parts to be imaged). During the final scan or the final read of the IP, the scanned histogram is compared with the pre-programmed histogram.

This adjustment of the sensitivity of the PMT shows the amount of amplification that the system applies to the image signal to produce the proper image in order to match the scanned histogram to the correct pre-stored histogram for the body part under investigation.

The relationship S = 200/exposure (mR) means that an exposure of 1mR {0.258×10^{-3} millicoulombs/kilogram (mC/kg)}, a known incident exposure to the IP, will result in an S-number of 200. A low exposure of 0.1mR (0.258×10^{-4} mC/kg) will result in an S-number of 2000, while a high exposure of 10mR (0.258×10^{-2} mC/kg) will result in S-number of 20. Figure 3-14 shows the effect of S-numbers of 1000 (low exposure), 200 (optimum exposure), and 50 (high exposure) on image quality. The challenge imposed by the CR imaging system is for the technologist to optimize the exposure indicator (in this case, the S-number) to reduce the dose to the patient, while maintaining optimum image quality so as not to compromise the diagnostic interpretation of the image.

The S-number can be thought of as being equivalent to the speed of the IP. If the exposure is low, the speed is increased (hence the S-number is large, say S = 1000, as shown in Figure 3-14) and the image will be noisy. If the exposure is high, the speed will be decreased (low S-number, say S = 50, as shown in Figure 3-14) and the image will be very good, but at the expense of higher dose to the patient.

Exposure Index (EI) of the Kodak CR System

Kodak's exposure index (EI) also provides information about the average exposure to the IP and it is calculated using the following relationship:

$$EI = Log \text{ (Exposure in mR)} \times 1000 + 2000$$

This relationship shows that the EI is directly proportional to the exposure; hence a high exposure will result in a high EI and a low exposure will generate in a low EI. The relationship also shows that a 1 mR exposure (under certain conditions) will produce an EI of 2000. Exposures of 0.1 mR (low) and 10 mR (high) will result in EIs of 1000 and 3000 respectively. If the exposure is doubled, the EI will increase by 300. On the other hand, a reduction of the exposure by 0.5 (one-half) will reduce the EI by 300 (Seibert, 2004).

Log of Median (LgM) Values of the Agfa CR System

The Agfa CR system uses an exposure indicator called the log of median (lgM) that is related logarithmically to the median value of the histogram from exposed IP. Under certain conditions, the relationship is given as

$$lgM = 2.2 + \log \text{ (Exposure in mR)}$$

If the exposure to the IP is 1mR, then the LgM would be 2.2, and "each increment of 0.3 in LgM corresponds to doubling or halving of the exposure level at the plate." (Goldman, 2004). As noted by the AAPM (2006), "every Agfa PSP examination is assigned a Speed Class, and the system compensates for exposure variations of a factor of 4 around the intended speed. The lgM value indicates the actual exposure to the IP by a mathematical relationship to the Scanned Average Level (SAL), which is just the average grayscale value. A 2.2 mR (20 µGy) exposure to the IP using 75 kVp and 1.5 mm added Cu developed with a Speed Class of 200 results in an SAL of 1800"

$$SAL200 = 1214 \times [\text{exposure (mR)}]$$

Agfa CR systems feature an option described appropriately by Seibert (2004) as follows: "After ~50 images of the same examination, the lgM mean value of 'acceptable' exposures is stored as a reference value. Subsequent lgM values are compared to the reference value, and a graphical indicator is displayed in the text fields of each image. If a given exposure exceeds a predetermined threshold limit, a visible warning bar is printed and warning messages are logged into a database file. This procedure provides an exam-specific feedback indicator that allows variable-speed characteristics of the CR system to be used to advantage."

Exposure Indicator Standardization

At the time of writing this chapter, two groups have been working on the standardization of exposure indicators in digital radiography. These two include the AAPM and the International Electrotechnical Commission (IEC). The IEC hopes to publish such standardization in August 2008. Appendix A highlights the fundamental elements of the AAPM standardization report.

Exposure Indicator Guidelines for Quality Control

Exposure indicators can be used as a means of monitoring the dose to patients while maintaining acceptable image quality. This task is an essential component on a quality assurance/quality control

TABLE 3-2. Guidelines for the use of exposure indicators for quality control in CR imaging of adults[a]

Sensitivity (Fuji)	LgM Index (Agfa)	Exposure Index (Kodak)	Incident Exposure (mR)	QC Indicator
> 1000	< 1.45	< 1250	< 0.2	Severely underexposed. Repeat
601 – 1000	1.45 – 1.74	1250 – 1549	0.33 – 0.2	Underexposed. QC exception
301 – 600	1.75 – 2.04	1550 – 1849	0.67 – 0.33	Underexposed. QC review
150 – 300	2.05 – 2.35	1850 – 2150	1.33 – 0.67	Acceptable range
75 – 149	2.36 – 2.65	2151 – 2450	2.66 – 1.33	Overexposed. QC review
50 – 74	2.66 – 2.95	2451 – 2750	4.0 – 2.66	Overexposed. QC exception
< 50	> 2.95	> 2750	> 4.0	Overexposed. Repeat

a. Does not include extremities or pediatric imaging and assumes proper collimation, positioning, and examination code
b. In this table, the estimated average exposure incident on the IP is correlated with the sensitivity number for a Fuji CR system as exposure (mR) = 200/sensitivity number (Willis et al, 1998)
Source: Seibert, 2004. Performance testing of Digital Radiographic Systems: Computed Radiography[b]. In Goldman LW and Yester MV (Eds) *Specifications, Performance, and Quality Assurance of radiographic and Fluoroscopic Systems in the Digital Era.* American Association of Physicists in Medicine (AAPM). College Park, Maryland. (*Reproduced by permission*)

(QA/QC) program (Chapter 10). The exposure indicator depends on a number of factors, such as the kVp, filtration, patient positioning, source-to-image receptor distance (SID), collimation, beam centering, image processing algorithms, and so forth. Therefore, guidelines for the QC of the exposure indicator are necessary. An example of such guidelines for QC image evaluation for general CR imaging of adults is given in Table 3-2.

 ## Image Quality Descriptors

The image quality descriptors for a digital image such as a CR image, for example, are illustrated in Figure 3-15 and include spatial resolution (detail), density resolution, noise, quantum detective efficiency (DQE), and artifacts (Korner et al, 2007; Seibert, 2006). This chapter will not describe these in any detail; however, the essential elements of each will be highlighted.

Spatial Resolution

The spatial resolution of a digital image is related to the size of the pixels in the image matrix. Different sizes of IPs have different pixel sizes. For example, IP sizes of 35 cm × 43 cm (24" × 17"), 23 cm × 30 cm (10" × 12"), and 18 cm × 24 cm (8" × 10") for one manufacturer, have pixel sizes of 0.2 mm, 0.14 mm, and 0.1 mm, respectively. The smaller the pixel size the better the spatial resolution of the image.

The pixel size (PS) can be calculated using the relationship

$$PS = \text{Field of View (FOV)}/\text{matrix size}$$

Thus, for the same FOV, the greater the matrix size, the smaller the pixels and the better the image sharpness. A typical CR image matrix size is 2048 × 2048. There are other factors affecting the sharpness of the digital image but they will not be described here.

Density Resolution

The density resolution of a digital image is linked to the bit depth, which is the range of gray levels per pixel (see Chapter 2). An image with a bit depth of 8 will have 256 (2^8) shades of gray per pixel. In general, the greater the bit depth, the better the density resolution of the image.

Noise

Noise on the other hand can be discussed in terms of electronic noise (system noise) and quantum

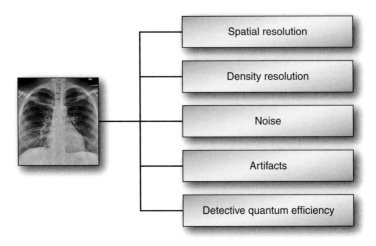

FIGURE 3-15. Five image quality descriptors for a digital image such as a CR image.
Source: *Delmar, Cengage Learning*

noise (quantum mottle). The quantum noise is determined by the number of X-ray photons (often referred to as the signal, S) falling upon the detector to create the image. Low exposure factors (kVp and mAs) will produce few photons at the detector (less signal and more noise, N) and higher exposure factors will generate more photons at the detector (more signal and less noise). The former will result in a noisy image (grainy image) that is generally a poor image, and the latter will produce a better image at the expense of increased dose to the patient. The noise increases as the detector exposure decreases.

Detective Quantum Efficiency

The final descriptor of digital image quality is the detective quantum efficiency (DQE). The overall concept of the DQE for a digital detector is illustrated in Figure 3-16. As can be seen, the detector receives an input exposure (incident quanta) and converts it into a useful output image. The DQE is a measure of the efficiency and fidelity with which the detector can perform this task. Note that in addition the DQE takes into consideration not only the signal-to-noise ratio (SNR) but also the system noise and therefore includes a measure of the amount of noise added.

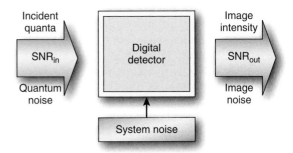

FIGURE 3-16. The concept of the detective quantum efficiency (DQE). The digital detector takes an input exposure and converts it into a useful output image. The DQE is a measure of the efficiency with which the detector performs this task.
Source: *Delmar, Cengage Learning*

The DQE can be calculated using the following relationship:

$$DQE = SNR^2_{out}/SNR^2_{in}$$

The DQE for a perfect digital detector is 1, or 100%. This means that there is no loss of information. Since SNR_{in} takes into consideration the amount of exposure used and the SNR_{out} considers the resultant image quality, the DQE indicates the detector performance in terms of output image quality and input radiation exposure used.

The DQE for CR is much better than film-screen (F-S) image receptors. This means that CR can convert an input exposure into a useful output image over a much wider range of exposures compared to F-S radiography. Seibert (2004) points out that for "conventional CR detectors" the DQE is "typically less than 30%." Different manufacturers will report different DQE values for their respective CR systems. Interested readers should consult the CR specifications of the different manufacturers for their reported values.

 ## Image Artifacts Overview

The notion of artifacts in F-S radiography is not new to technologists, who can readily identify them, describe how they are produced, and even eliminate or reduce their impact on the image. In review, film-screen artifacts rise from radiographic exposures, processing of the film in a chemical processor containing developer and fixer solutions, and handling and storage of films (Bushong, 2009).

Definition

An artifact can be defined as "a distortion or error in an image that is unrelated to the subject being studied" (Morgan, 1983). A more recent definition of an artifact is provided by Willis and others (2004), who state that "an artifact is a feature in an image that masks or mimics a clinical feature." Artifacts therefore can be disturbing to radiologists and may even result in an inaccurate diagnosis. For CR, it is important that both radiologists and technologists be able to not only identify artifacts but also understand how they arise and how they can be reduced or removed from the image.

Sources of Artifacts

In CR, artifacts arise from a number of sources, including the imaging hardware (equipment), image processing software, and objects that are imaged and linked to the operators (AAPM, 2006; Cesar et al, 2001; Willis et al, 2004). It is not within the scope of this chapter to describe in detail the

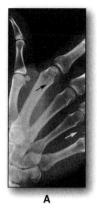 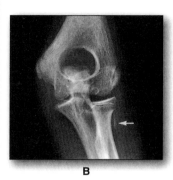

A   **B**

FIGURE 3-17. Two imaging plate (IP) artifacts. (A) Thumb radiograph showing cracks (white arrow), which usually first become visible on the IP edges. As deterioration progresses, cracks appear closer to the clinically used areas of the IP (black arrow) as shown in (B). In some instances, early cracking along the edge of the IP does not occur. This crack appears as a lucency near the radius, which could be confused with a foreign body. *Artifact remedy:* an IP must be replaced when cracks occur in clinically useful areas.
Source: L. J. Cesar, RT(R)(QM), B. A. Schueler, PhD, F. E. Zink, PhD, T. R. Daly, RT(R)(QM), J. P. Taubel, RT(R) (QM), and L. L. Jorgenson, RT(R). (2001) Artefacts found in computed radiography. *British Journal of Radiology, 74,* 195–202. (Reproduced by permission of the British Institute of Radiology)

various artifacts in CR; however, it is noteworthy to highlight a few artifacts that are commonplace in a CR environment. These artifacts are illustrated in Figure 3-17 to Figure 3-24.

Artifacts can arise from the IP, and they are somewhat common simply because the IP is frequently used and handled by technologists. The IPs must be handled properly and with great care; they must be stored correctly; and they must be cleaned routinely in order to avoid artifacts caused by the presence of dirt, dust, cracks, and scratches on the phosphor plate. An exposed IP must be stored safely to prevent scattered radiation from reaching it and causing scatter artifacts.

The CR reader is another source of artifacts, as illustrated in Figure 3-19 and Figure 3-20. CR artifacts can also arise from digital image processing. For example, incorrect use of the various image-processing algorithms (software) will

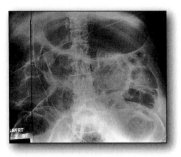

FIGURE 3-18. This image shows a dark line along the lateral portion of this upper abdomen caused by back-scatter transmitted through the back of the cassette. The line corresponds to the cassette hinge where the lead coating was weakened or cracked. *Artifact remedy*: to reduce backscatter, the radiographer should collimate when possible. Since backscatter cannot be eliminated in every case, knowledge of the radiographic appearance of cassette backs is useful.
Source: L. J. Cesar, RT(R)(QM), B. A. Schueler, PhD, F. E. Zink, PhD, T. R. Daly, RT(R)(QM), J. P. Taubel, RT(R) (QM), and L. L. Jorgenson, RT(R). (2001) Artefacts found in computed radiography. *British Journal of Radiology, 74*, 195–202. (*Reproduced by permission of the British Institute of Radiology*)

produce several kinds of artifacts, two of which are shown in Figure 3-21. Automatic image processing involves assumptions about the radiographic technique, the composition of the anatomic region imaged and the use of collimation. A number of factors can interfere with the automatic detection of the boundaries of the radiation field, including nonparallel collimation, use of multiple fields on a single imaging plate, poor centering, implants (especially when they overlie the boundary) and violation of collimation rules provided by the vendor."

Object artifacts are linked to operator errors during imaging that result in image artifacts. Typical errors includes incorrect storage of IPs, use of the incorrect grids, improper orientation of the cassette for the anatomy under examination, poor radiographic technique selection, and incorrect use of image processing, to mention only a few (Cesar et al, 2001; Willis et al, 2004). Several examples of artifacts caused by operator errors are shown in Figure 3-22 to Figure 3-24.

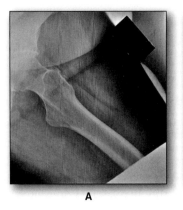

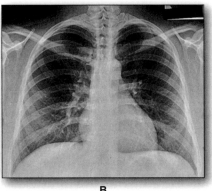

A   B

FIGURE 3-19. Two CR reader artifacts. In A, the pattern of lines seen on this oblique hip view occurred intermittently. The artifact was traced to the plate reader's electronics. *Artifact remedy*: the electronic board that controlled the photomultiplier tube was replaced. In B, the horizontal white line (arrow) shown on this upright chest radiograph was caused by dirt on the light guide in the plate reader. The light guide collects light emitted from the imaging plate when it is scanned by the laser. *Artifact remedy*: the light guide of the photomultiplier tube was cleaned by service personnel.
Source: L. J. Cesar, RT(R)(QM), B. A. Schueler, PhD, F. E. Zink, PhD, T. R. Daly, RT(R) (QM), J. P. Taubel, RT(R)(QM), and L. L. Jorgenson, RT(R). (2001) Artefacts found in computed radiography. *British Journal of Radiology, 74*, 195–202. (*Reproduced by permission of the British Institute of Radiology*)

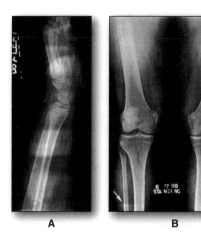

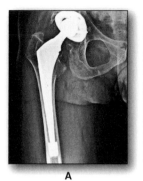

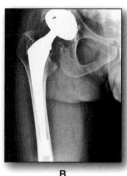

A   B

FIGURE 3-21. Image processing artifact. A. When too large a kernel size is selected for image enhancement, artifacts like the black halo surrounding the prosthesis can create the appearance that the prosthesis is loose. B. The same image as A processed with a smaller kernel size.
Source: L. J. Cesar, RT(R)(QM), B. A. Schueler, PhD, F. E. Zink, PhD, T. R. Daly, RT(R)(QM), J. P. Taubel, RT(R)(QM), and L. L. Jorgenson, RT(R). (2001). Artefacts found in computed radiography. *British Journal of Radiology, 74,* 195-202. (*Reproduced by permission of the British Institute of Radiology*)

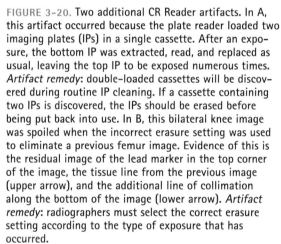

A   B

FIGURE 3-20. Two additional CR Reader artifacts. In A, this artifact occurred because the plate reader loaded two imaging plates (IPs) in a single cassette. After an exposure, the bottom IP was extracted, read, and replaced as usual, leaving the top IP to be exposed numerous times. *Artifact remedy*: double-loaded cassettes will be discovered during routine IP cleaning. If a cassette containing two IPs is discovered, the IPs should be erased before being put back into use. In B, this bilateral knee image was spoiled when the incorrect erasure setting was used to eliminate a previous femur image. Evidence of this is the residual image of the lead marker in the top corner of the image, the tissue line from the previous image (upper arrow), and the additional line of collimation along the bottom of the image (lower arrow). *Artifact remedy*: radiographers must select the correct erasure setting according to the type of exposure that has occurred.
Source: L. J. Cesar, RT(R)(QM), B. A. Schueler, PhD, F. E. Zink, PhD, T. R. Daly, RT(R)(QM), J. P. Taubel, RT(R)(QM), and L. L. Jorgenson, RT(R). (2001). Artefacts found in computed radiography. *British Journal of Radiology, 74,* 195-202. (*Reproduced by permission of the British Institute of Radiology*)

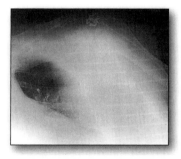

FIGURE 3-22. An artifact caused by operator error, where a wire mesh cart loaded with unexposed imaging plates (IPs) was placed too near a source of scatter radiation. Because of the high sensitivity of the phosphor to scatter, exposure that may have been minimally seen on a film-screen image was well demonstrated on this portable image. *Artifact remedy*: protect IPs from sources of scatter radiation. Erase IPs that have been unused for an unknown period of time. One vendor recommends that IPs be erased if left unused for more than 8 h. We have had good results using 1 week as the time limit.
Source: L. J. Cesar, RT(R)(QM), B. A. Schueler, PhD, F. E. Zink, PhD, T. R. Daly, RT(R)(QM), J. P. Taubel, RT(R)(QM), and L. L. Jorgenson, RT(R). (2001). Artefacts found in computed radiography. *British Journal of Radiology, 74,* 195-202. (*Reproduced by permission of the British Institute of Radiology*)

Continuous Quality Improvement Overview

The maintenance of equipment is an integral part of the daily activities in radiology since it is considered a component of a continuous quality improvement (CQI) program. The notion of CQI was developed by the Joint Commission, formerly known as the Joint Commission on the Accreditation of Healthcare Organizations (JCAHO), in 1991. CQI

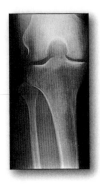

FIGURE 3-23. Artifact due to operator error. The Moiré pattern seen in this knee image was caused by using a grid with a frequency of 33 lines cm^{-1}, which was oriented with the grid lines parallel to the plate reader's scan lines. *Artifact remedy*: use grids with no less than 60 lines cm^{-1}. In addition, grid lines should run perpendicular to the plate reader's laser scan lines.
Source: L. J. Cesar, RT(R)(QM), B. A. Schueler, PhD, F. E. Zink, PhD, T. R. Daly, RT(R)(QM), J. P. Taubel, RT(R)(QM), and L. L. Jorgenson, RT(R). (2001). Artefacts found in computed radiography. *British Journal of Radiology*, 74, 195–202. *(Reproduced by permission of the British Institute of Radiology)*

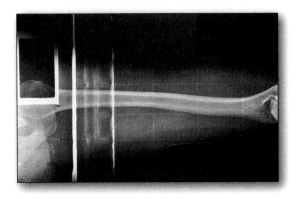

FIGURE 3-24. Artifact due to operator error. This axillary shoulder was exposed through the back of a cassette. *Artifact remedy*: be sure that radiographers are well educated about how to use the entire computed radiography system.
Source: L. J. Cesar, RT(R)(QM), B. A. Schueler, PhD, F. E. Zink, PhD, T. R. Daly, RT(R)(QM), J. P. Taubel, RT(R) (QM), and L. L. Jorgenson, RT(R). (2001). Artefacts found in computed radiography. *British Journal of Radiology*, 74, 195–202. *(Reproduced by permission of the British Institute of Radiology)*

ensures that every employee plays a role in creating a quality product.

In radiology in particular, quality assurance (QA) and quality control (QC) programs are essential not only for optimizing the assessment and evaluation of patient care, but also for monitoring the performance of equipment.

Quality Assurance

Quality assurance (QA) is a term used to describe systems and procedures for assuring quality patient care. It deals specifically with quality assessment, continuing education, the usefulness of quality control procedures, and the assessment of outcomes. QA deals with the administrative aspects of patient care and quality outcomes.

Quality Control

Quality control (QC) is a component of QA and refers specifically to the monitoring of important variables that affect image quality and radiation dose. QC deals with the technical aspects (rather than administrative aspects) of equipment performance. The purpose of the procedures and techniques of CQI, QA, and QC is three-fold: to ensure optimum image quality for the purpose of enhancing diagnosis, to reduce the radiation dose to both patients and personnel, and to reduce costs to the institution.

Quality control involves a number of activities that are of significance to the technologist, particularly if the technologist is in charge of the QC program. Such activities range from acceptance testing; routine performance, including analysis of reject rates (Foos et al, 2009); and error correction (Bushong, 2009). Acceptance testing (AT) is the first major step in a QC program and it ensures that the equipment meets the specifications set by the manufacturers. Routine performance involves conducting a QC test on the equipment on a regular basis with varying degrees of frequency (annually, semiannually, monthly, weekly, or daily). Error correction ensures that equipment not meeting the performance criteria or tolerance limit established for specific QC tests must be replaced or repaired to meet specifications.

Tools for CR QC Testing

Test tools for CR have evolved through the years and range from simple tools to more sophisticated tools provided by various CR vendors. For example, a tool from Fuji uses one exposure to provide information on a number of parameters. The Fuji "FCR 1 shot Plus System," for example, will provide automated QC tests for noise, linearity, relative "S" number, laser jitter, erasure, and shading and so forth. Furthermore, the tool will also provide visual evaluation of high contrast resolution, low contrast resolution, and artifacts, using appropriate QC software.

In addition, the AAPM (2006) has recommended a number of tools for CR QC, including a densitometer, copper and aluminum filters, calibrated ion chambers, screen contact wire mesh patterns, antiscatter grid (10:1 or 12:1 at 100 lines/inch), high contrast resolution line pair phantoms (40 sector type up to 5 line pairs/mm), low contrast phantoms, and anthropomorphic phantoms, to mention only a few.

Parameters for QC Monitoring in CR

QC for CR has evolved from simple to more complex tests and test tools for use by radiology personnel to ensure that the CR equipment is producing optimum image quality within the "as low as reasonably achievable" (ALARA) philosophy in radiation protection. It is not within the scope of this chapter to describe the elements of these QC programs; however, a few important points will be highlighted and a more detailed description will be presented in Chapter 10.

The AAPM has recommended several testing procedures for CR QC (AAPM, 2006), using specific tools developed for the purpose. These testing procedures include physical inspection of the IP, dark noise and uniformity, exposure indicator calibration, laser beam function, spatial accuracy, erasure thoroughness, aliasing/grid response, and positioning and collimation errors, to mention only a few. Examples of QC tools include screen-contact wire mesh pattern, antiscatter grid, calibrated ion chamber, densitometer for hard copy film evaluation (in cases where film is used), manufacturer-approved cleaning solutions and cloths, two metric-calibrated 30-cm steel rulers, and low-contrast phantom, to mention only a few.

Tolerance Limits or Acceptance Criteria

The AAPM has also established acceptance criteria for the recommended tests. They offer both qualitative and quantitative criteria. For example, they state that for CR IP uniformity response, the qualitative criteria be a "uniform image without any visible artifacts with window/level adjustments." For details of the criteria and tests, the interested reader should refer to the AAPM Report No 93.

Examples of CR QC Tests

The following CR QC tests recommended by the AAPM (2006) will be briefly described in this subsection as examples using only qualitative acceptance criteria: Dark Noise, CR Screen Test for Uniformity, Spatial Accuracy, and Erasure Thoroughness. For details of quantitative criteria, the reader should refer to the AAPM Report (2006).

QC Test 1: Dark Noise

Purpose: To assess the level of noise present in the system (intrinsic noise)

Exposure Condition: No exposure. Erase a single screen and read it without exposing it

Process in the Image Reader: Use the appropriate QC image-processing tool

Qualitative Criterion for Acceptance: Uniform image without artifacts, as shown in Figure 3-25A

QC Test 2: CR Imaging Plate Test = Uniformity

Purpose: To assess the uniformity of the recorded signal from a uniformly exposed imaging plate (a nonuniform response could affect clinical image quality)

Exposure Condition: Expose imaging plate using appropriate exposure factors

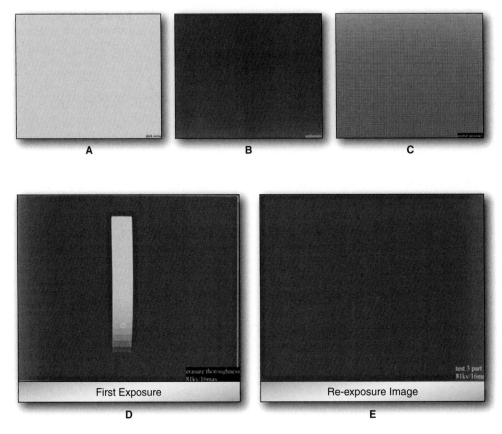

A   B   C

First Exposure   Re-exposure Image

D   E

FIGURE 3-25. (A) Results of CR QC tests for dark noise, (B) CR screen test or uniformity, (C) spatial accuracy, and (D) erasure thoroughness
Source: *Delmar, Cengage Learning*

Process in the Image Reader: Use the appropriate QC image processing tool

Qualitative Criterion for Acceptance: Uniform image without artifacts, as shown in Figure 3-25B

QC Test 3: Spatial Accuracy

Purpose: To check that there is no spatial distortion in the image

Exposure Condition: Place a regular wire mesh screen-film contact test tool over the CR imaging plate and expose the imaging plate to appropriate exposure technique

Process in the Image Reader: Use the appropriate QC image processing tool

Qualitative Criterion for Acceptance: The grid pattern spacing of the wire mesh should be uniform without any distortion across the CR image as shown in Figure 3-25C

QC Test 4: Erasure Thoroughness

Purpose: To test that minimal residual signal (ghosting) on a CR imaging plate after readout and exposure

Exposure Condition: Place a step-wedge at the center of a 14×17 CR IP and expose using appropriate exposure technique (to image the stepwedge) and process in the image reader (Figure 3-25D). Re-expose the same IP a second time without the step-wedge using the appropriate exposure technique. Collimate in by about 5 cm on each side of the CR IP

Process in the Image Reader: Use the appropriate QC image processing tool

Qualitative Criterion for Acceptance: Absence of a ghost image of the step-wedge from the first exposure in the re-exposed image, as is clearly shown in Figure 3-25E. Other major aspects of CR QC are described in detail in Chapter 10.

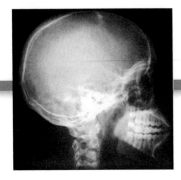

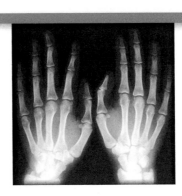

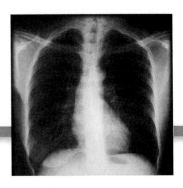

REVIEW QUESTIONS

1. What is meant by the term "computed radiography"?
2. What other terms are used to refer to computed radiography (CR)?
3. Identify three basic steps in the creation of a CR image.
4. Explain briefly the function of each of the four primary steps in the CR imaging process.
5. Describe a photostimulable storage phosphor (PSP) and provide examples.
6. What is photostimulable luminescence (PSL)? Explain the formation of the latent image when using a CR imaging plate (IP).
7. Draw and label the components of a CR IP and describe the purpose of each component.
8. Explain the steps involved in the IP imaging cycle.
9. Compare and contrast cassette-based and cassette-less CR systems.
10. Explain how a latent image is rendered visible in CR imaging.
11. What are the main features of a CR workstation?
12. What is meant by "preprocessing" in CR? Describe the details of exposure field recognition.
13. State the purpose of post-processing in CR and list several post-processing operations and the purpose of each.
14. What is the difference between the response of film and CR IP to X-ray exposure?
15. What is an exposure indicator?

16. List several exposure indicators and explain the difference between each of them.

17. Explain what is meant by "exposure creep."

18. Explain briefly the elements of each of the following as applied to CT imaging:
    - Spatial resolution
    - Density resolution
    - Noise
    - Detective quantum efficiency

19. What is an artifact? List several sources of artifacts in CR.

REFERENCES

American Association of Physicists in Medicine (AAPM), (2006). *Acceptance Testing and Quality Control of Photostimulable Storage Phosphor Imaging systems.* Report No 93. College Park, MD.

Andriole, K. (2006). Image Acquisition. In B. Dreyer, A. Metha, & J. Thrall (Eds.), *PACS: A Guide to the Digital Revolution* (pp. 131–144). New York: Springer-Verlag.

Andriole, K. (1996). Computed Radiography Technology Overview. *Radiological Society of North America (RSNA) Categorical Course in Physics.* Illinois, RSNA.

Arakawa, S., Hiroak, T., Kuwabara, H., Suzuki, H., Suzuki, T., & Hagiwara, T. (2004). Compact high speed computed radiography (CR) system using a linear CCD with large-area photodiode (PD) and dual transfer lines. *Proceedings of the Society of Photo-Optical Engineers (SPIE), 5030,* 778–787.

Cesar, L. J., Schuelar, B. A., Zink, F. E., Daly, T. R., Taubel, J. P., & Jorgenson, L. L. (2001). Artefacts in Computed Radiography. *British Journal of Radiology, 74,* 195–202.

Flynn, M. J. (2003). Processing digital radiographs of specific body parts. In E. Samei (Ed.), *Advances in Digital Radiology, Categorical Course in Diagnostic Radiology Physics.* Illinois: RSNA.

Foos, D. H., Sehnert, W. J., Reiner, B., Siegel, E. L., et al. (2009). Digital radiography reject rates: Data collection Methodology, results, and recommendations from in in-depth investigation at two hospitals. *Journal of Digital Imaging, 23*(1), 89–98.

Fuji Photo Film Company. (2002). *Fuji Computed Radiography Technical Review. No 14, Imaging Plate (IP)* (pp. 1–23). Tokyo: Japan.

Korner, M., Weber, C. H., Wirth, S., Klaus-Jürgen Pfeifer; Maximilian F. Reiser; and Marcus Treitl (2007). Advances in digital radiography: Physical principles and system overview. *Radiographics, 27,* 675–686.

Lanca. L., & Silva, A. (2009). Digital radiography detectors: A technical overview. *Radiography, 15*(1), 23–35.

Neitzel, U. (2005). Status and prospects of digital detector technology for CR and DR. *Radiation Protection Dosimetry, 14*, Nos 1-3, 32–38.

Rowlands, J. A. (2002). The physics of Computed radiography. *Physics in Medicine and Biology, 47*, R123-R166.

Schaetzing, R. (2003). Computed radiography technology. In E. Samei & M. J. Flynn (Eds.), *Advances in Digital Radiology, Categorical Course in Diagnostic Radiology Physics.* Illinois: RSNA.

Seeram, E., & Seeram, D. (2008). Image postprocessing in digital radiology: A primer for technologists. *Journal of Medical Imaging and Radiation Sciences, 39*(1), 23–44.

Seibert, J. A. (2004). Computed radiography technology 2004. In L.W. Goldman & M. V. Yester (Eds.), *Specifications, Performance, and Quality Assurance of Radiographic and Fluoroscopic Systems in the Digital Era.* American Association of Physicists in Medicine (AAPM): College Park, Maryland.

Seibert, J. A. (2006). Computed radiography/Digital radiography: Adult. *Invisible to Visible: The Science and Practice of X-Ray Imaging and Radiation Dose. RSNA Categorical Course in Diagnostic Radiology Physics* (pp. 57–71). Illinois: RSNA.

Willis, C. E. (2006). Computed radiography/Digital radiography: Pediatric. *Invisible to Visible: The Science and Practice of X-Ray Imaging and Radiation Dose. RSNA Categorical Course in Diagnostic Radiology Physics.* RSNA, Illinois, 73–83.

Willis, C. E., Thompson, S. K., & Shepard, S. J. (2004). Artifacts and misadventures in digital radiography. *Applied Radiology, Jan,* 11–20.

Willis, C. E., Parker, B. R., Orand, M., & Wagner, M. L. (1998) Challenges for Pediatric Radiology using Computed Radiography. *Journal of Digital Imaging, 11*(1), 156–158.

CHAPTER 4

Effective Use of Computed Radiography

by Barry Burns

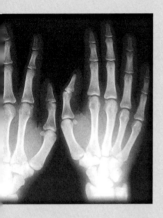

OBJECTIVES

Upon completion of this chapter, the student should be able to:

1. Explain the response of the computed radiography (CR) imaging plate to radiation exposure.

2. Explain the meaning of the term "speed class."

3. Describe the use of exposure indicators in clinical practice.

4. Identify several sources of suboptimal images in CR.

5. Explain several criteria in the selection of technical factors in CR.

6. Describe other factors that play a role in affecting the quality of the CR image.

KEY TERMS

Dynamic range
Histogram analysis
Histogram analysis errors
Multiple exposure fields

Sampling frequency
Saturation
Speed class

Introduction

The physical principles of computed radiography (CR) were described in detail in Chapter 3. To summarize, the CR imaging process is divided into discrete steps: image acquisition, image extraction (reading the imaging plate), image processing, and image display. The initial image acquisition and extraction must provide quality data that will allow for appropriate image manipulation.

Despite CR's flexibility, it still requires a high level of technical skill from the technologist to produce the optimal image during the acquisition stage. This chapter will focus on the effective use of CR in the clinical environment required to produce images of optimum clarity.

CR Cassettes

The CR cassettes (or imaging plates (IP), as they are often referred to) are employed in the same manner as screen/film cassettes in existing radiographic units designed to accommodate cassettes. The plates are exposed using conventional radiographic techniques similar to those one would use for the appropriate film-screen systems. The dynamic range of the IP is much greater than the 10- or 12-bit contrast resolution currently used by most CR systems. The greater amount of image information on the plate must be mapped onto bit depth of the system. In order to visualize the anatomical structures of interest, some initial preprocessing must occur during imaging data extraction. Since the entire plate is scanned, all of the exposure data on the plate is captured. This includes background captured before exposure, the actual image data, and off-focus and scattered radiation captured during exposure. The first, and perhaps the most critical step, is locating or identifying the data within the exposure field. If the exposure field (collimation margins) is not correctly located, the histogram analysis will be performed on all the exposure data. If there is substantial extraneous exposure on the plate, a histogram analysis error is likely to occur. If a histogram analysis error occurs, then the exposure index will be improperly determined and the rescaling

of the values of interest (VOI) will result in a dark, light, or low contrast image.

Various CR vendors employ different terms to describe how the systems extract the relevant exposure data. During this discussion, generic terminology will be employed wherever possible. In some cases, vendor-specific terminology will be employed to address particular issues.

In most cases, the software automatically detects the exposure field, extracts the data, performs the histogram analysis of the extracted data, determines the exposure index, and rescales the data to provide the default display brightness. Some vendors provide for determination of an operating speed class that affects the exposure indicator determination, the rescaling, and the image appearance.

If a vendor provides a fixed-speed class operation, the system operates as a screen/film system of the selected speed. There is no histogram analysis or rescaling. With fixed-speed class operation the brightness depends on the selected technique. If the receptor exposure is high, the image is dark, if the receptor exposure is low, the image is light. Unlike film, where the density is fixed, the digital image allows one to adjust the brightness after acquisition at the QC workstation. However, if the receptor exposure is >50% below the optimal level, the image may exhibit objectionable mottle. Although histogram analysis and rescaling can overcome some of the limitations of screen/film imaging, they present their own sources of limitations and potential errors in the appearance of the final image.

The large dynamic range of the imaging plates provides a very low contrast initial image. Therefore processing algorithms are applied to the raw digital data to render the image appearance acceptable.

Image Plate Response and Exposure

The use of the photostimulable phosphor plates provides an exposure-to-response range, which is essentially linear with a large dynamic range (as described in Chapter 3). Figure 4-1 compares the dynamic range of a mid-contrast film to that of a digital receptor, such as the CR imaging plate. Increased dynamic range allows more data to be

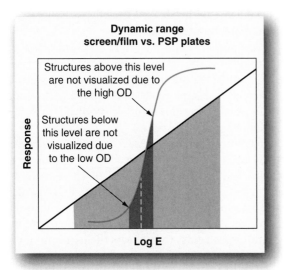

FIGURE 4-1. A comparison of the dynamic range of film to a digital detector. One of the advantages of digital radiography is the increase in dynamic range by ~50×. The dark gray area represents the delimited dynamic range of film and the light gray area represents the dynamic range of a digital acquisition system.
Source: *Delmar, Cengage Learning*

captured during acquisition. In order to visualize all of the captured information, the image must be sent to the PACS so the radiologist can change the display brightness. If the image is printed to film, the visibility of the structures is again limited by the dynamic range of the film. Large dynamic range is of great benefit when imaging structures such as the chest, where the remnant beam intensities will differ by factors of 1000. The increased dynamic range provides visualization of structures, such as the mediastinum and lateral rib margins (where the exposure is low), without loss of lung structures due to overexposure. The increased dynamic range combined with automatic rescaling provides an apparent increase in exposure latitude for a specific imaging application. It is vital to remember that classically the terms overexposure and underexposure have been used to describe image optical density. Overexposure implies dark images and underexposure implies light images. However, the image density may be high or low because of a number of factors

other than exposure. With digital imaging, automatic rescaling of the image provides images that have similar brightness (density) over an exposure range greater than 50X. Therefore, the terms overexposure and underexposure correctly refer to the actual exposure (mR) to the image receptor. Overexposure means that the photon intensity reaching the receptor is higher than that required to produce an optimal image. The resultant image exhibits lower contrast because of the extra scatter produced by the higher photon intensity, and the patient is overexposed. Underexposure means that the photon intensity reaching the receptor is lower than that required to produce an optimal image. The resultant image exhibits quantum mottle, with the noise level increasing as the exposure to the receptor decreases.

Because of the wide dynamic range of the PSP plate and automatic rescaling the relationship between exposure and image brightness is decoupled. One can no longer examine the image for brightness (density) to evaluate the appropriateness of the receptor exposure.

Speed Class

Because of automatic rescaling, digital systems may be employed at a wide rage of exposure, but it is inappropriate to use the term "speed" to describe the response of a digital radiography system. With screen-film systems the speed of the receptor determines the appropriate level of receptor exposure required to achieve the optimal image density. With digital systems, the receptor exposure (technical factors) determines the speed class at which the system is operated. Figure 4-2 shows three knee images recorded at exposure levels between 250 and 60 speed class exposure levels, yet all images have similar display brightness. However, the noise characteristics of the images are quite different. The 2 mAs image exhibits objectionable mottle and the 32 mAs image exhibits reduced contrast due to scatter fogging. Because automatic rescaling produces images with similar brightness, this is viewed as the exposure latitude of the system. The exposure latitude of a digital detector is substantially higher than screen-film. If the digital exposure is >50% below the optimal signal level, quantum

Automatic rescaling

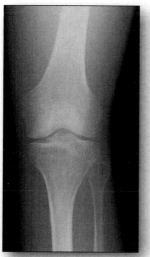 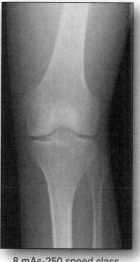 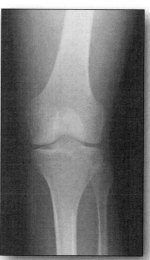

| 2 mAs-100 speed class | 8 mAs-250 speed class | 32 mAs-60 speed class |

FIGURE 4-2. The impact of rescaling. The software rescales the image brightness to a preset level over an exposure range of 100×. These images show the effect from 2 mAs to 32 mAs. All images have the same brightness. The 8 mAs is the correct exposure level. The 2 mAs image is very noisy, and the 32 mAs exhibits reduced contrast from the extra scatter produced by the 10× overexposure. Source: *Delmar, Cengage Learning*

mottle may be objectionable to the viewer. If the exposure is >100% above the optimal signal level, the ALARA principle is violated, and the extra scatter generated will degrade the contrast. Figure 4-2 is an excellent example of the ability of automatic rescaling to provide an image with appropriate brightness over a very large exposure range. Figure 4-3 is an abdomen image acquired at 3000 speed class as part of a research study. Although the image is very noisy, the metal targets in the gastric tube are clearly visible.

Exposure Indicators

Digital image acquisition decouples the relationships between exposure and image appearance via automatic rescaling and image processing algorithms. One can no longer use image density (brightness) to evaluate the accuracy of the receptor exposure.

To evaluate the appropriateness of the receptor exposure for a CR image, all the CR vendors provide an exposure indicator, determined during histogram

3000 speed class operation

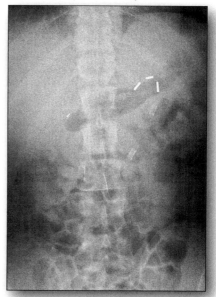

ESE–12 mR

FIGURE 4-3. A digital imaging system can be operated at a very high speed class exposure level. Although this image is very noisy, the objects of interest in the nasogastric tube are visible to the researchers. A typical ESE for this projection is >300 mR. Source: *Delmar, Cengage Learning*

analysis. These exposure indicators express the receptor's exposure. If the receptor is overexposed by a factor of 2X, one would assume that the patient received an equally high exposure. If there are histogram analysis errors, the exposures indicator may be misdetermined and a rescaling error is likely to occur, producing a dark or light image. Figure 4-4 shows four images that have inappropriate rescaling due to exposure field recognition errors. If a rescaling error has occurred, producing a light or dark image, one can be certain that the exposure indicator is not accurate. The problem is compounded by an overexposure. If the exposure field is not recognized, the off-focus radiation and scatter outside the exposure field become part of the histogram. This low-intensity exposure causes the system to rescale the image as if the plate is actually underexposed, producing a dark image and an incorrect exposure indicator due to the resulting widened histogram.

Unfortunately, there is no standardization of these exposure indicators at this time. However, as described in Chapter 3 (and at the time of writing this chapter), several agencies are working to establish a standard method of expressing the receptor exposure. All the vendors determine the exposure indicator during histogram analysis, and the accuracy of the exposure indicator requires that the CR reader be calibrated using an accurate dosimeter.

Currently, each major vendor uses a unique exposure indicator whose values indicate the exposure delivered to the plate. Each of the exposure indicators is derived during the histogram analysis. The accuracy of the exposure indicators depends on accurate reader calibration and appropriate exposure field recognition. If the reader is not routinely

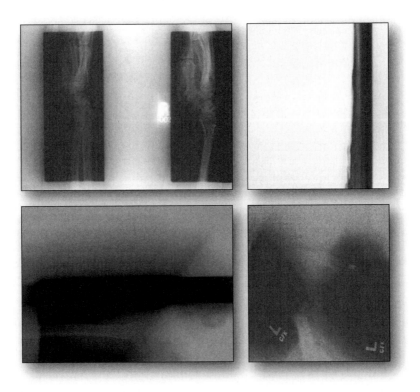

FIGURE 4-4. Four images with rescaling errors. Because the exposure margins were not recognized, the result is a widening of the histogram, producing the rescaling error and an incorrectly determined exposure indicator.
Source: *Delmar, Cengage Learning*

calibrated using a dosimeter and if the histogram contains exposure data from outside the irradiated fields (off-focus and scatter), the exposure indicator will not accurately indicate the exposure.

Generally, the reader calibration is performed using 1 mR to the plate. When that plate is processed using a special menu, the 200 speed class exposure indicator is achieved. While vendors typically use the 200 speed class exposure indicator as the aim, most CR systems are capable of producing quality, low-noise images at 300 to 350 speed class exposure levels. There is no need to reach the 200 speed class exposure level for any body trunk exam. However, distal extremities should be routinely exposed at the 100 speed class level to minimize quantum mottle due to the lower mAs used for the thinner structures.

Although vendors may tout the wide range of exposure indicators allowed, one must realize that wide exposure indicator range only provides an image with appropriate display brightness. If the exposure is >30–40% below the 300 speed class level the image is likely to exhibit objectionable mottle. If the exposure is >200% above the 300 speed class, the contrast will be degraded by the extra scatter produced by the over exposure and clearly violates the ALARA principle. Under certain conditions prescribed by the radiologist, such as line placements, one may choose to dramatically lower the exposure to the patient, obtaining an image with satisfactory display brightness, albeit one with high mottle.

To achieve the correct range of exposure indicator values with CR, it is vital that the exposure factors be selected with the same level of precision as those for screen-film systems. When CR systems are matched with properly operating automatic exposure control systems, the exposure indicator values are very consistent, generally requiring no repeat exams due to exposure errors.

Causes of Suboptimal Images

As with any radiographic imaging system, three important factors contributing to high image clarity and visualization of desired anatomical structures are (1) selection of technical exposure factors;

(2) correct positioning of part; and (3) precise alignment of part, beam, and receptor.

With film-screen systems, technique selection appropriateness is judged by the resulting image density and contrast. Digital systems decouple the relationships between exposure and brightness (density) and kV and contrast via automatic rescaling and image processing algorithms that provide a specific image appearance. However, the digital system cannot adjust for poor positioning or part centering; incorrect beam, part, and receptor alignment; low photon intensity leading to high mottle; and low contrast due to excessive scatter radiation or grid cutoff.

There are a number of factors that may produce suboptimal digital images:

1. Excessive mottle/noise
   a. >50% below the optimal receptor exposure
2. Low contrast
   a. >200% overexposure of the plate
   b. Background buildup on plate
   c. Grid cutoff
   d. Nongrid images
   e. Insufficient contrast improvement of grid
   f. Incorrect menu for anatomy imaged
3. Dark or light images
   a. Rescaling errors due to histogram analysis errors
   b. Inappropriate exposure field alignment or collimation leading to exposure field recognition failure

Effective use of CR systems requires that appropriate technical practices be followed to avoid suboptimal images and to minimize patient exposure increases. Due to the slightly lower DQE (Chapter 3) of PSP materials, most CR systems need to operate at around the 300 speed class to achieve the appropriate receptor signal level, avoiding objectionable image mottle. If a facility is converting from a 400 speed S/F system to CR, the receptor exposure needs to be increased by about 40%. By careful selection of the technical factors, a facility may be able to convert from S/F to CR with little or no increase in patient exposure. The various technical factors employed for CR imaging should be selected with the same care and accuracy as factors for screen-film image acquisition.

One unique characteristic of CR imaging that may complicate technical factor selection is the increased response of the PSP material to low-intensity radiation. PSP storage phosphor plates store exposure and have a very large dynamic range (Figure 4-1), responding to exposures below 100 µR. With a typical background level of 60–80 µR/day, a plate could store 180–240 µR over a weekend. This problem does not occur with film due to the long "foot" section of the D-log E response curve of the typical film. Figure 4-5 compares the relative response of a PSP plate to the response of a typical mid-contrast film. There is a large segment of the D-log E curve that exhibits no increase in OD while the PSP is responding to the low-intensity radiation. This background exposure will degrade the contrast, especially for structures that have low anatomical contrast, such as pediatrics. Most vendors recommend that plates not used and erased within 48 hours should be erased prior to image

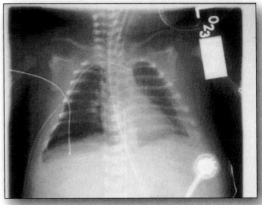

A. Image on plate that has been erased

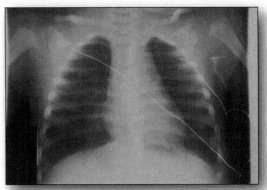

B. Image on plate not erased after four-day weekend

FIGURE 4-6. The effect of not erasing a plate after 86 hours of nonuse. Image A is done on a fresh plate because it is second image on that plate. Image B is the first image taken on that plate on Tuesday morning after a four-day holiday weekend. The contrast reduction to the accumulated background is clearly shown.
Source: *Delmar, Cengage Learning*

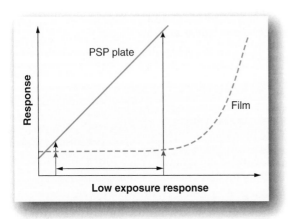

FIGURE 4-5. The response of a PSP plate and a mid-contrast film. The film H and D curve had a long "foot" section that did not respond to low levels of exposure. The PSP plate has a linear response that registers the low exposure levels, to which film did not respond. This, along with the fact the PSP material is a "storage" phosphor, accounts for the enhanced repose of PSP materials to background and scatter radiation.
Source: *Delmar, Cengage Learning*

acquisition. Figure 4-6 illustrates the results of not erasing a plate unused from 5:00 pm Friday to 7:00 am Tuesday following a four-day holiday weekend. Image A is the first image acquired on the unerased plate. The plate was then processed and erased. Image B is the second image acquired on the same plate. Note the dramatic loss of contrast due to the collection of 86 hours of background. If the plate is going to respond to background that was not an issue with S/F receptors, imagine the response to scatter that is hundreds of times more intense than background. Figure 4-7 shows an image recorded by taping a hand phantom on a CR

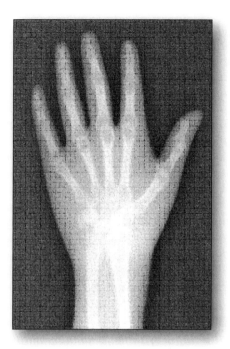

FIGURE 4-7. This figure shows an image of a hand phantom taped to a standard CR cassette that was placed in the control–booth window facing an abdomen phantom on the radiographic table 8 feet from the cassette while the abdomen phantom was exposed twice using 5 mAs@ 90 kVp.
Source: *Delmar, Cengage Learning*

cassette located 8 feet from an abdomen phantom that was exposed two times at 5 mAs—90 kVp. Controlling scatter is a critical consideration in optimizing image quality with CR systems.

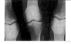

Selection of Technical Factors

To achieve the desired range of receptor exposure values, it is vital the technical factors be selected with the same care and precision as used for screen-film systems. One should use an accurate technique chart or a properly functioning automatic exposure control (AEC) system. Substantial clinical experience has indicated that the use of CR combined with an ion chamber AEC, which is centering critical, will yield a very low repeat rate due to exposure errors. The normal exposure variation associated with equipment performance fluctuation, patient

attenuation variations, and so on, are generally hidden by automatic rescaling. Each exposure factor should be selected considering specific criteria that meet the needs of the examination.

Source to Image Receptor Distance (SID)

The SID is generally in the same ranges as for screen/film due to the fact that facilities rarely change grids when making the transition from S/F to CR. The SID is essentially limited by the grid's focal range. However, one can reduce the patient exposure by 12–15% by doing routine radiography at a 48" (122 cm) SID rather than the typical 40" (100 cm) SID. Care must be taken to avoid violation of the focal range or other situations that would result in grid cutoff. With CR, grid cutoff does not result in a light image, due to the automatic rescaling of the image. Grid cutoff results in flattening of the luminance from the plate and loss of contrast. This will be discussed again under grid selection criteria. Figure 4-8 is a CR lateral spine acquired at 100 cm using a 17:1 grid with a focal distance of 150 cm. The grid cutoff produced

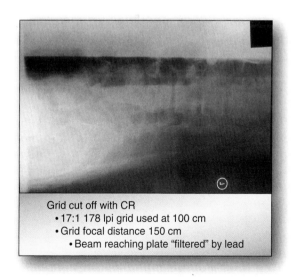

Grid cut off with CR
• 17:1 178 lpi grid used at 100 cm
• Grid focal distance 150 cm
  • Beam reaching plate "filtered" by lead

FIGURE 4-8. Low contrast resulting from grid cutoff. The image was acquired using a new grid. This is a 17:1 70 line/cm with a focal distance of 150 cm (60 in.). When the image was acquired at a 40" SID, off–focus cutoff occurred. The beam was "flattened" by the cutoff, resulting in flattening of the luminance from the plate.
Source: *Delmar, Cengage Learning*

a flattening of the plate luminance, reducing the contrast. An S/F image acquired with a focal range violation would be light and exhibit low contrast. A digital image acquired with a focal range violation will be rescaled, providing the appropriate brightness but exhibiting low contrast.

Scattered Radiation Grids

With the increased sensitivity of the PSP plate to low intensity radiation, scatter control becomes an important consideration. As with S/F imaging beam size and the water content have a vital role in determining the amount of scatter generated. Limiting the beam to the anatomy of interest is practiced in the same way as S/F imaging. However, there is a common belief that one cannot collimate with CR systems. This myth is well established and has its foundations in that if the beam is inappropriately collimated, the exposure field may not be recognized and the image is rescaled dark or light. If no

collimation occurs then there is no exposure field to recognize and rescaling is more likely to occur correctly. The lack of collimation generates more scatter that reduces the contrast. Many technologists believe that post-processing contrast adjustments can make up for any acquisition error. No processing currently available can correct for the low signal difference that occurs due to scatter exposure to the plate. Figure 4-9 compares a nongrid chest to a grid chest to demonstrate the effect of scatter on signal difference (contrast).

Two of the problems associated with grid selection for bedside radiograph are grid cutoff and Moiré artifacts, also referred to as aliasing artifacts. When performing a mobile chest scan the cassette is normally oriented crosswise (landscape). If one uses the generally available long dimension (LD) grids, the risk of grid cutoff due to off-center and off-level violations is more likely to occur (Figure 4-10). To reduce the risk of off-level grid cutoff one should employ short dimension (SD)

Grid vs non-grid

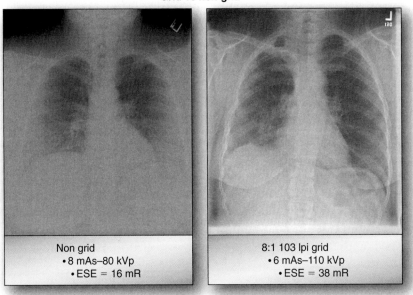

Non grid	8:1 103 lpi grid
• 8 mAs–80 kVp	• 6 mAs–110 kVp
• ESE = 16 mR	• ESE = 38 mR

FIGURE 4-9. The effect on a grid image of signal difference and image contrast. Due to the higher signal difference, the grid image exhibits many more anatomical structures. Since the scatter was removed by the grid, the applied equalization processing demonstrates structures behind the heart and below the diaphragm. Even though the ESE is higher for the grid image, it is acceptable because of the improved diagnostic information available.
Source: *Delmar, Cengage Learning*

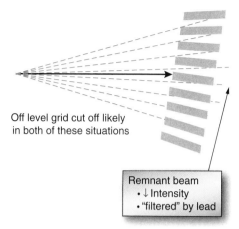

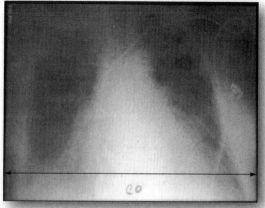

Grid cut-off 6:1/103 lpi SD grid

FIGURE 4-10. The effect of grid cutoff when using a typical LD for crosswise beside–chest radiographs. The same that happens as with the focal range violation in Figure 8. The beam intensity is flattened, reducing signal difference. Source: *Delmar, Cengage Learning*

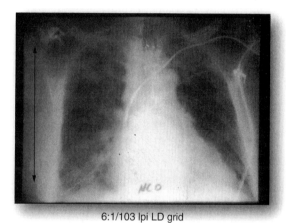

6:1/103 lpi LD grid

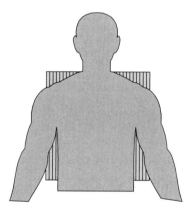

Mobile chest with cassette crosswise
SD grid
Off level cut-off less likely to occur

FIGURE 4-12. The top image shows the results of off–level cutoff with an LD grid. The bottom image is from the same patient done two hours later with a new SD grid that had just been delivered. Source: *Delmar, Cengage Learning*

FIGURE 4-11. This diagram shows the use of an SD grid for performing beside–chest radiographs. Because the grid strips are vertical, the risk of off–level cutoff is reduced. Source: *Delmar, Cengage Learning*

or "decubitus" grids (Figure 4-11). Since the grid strips are oriented in the direction of grid tilt, grid cutoff is much less likely to occur. Figure 4-12 compares the image quality of two chests, one exhibiting grid cutoff using an LD grid and the other without grid cutoff using a SD grid. The images were acquired about two hours apart using the same technical factors.

When selecting the appropriate grid for use with CR, the grid frequency (lines per inch = lp/in) is important because the image is scanned line by line. If the grid used has a frequency near the scan frequency and the grid strips are oriented in the same direction as the scan, one will observe a Moiré effect. Because of the different sampling frequencies of the plates according to receptor size, the only universally recommended grid frequency is 178 lp/i or 70 lines/cm. The problem with the high frequency grids is that as the frequency increases the lead content decreases. A 12:1 103 lp/i grid and a 17:1 178 lp/i grid will have similar lead content. However, the 17:1 grid will exhibit much less alignment latitude. For most CR systems, an 8:1 103 lpi stationary grid hold will not produce Moiré patterns on 35 × 43 and 24 × 30 receptors. Moiré may occur with flat panel DR detectors if the grid frequency is near the Nyquist frequency of the detector array.

Using a grid does increase the ESE, but grid images are acquired at higher kV levels, so the ESE does not follow the grid factor. Figure 4-9 illustrates the effect on the ESE of switching from nongrid to grid for chest radiography and then increasing the kV above the 80 kV used for the nongrid imaging. Because the grid image acquired at 110 kV employed a grid, the remnant beam had much higher signal difference, so the grid image exhibits much higher contrast than the nongrid image at 80 kV. Due to the higher signal difference, the grid image exhibits many more anatomical structures. Since the scatter was removed by the rid, the applied equalization processing demonstrates structures behind the heart and below the diaphragm.

Selection of kVp

Because the digital detector response is essentially linear (Figure 4-1), the initial contrast is very low and the processing algorithm must be applied to achieve the desired level of image contrast. Since the image contrast is generally determined more by the processing algorithm, the kVp does not have the impact on final image contrast as with screen/film systems. However, kVp still controls the differential attenuation, signal difference or subject contrast, so kVp selection with digital systems is just as important as with conventional film-screen systems. The kVp should be elected for the desired level of subject contrast and the selectivity of the grid used. For example, if performing an IVU, one should employ 75–80 kVp to optimize the incident beam absorption by the diluted iodinated contrast medium.

Unfortunately, many technologists and radiologists still think in film mode and use the kVp to alter the contrast. In fact, the processing algorithm has more effect on image contrast than the kVp. One may use 10–20 kVp more for digital systems to limit the patient dose. One may also use higher kVp when using a high efficiency grid. For

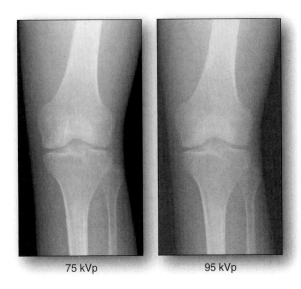

75 kVp   95 kVp

FIGURE 4-13. Two images acquired using the same processing algorithm. One image was taken at 75 kVp and one was taken at 95 kVp. While there is a slight difference in contrast, it is not the difference one would expect with film. This effect is primarily due to the very low (flat) contrast of the "raw" for-processing image. We depend on the processing algorithm to provide the desired contrast. Thus, altering the kVp 10–20 does not have a large effect on the image contrast.
Source: *Delmar, Cengage Learning*

example, 75 kVp with an 8:1 grid and 95 kVp with a 12:1 grid will yield comparable image contrast (Figure 4-13).

The use of higher kVp may have a dramatic effect on patient exposure. Table 4-1 shows the effect of increasing the kVp from 90 to 120 for routine chest radiography. Figure 4-14 shows the two images taken at 90 and 120 kVp. While there is a small difference in the contrast, it is minimal. Figure 4-15 shows the contrast detail patterns in the phantom. One can see that the noise level of

TABLE 4-1. The impact of kVp on patient exposure.

kVp vs ESE		
13:1 178 lpi grid		
Constant receptor exposure		
kVp	MAs	ESE-mR
90	14	67
120	5.0	40

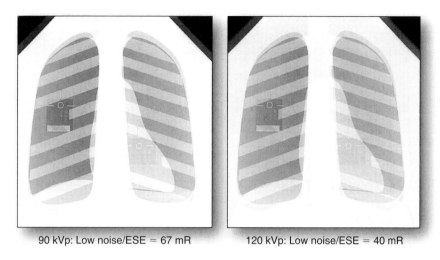

| 90 kVp: Low noise/ESE = 67 mR | 120 kVp: Low noise/ESE = 40 mR |

FIGURE 4-14. A comparison of the images acquired using the data provided in Table 4-1.
Source: *Delmar, Cengage Learning*

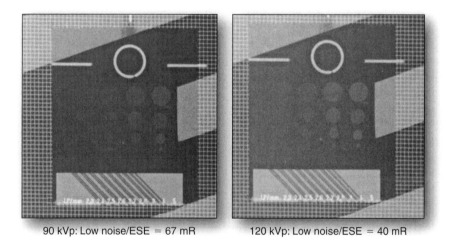

| 90 kVp: Low noise/ESE = 67 mR | 120 kVp: Low noise/ESE = 40 mR |

FIGURE 4-15. A comparison of the contrast-detail pattern in the two images in Figure 4-14.
The visibility of the low contrast masses is essentially the same in both images.
Source: *Delmar, Cengage Learning*

both images is similar, with a 30% reduction in ESE with no loss of information. One should use the highest kVp practical for the available grid, but avoid a kVp of more than 130 because the image is likely to become noisy.

Using a higher kV also reduces the width of the acquired data due to the simple relationship between the kVp and signal difference, as illustrated by Figure 4-16. This relationship is particularly difficult

for the technologist who uses film-based imaging to comprehend. With screen/film imaging, the consideration of the effect of technical factors is normally based on the image appearance rather the physics behind the appearance. Using screen/film systems, increasing the kVp increases the grayscale (wider). With this concept so firmly implanted, it is difficult to get technologists to accept the data width reduction produced by increasing the kVp. One has to consider

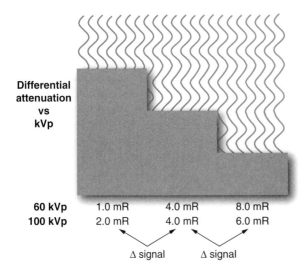

FIGURE 4-16. The differential attenuation resulting from a large kVp changes. As the kVp increases the differential attenuation decreases and the signal difference from max to min is dramatically reduced.
Source: Delmar, Cengage Learning

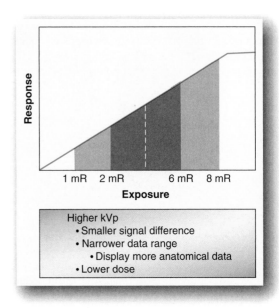

FIGURE 4-17. The values from Figure 4–16 applied to a diagram shows that as the kVp increases the data width acquired is less, so that more anatomical information may be visible on an image without having to change the brightness.
Source: Delmar, Cengage Learning

the differential attenuation to see the actual effect of a kVp change. In Figure 4-17, one can see that increasing the kVp reduces the differential attenuation, narrowing the signal difference between the thickest step and the thinnest step. By reducing the acquired data width, more of the anatomy may be visualized for a single image display setting.

Because of the increased sensitivity to scattered radiation, the kVp should not exceed 80 for any nongrid radiography, including chest. If the structure provides a remnant beam where scatter ratio is more than 50% of the beam reaching the receptor, an appropriate grid should be used. Failure to do so will result in substantial loss of contrast due to scatter fogging.

Selection of mAs

The actual exposure latitude of the typical digital system is about double that of the typical film-screen radiographic system. However, in the interest of patient dose and image quality, the mAs should be selected with the same care and precision used for film-screen systems. One should use an accurate technique chart or a properly functioning automatic exposure control system. Our experience has indicated that the use of digital systems combined with

an ion chamber automatic exposure control, which is centering critical, will result in very low repeat rates due to exposure errors. The small inherent exposure variation associated with equipment performance fluctuation, patient attenuation variations, and so on, is corrected by automatic rescaling.

Exposure levels >50% below the optimal level will produce images that exhibit excessive mottle. The objectionable level of mottle is determined by the radiologist. Exposure levels >100% above the optimal level will be properly rescaled, but this level has to be considered an ALARA violation. Once the exposure is >200% above the optimal level, the extra scatter generated will begin to degrade the image. At some point of overexposure, sections of the detector will become saturated and anatomical structures in this region will not be visualized due to the lack of signal difference in the region.

Part, Beam, and Receptor Alignment

The entire PSP plate is scanned during the reading process. With the cassette-based systems, before the initial image processing can occur, the system must locate the exposure field(s) and only use data from that region for the histogram analysis. If extraneous data is included in the histogram because the exposure fields were not located, histogram analysis errors are likely. Histogram analysis errors generally result in rescaling errors and exposure indicator determination errors. The most common reason for histogram analysis errors is exposure field recognition failure. The inclusion of the off-focus radiation and the scatter outside the collimation margin will widen or skew the histogram.

If the histogram data is skewed relative to the values of interest (VOI) of the histogram analysis used for that exam, any number of processing errors may occur, resulting in image degradation. If the anatomical structures are not centered to the plate or if the X-ray beam is not correctly aligned to the edges of the plate, the exposure field may not be correctly identified and the off-focus radiation and scatter outside the exposure field will widen the histogram, resulting in a processing error. The final image will show one or more image problems, including low contrast. The same effect may occur if the beam edge is irregular because of the overlap of the radiopaque shadow, such as gonadal shield, or if the beam edge is irregular or incorrectly aligned

to the edges of the plate, the image degradation effects may be minimized.

There are unique beam alignment precautions for both single field and multiple field exposures. Each vendor should be able to provide information on beam alignment precautions and rules for beam distributions. The optimal alignment for all digital detectors is to have the part and beam centered to the receptor, with four collimation margins parallel to the cassette edges. In clinical practice this is not going to be achievable for every exam, so one needs to be aware of the limitations of the systems. Generally, a centered field with two margins parallel to the cassette edge will be recognized. The optimal alignment is field-centered to the plate with four collimation margins parallel to the cassette edges. Some exams, such as tibia/fibula, cross-table lateral hip, and axial shoulders, may cause some problems. For the tibia/fibula, the exposure field should extend from corner to corner and the collimation margins should be parallel. The problem with CR lateral hips and axial shoulders is that there is only one collimation margin between the exposure field and the edge of the plate, as shown in Figure 4-18. Some vendors have special acquisition

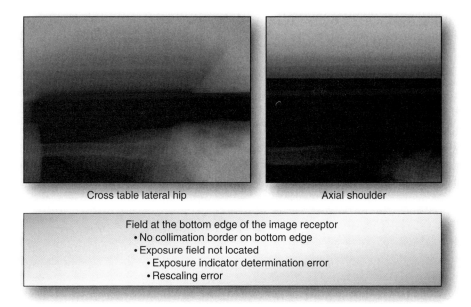

Cross table lateral hip | Axial shoulder

Field at the bottom edge of the image receptor
- No collimation border on bottom edge
- Exposure field not located
  - Exposure indicator determination error
- Rescaling error

FIGURE 4-18. Two images with rescaling errors as a result of one collimation margin. Because there is not a collimation margin at the bottom of the image, an exposure–field recognition error occurred, resulting in an histogram analysis error that in turn led to the rescaling error. Source: *Delmar, Cengage Learning*

**Create "collimation margin"
with lead strip**

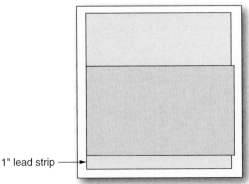

1" lead strip

FIGURE 4-19. A universal solution to the exposure-field recognition error in Figure 4-18. A strip of lead is placed at the bottom of the receptor, creating a collimation margin so that the software will locate the exposure field. Source: *Delmar, Cengage Learning*

modes or post-processing ROI adjustments to ideal with this problem. Figure 4-19 illustrates a universal solution. One may create a second collimation margin by using a narrow (~1 inch) lead strip at the bottom of the cassette to generate a "margin" between the exposure field and the edge of the plate. When the lead strip is employed, one acquires images like the one shown in Figure 4-20. Fuji and

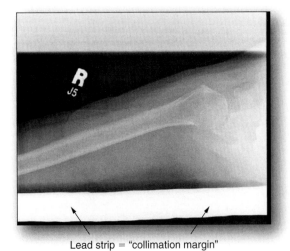

Lead strip = "collimation margin"

FIGURE 4-20. An image without a rescaling error. Source: *Delmar, Cengage Learning*

Philips CR systems have a Semi-X image processing mode. With Semi-X, the plate is divided into nine regions. The technologist may select the region where the exposure field is located. If technologist forgets where the exposure field is located and selects the wrong area, a histogram analysis and rescaling error will occur.

Many of the beam alignment debates with cassette-based CR systems are related to multiple exposure fields on one plate for distal extremities. This is not an issue with cassetteless systems, where the image is read as soon as the exposure terminates. With CR systems one may acquire any number of images on one plate before the plate is placed in the reader. However, if the decision is made to acquire multiple exposure fields on one plate, very strict alignment rules must be followed to ensure that exposure field(s) is(are) recognized and that a histogram analysis failure does not occur. One of the major decisions a radiology department must make is whether multiple exposure fields will be acquired on a plate. To avoid an exposure field recognition error, the safe approach is to acquire one image on the smallest plate available. However, for those facilities that only have 43 × 35 and 24 × 30 plates, acquiring images such as a single finger or a tightly coned beam navicular bone on a 24 × 30 is likely to result in an exposure field recognition error, because most sytems cannot recognize a field less than 1/3 the area of the plate. Figure 4-21 shows a navicular bone projection on a 24 × 30 with the resulting rescaling error. In addition, some vendors do not provide the highest sampling frequency (spatial resolution) until the smallest plate is employed. With very small fields, such as premature infant mobile chests or special navicular and temporomandibular joint (TMJ) projections, it is imperative that these images be acquired on the smallest plate available. Routine hands and feet should be acquired one image per plate. Simultaneous acquisition of bilateral hands may be acquired on a plate with no problem. Most vendors recommend that extremities be acquired one image per plate. The main reason for this recommendation is the vendors know that histogram analysis errors are more likely to occur with multiple field exposures and the vendors want their product to look good. Some have suggested that by limiting all extremities to one image per plate, the

FIGURE 4-21. The navicular bone image acquired on a 24 × 30 receptor. The very small exposure field was not recognized, resulting in a rescaling error. One should use an exposure field that is about one-third the area of the receptor. In addition, one should use the smallest plate possible to ensure the highest sampling frequency for those systems that alter the sampling frequency as a function of receptor size.
Source: *Delmar, Cengage Learning*

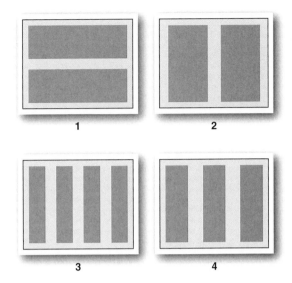

FIGURE 4-22. Recommended split-field patterns. It is very important that the fields be symmetrically distributed across the plate with collimation margins parallel to the plate edges.
Source: *Delmar, Cengage Learning*

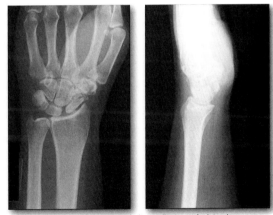

Split field failure/no technique adjustment for lateral

FIGURE 4-23. A split-field error (failure). The technologist did not adjust the technique for the lateral projection. Even though digital systems rescale the images for single projections on a plate, one must adjust the technique for the projection to maintain the correct receptor exposure.
Source: *Delmar, Cengage Learning*

plates will have to be replaced more frequently. One reason to collect only one image per plate is the ability of the radiologist to then split the PACS monitor and display the current image and the prior image side by side for comparison.

Figure 4-22 illustrates appropriate multiple exposure field placement on a single plate. The keys to multiple fields on a plate are symmetry, and uniform distribution. One should only use 3-on-1 distribution for fingers and toes where the amount of intrafield scatter is low. If larger body structures are done 3 on 1, the intrafield scatter will reduce the contrast unless the unexposed areas are shielded between exposures. It is also critical to adjust the exposure for the projection. Figure 4-23 illustrates a PA and lateral wrist without technique adjustment for the lateral projection.

An oblique and lateral foot may be acquired on one plate without risk of a rescaling error, but an AP foot and any other image on the same plate is likely to result in improper display. The toes are likely to be dark and the hindfoot light. Figure 4-24 illustrates an AP and oblique foot protections on

one plate. Note the loss of information at the toes and the hindfoot. One image per plate is illustrated by Figure 4-25. Note that the hindfoot and the

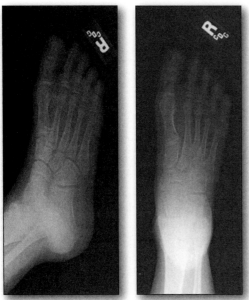

Two images on one plate/hind foot = light and toes = dark?

FIGURE 4-24. Typical results of acquiring two projections of a foot on a single plate. The wide range of digital values makes accurate rescaling difficult. The toes tend to be dark and the hindfoot tends to be light.
Source: *Delmar, Cengage Learning*

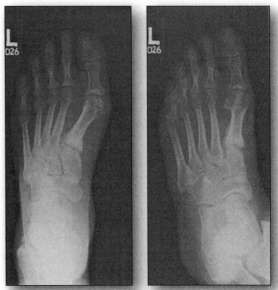

One image per plate—more consistent images

FIGURE 4-25. Improvement resulting from acquiring a single projection foot on a single plate. The image brightness tends to be more consistent from hind foot to the toes because the software doesn't have to deal with complex histogram created by two images on a plate.
Source: *Delmar, Cengage Learning*

toes have a more appropriate brightness. One foot per plate has become easier now that at least one vendor has provided a 15 cm × 30 cm (6" × 12") plate.

Collimation

Many myths abound that one cannot collimate with digital imaging, especially CR. This is largely due to the early systems in which some histogram analysis models required raw radiation beyond the skin margin. If the collimation is not aligned to the plate margin a histogram analysis error may occur. Collimation is still critical for optimal image acquisition. Collimation limits the irradiated volume and reduces undercutting. Unfortunately, images light that in Figure 4-26 are very commonly mishandled in the average radiology department. Due to the high sensitivity of digital detectors to low

intensity radiation (background and scatter and off-focus), there is likely to be scatter and off-focus radiation contributing to the image outside the collimation margins (Figure 4-27). Many radiologists find this distracting while viewing images, and technologists respond by not collimating. This increases the patient's effective dose and increases the amount of scatter, which will degrade the contrast. The appropriate response to scatter and off-focus exposure outside the collimation margin is to apply black border to the image before it is printed or sent to PACS (Figure 4-28). Another beam-limiting issue is related to acquisition of images. If the exposure field extends well beyond the edge of the structure, the intense raw radiation produces undercutting radiation that degrades structure visibility along the margin of the structure. This is very well illustrated by Figure 4-29. Adjusting the image brightness will not restore the

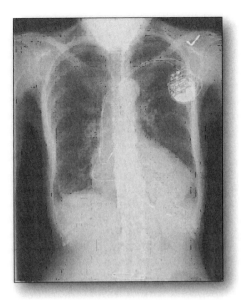

FIGURE 4-26. Typical CR chest image. There is a common belief that one cannot collimate with CR because it may cause a histogram–analysis error. If the collimation is symmetrical and parallel to the plate margins, histogram-analysis errors should not occur. This area may be even darker if the image is overexposed due to low grid efficiency.
Source: *Delmar, Cengage Learning*

To avoid distracting radiologist, apply back border.

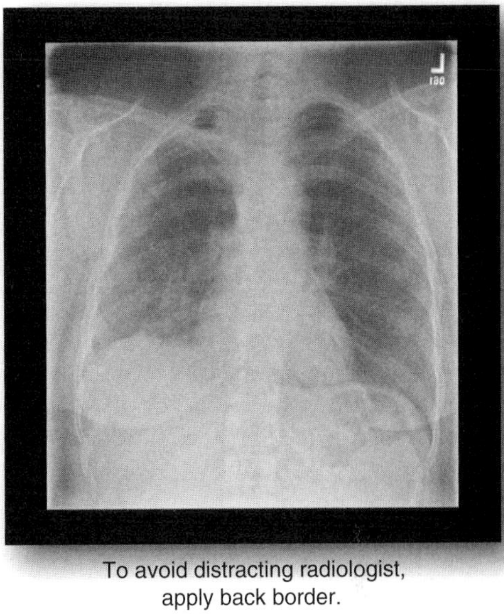

FIGURE 4-28. Activating the automatic black border feature, as seen in this image, removes the distraction faced by the radiologist interpreting the image.
Source: *Delmar, Cengage Learning*

Collimated image

If grid efficiency is low or image is overexposed, scatter and off focus radiation degrades "clear zone."

Produces distraction for radiologist

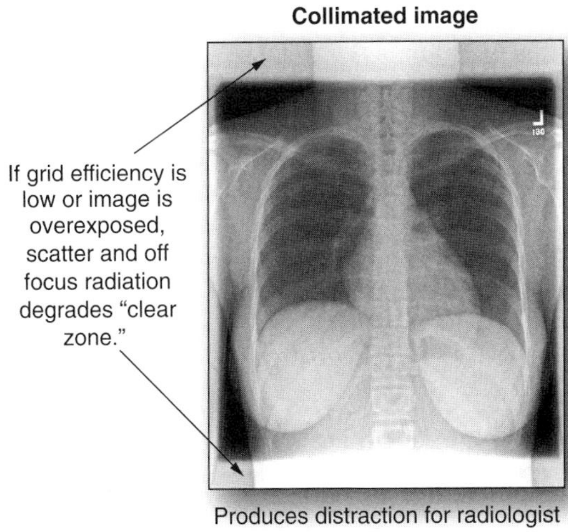

FIGURE 4-27. Owing to the low-intensity radiation sensitivity, off-focus and scattered radiation are recorded beyond the collimation margin.
Source: *Delmar, Cengage Learning*

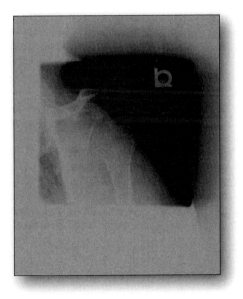

FIGURE 4-29. Results of poor centering. The excessive "raw" radiation field beyond the anatomical structures results in undercutting.
Source: *Delmar, Cengage Learning*

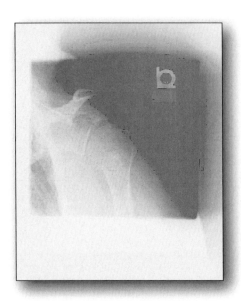

FIGURE 4-30. In changing the image brightness, the soft tissue peripheral structures are lost.
Source: *Delmar, Cengage Learning*

anatomical structure because that portion of the image is saturated (Figure 4-30).

 ## Other Considerations

Low-Contrast Images

Many of the factors that cause low contrast in film-screen systems also cause low contrast in CR images: (1) high kVp, (2) inadequate grid efficiency or no grid, and (3) insufficient beam limiting. In addition to these common causes, low contrast in CR may be the result of incomplete erasure of the IP after reading and several days of exposure to background radiation without being used or erased.

Because of their wide dynamic range, PSP plates are much more susceptible to fogging than are conventional film-screen systems. Therefore, extra care must be taken to minimize scatter fogging by proper use of beam limiting, avoidance of substantial overexposure, careful attention to grid use, and increased awareness of the necessity of erasing plates that have not been used for 48 hours. If there is any question about how long it has been since the plate has been though the read/erase cycle, one

should erase the plate, especially if pediatric images are being performed. One should also be aware if images suddenly begin to exhibit low contrast; the erasure system may have failed. Erasure thoroughness must be a routine QC test for all CR systems.

Substantial (>2x) overexposure of a body part generates additional scatter in proportion to the overexposure. Non-grid exposures are dramatically affected by the additional scatter and even a grid may not be able to remove it. For standard CR plates, exposure levels of more than 100 speed class will manifest lower contrast.

If the plate has been substantially overexposed at >50 speed class levels, there is a good chance the post-read erasure will not restore the plate to an unexposed state. In consequence, the residual charge may produce a fogging effect on the next examination, lowering the contrast. In these cases, an additional erasure should be performed on the plate used for that examination. If one processes that plate using the normal protocol, the image will show a very clear outline of the previous examination.

Image Loss due to Overexposure (Saturation)

Even though the digital detectors have a very large dynamic range, it is not limitless. If the image is overexposed by more than 4X to 5X, a portion of the image may be saturated. Saturation means that beyond a certain exposure level, a large number of the pixels will be at the maximum digital value (black) so that there is no signal difference in the very high exposure areas, resulting in a loss of anatomical structures in that region. Saturation and ALARA violations are the primary reasons to use appropriate exposure level. Figure 4-31 shows an overexposed lateral thoracic spine with a large area of saturation in the lower lung. Note the lack of anatomical information in the area. This kind of image must be repeated, since there is no way to recover a saturated image.

Recorded Detail with Digital Radiographic Systems

Recorded detail refers to the fidelity with which the structure being imaged is recorded by the receptor and is determined by a complex interrelationship of

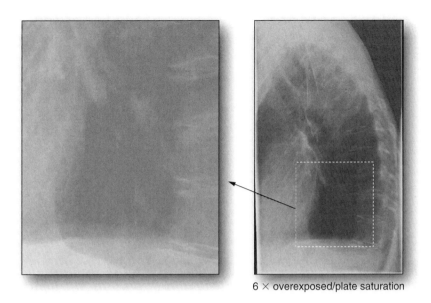

6 × overexposed/plate saturation

FIGURE 4-31. This illustration shows saturation due to an overexposure of >5X. Saturation means that the detector is so overexposed in an area that all the pixel values in that area are at the maximum (black). Saturated images must be repeated, since that area cannot be lightened.
Source: *Delmar, Cengage Learning*

many factors. Another way to describe the level of recorded detail is to identify the level of the "blur." Low blur equals high recorded detail and high blur equals low recorded detail. The factors determining recorded detail included motion factors, geometric factors, and the spatial resolution of the receptor unit (line pair/mm). Spatial resolution is the standard expression for the receptor's contribution to recorded detail. With screen/film systems the spatial resolution is related to the light diffusion from the intensifying screen relative to its "speed." Slower speed screens exhibit less light diffusion, which provides higher spatial resolution. With screen-film systems, quantum mottle is a rare contributor to loss of recorded detail because mottle is associated with screen speeds greater than 600. With digital systems, the motion and geometric components are the same. Longer exposure times are more likely to result in motion blur. Short SIDs, longer object image distances (OID), and larger focal spots yield increased geometric blur. The major difference in recorded detail contributors is the receptor. Speed no longer has an effect because digital detector

generally has a fixed spatial resolution that is dependent on the pixel pitch. With digital systems, if the exposure is >50% below the ideal, objectionable quantum mottle will occur, which degrades edge smoothness. Therefore, it is important that the optimal exposure be employed in order to reduce mottle. For distal extremities, one should use 100 speed class exposures to avoid mottle for those exams that would require very low mAs for a 400 speed class exposure.

With digital systems, the spatial resolution is related to the pixel pitch (Figure 4-32). The maximum spatial resolution is equal to the Nyquist frequency, 1/2X the pixel pitch (mm). A 0.050 mm pixel pitch would yield a Nyquist of 10 lp/mm while a 0.100 mm pixel pitch would yield a Nyquist of 5 lp/mm.

Cassetteless digital systems have a fixed spatial resolution determined by the thin film transistor (TFT) detector element (DEL) size. The larger the DEL, the lower the spatial resolution. TFT DEL sizes range from 100 microns to 200 microns. 100 microns provides a spatial resolution of ~5 lp/mm

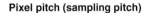
Pixel pitch (sampling pitch)

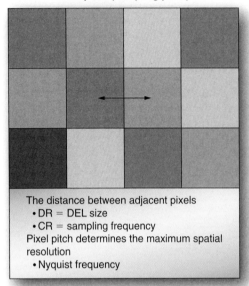

The distance between adjacent pixels
- DR = DEL size
- CR = sampling frequency

Pixel pitch determines the maximum spatial resolution
- Nyquist frequency

FIGURE 4-32. A diagrammatic illustration of pixel pitch, or sampling pitch, which is the primary factor determining the spatial resolution of a digital detector. The pixel pitch is determined by the DEL size for a cassetteless DR stem and by sampling frequency for a cassette-based CR stem. Some CR stems have a fixed sampling frequency and others vary the sampling frequency as a function of receptor size.
Source: *Delmar, Cengage Learning*

while the 200 micron DEL systems provide ~2.5 lp/mm. The only detectors with 100 micron DELs are small area detectors used for digital mammography. Large area TFT detectors range from 140 microns (3.7 lp/mm) to 200 microns (2.5 lp/mm), which is less than the 400-speed screen. No TFT digital detector approaches the 10 lp/mm of the 100-speed screen. Because digital detectors have lower spatial resolution than screen/film systems, it is important to control the other sources of blur.

With Cassette-based PSP systems (CR) spatial resolution becomes a bit more complicated. With CR systems the spatial resolution is determined by the pixel pitch, which is determined by the sampling frequency as the laser scans the plate. Sampling frequency is expressed as pixels/mm, also referred to as pixel density. The higher the sampling frequency and the smaller the pixel pitch, the more pixels/mm and the higher the spatial resolution. Several vendors alter the sampling frequency with plate size so that the highest resolution is only achieved using the 8" × 20" plate. Thus the myth "smaller plates are slower than larger plates," because the smaller plate has higher resolution, as do slower screens. Except for special extremity plates from Kodak, all plates are basically made from the same barium fluorohalides and are coated to the same thickness. Generally, there is no difference in the response of the plates as a function of size; thus, there is no difference in the "speeds" of the plates. Because of the light spread between the plate and the light guide, the spatial resolution is less than the Nyquist frequency.

At the present time Agfa, Kodak, and Konica have variable sampling frequencies as a function of receptor size or a selectable option at the workstation before the plate is scanned.

Most new Fuji and Philips systems are sold with the HQ mode activated so that all plates are sampled at 10 pixels/mm, yielding a spatial resolution of ~4 /lp/mm for all plate sizes. However, the new units can be set for ST mode if the customer desires smaller file sizes and less resolution. Agfa offers an HR mode so that all plates may be sampled at 10 pixels/mm.

Kodak's new GP Plus software allows the sampling frequency to be encoded into the image acquisition menu so that the spatial resolution may be a function of the exam not the plate size. A tibia/fibula exam may be read at 10 pixels/mm and a KUB at 6 pixels/mm, because it is preferable to have more recorded detail for such an exam. Some of the newest PDP CCD scanning arrays will provide 20 pixels/mm. However, because of the large file sizes (14 × 17 = 120 MB), most facilities down sample 14 × 14, and 14 × 14 receptors. Except for the CCD scanning arrays, the highest frequencies (20 pixels/mm) are only available with CR systems approved by the Food and Drug Administration (FDA) for full-field digital mammography.

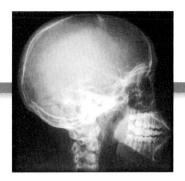

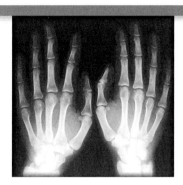

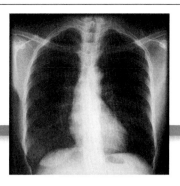

REVIEW QUESTIONS

1. Computed Radiography is considered a _____ digital acquisition system.

2. The ability of the CR system to provide images with consistent brightness over an exposure range of ~50X is due to a software feature termed _____

3. A dark or light digital image is most likely the result of _____

4. Rescaling error is most likely to occur because of _____

5. One of the major advantages of digital image acquisition is the increased _____ of the receptors.

6. If a digital image is acquired using an exposure > 50% below the ideal exposure, the image is likely to exhibit _____

7. If a bedside chest is acquired using a grid and grid cut-off occurs, the image will exhibit reduced _____

8. Because the relationship between exposure in image brightness is decoupled one has to rely on _____ to evaluate receptor exposure accuracy.

9. The exposure latitude for digital systems is about _____ that of screen film systems.

10. Because of rescaling the exposure latitude of digital systems is limited by ____ on the low end and _____ on the high end.

REFERENCES

American Association of Physicists in Medicine (AAPM). (2006). *Acceptance Testing and Quality Control of Photostimulable Storage Phosphor Imaging systems.* Report No 93. College Park, MD.

Huda, W. (2005, February 1). The Current Concept of Speed Should Not Be Used to Describe Digital Imaging Systems, *Radiology*, 234(2), 345–346.

Samei, E., & Flynn, D. (Eds.). (2005). Advances in Digital Radiography. Syllabus: *2005 RSNA Categorical Course in Diagnostic Radiologic Physics*, AAPM Report 93.

CHAPTER 5

Flat-Panel Digital Radiography

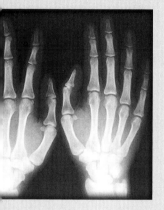

OBJECTIVES

Upon completion of this chapter, the student should be able to:

1. State the limitations of computed radiography.

2. State the meaning of the term flat-panel digital radiography and list the major system components of a flat-panel imaging system.

3. Compare and contrast the two types of flat-panel digital detectors.

4. Describe the major design characteristics such as the configuration, dimensions, and the fill factor of flat-panel detectors.

5. Outline the principles of operation of CCD digital detectors.

6. Outline the principles of operation of indirect and direct flat-panel digital detectors.

7. Discuss exposure latitude and exposure indicators for flat-panel digital detectors.

8. State the purpose of image processing in flat-panel digital radiographic imaging.

9. Describe the elements of preprocessing and postprocessing in flat-panel digital radiographic imaging.

10. Explain the effect of three factors that play a role in optimizing the image display in flat-panel digital radiographic imaging.

11. List three image processing optimization rules.

12. Explain briefly the following imaging performance characteristics of flat-panel digital detectors:

    • Spatial resolution

    • Modulation transfer function

    • Dynamic range

    • Detective quantum efficiency

    • Image lag

13. Identify several different kinds of artifacts that are common in flat-panel digital detectors.

14. State the other imaging application areas of flat-panel digital detectors not mentioned above.

KEY TERMS

Amorphous selenium (a-Se)
Amorphous silicon (a-Si) photodiode
Cesium iodide (CsI)
Charge-coupled device (CCD) digital detector
Direct detectors
Exposure latitude
Fill factor
Flat-fielding
"For-presentation" image

"For-processing" image
Image display optimization
Image lag
Indirect detectors
Modulation transfer function (MTF)
Pixel pitch
Scaling the histogram
Thin film transistor (TFT)
X-ray scintillator

Introduction

In Chapter 3, the physical principles and technology of computed radiography (CR) imaging systems were described in detail. In review, a CR imaging system consists of at least four fundamental steps, as shown in Figure 5-1. First, the CR imaging plate (IP) is exposed to X-rays, after which it is placed into the CR image reader for signal extraction. Third, a computer processes the signal and displays a digital image on a viewing monitor for diagnostic interpretation and image postprocessing, if required.

The physical basis for the CR image is the IP detector, which is made of a photostimulable phosphor (PSP) such as barium flourohalide (BaFX-X is the halide, which can be a bromide, chloride, iodide, or a combination of these). After X-ray exposure of the IP PSP, a latent image is formed on the IP. To render this latent image visible, the IP is taken to the image reader, which uses a laser beam to extract the image information signal. This signal is subsequently digitized and sent to a computer for preprocessing. The computer-generated image is then displayed on a monitor for viewing and interpretation.

Limitations of CR

Although CR has its advantages over film-screen (FS) radiography, the most conspicuous being a wider dynamic range (Chapter 3), it also has several limitations. These include the following:

1. The X-ray detection of CR is inefficient and this affects image quality and dose. The detection efficiency is also inferior to that of FS radiography (Koner et al., 2007).

2. The spatial resolution of CR is less than FS radiography. While the spatial resolution of CR is about 3–5 line pairs/mm (lp/mm) for a 35 cm × 43 cm IP (Korner et al., 2007), it is about 10–15 lp/mm for FS radiography (Bushong, 2009).

3. CR IPs (image plates) can easily be damaged. They can be dropped accidentally (during portable radiography or transported to the IP reader) and are susceptible to scratches and cracking. They can also be easily damaged when they are in the image reader (Hammerstrom et al., 2006).

4. CR IPs must be transported to a separate image processor (image reader) for image data extraction (Korner et al., 2007; Yorkston, 2003).

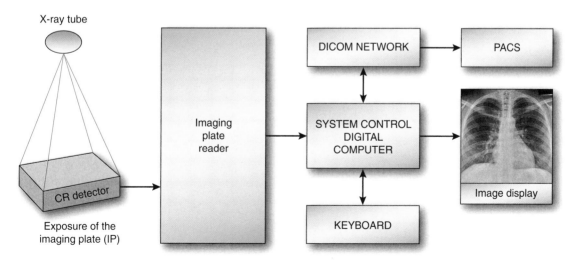

FIGURE 5-1. The four fundamental steps in the CR process. After the IP is exposed to X-rays, it is taken to the image reader for latent image extraction. The IP is scanned by a laser beam and the resulting signal is digitized and converted into an image. The image is displayed for viewing and interpretation and subsequently sent to the PACS. Source: *Delmar, Cengage Learning*

The above limitations are some of the important considerations that provided the motivation for the development of other digital radiography systems (Chotas et al., 1999; Kotter & Lauger, 2002; Korner et al., 2007; Yorkston, 2004; Neitzel, 2005). These systems are popularly referred to as digital radiography (DR) systems, which use flat-panel detector technology. In this book, the term flat-panel digital radiography (FPDR) will be used.

The purpose of this chapter is to describe the overall structure of flat-panel digital detectors and outline the physical principles and technology aspects of these detectors. In addition, several performance characteristics as well as other considerations will be highlighted.

What is Flat-Panel Digital Radiography?

Flat-panel digital radiography detectors were introduced as early as 1995 for use in radiographic imaging (Antonuk et al., 1995; Lanca & Silva, 2009; Zhao & Rowlands, 1995). One system was developed based on the use of amorphous silicon (Autonuk et al., 1995), and the other was an amorphous selenium detector (Zhao & Rowlands, 1995).

It is important to note here that other digital detectors for use in radiography were being used before 1995; however, they were not based on flat-panel detector technology. Two of these systems were a (CCD chip) slot-scan digital detector, which was introduced in 1990, and the selenium drum digital radiography system introduced in 1994 (Korner et al., 2007).

The selenium drum technology was developed as a dedicated system specifically for imaging the chest. The unit was called the Thoravision (Philips Medical Systems, the Netherlands). Selenium is a photoconductor, and it conducts electrons when struck by light or X-ray photons. Since there may still be a few systems currently in use, the fundamental principles will be reviewed briefly. Figure 5-2 shows how the selenium drum technology works. A positive charge is first placed on the drum, which is then exposed to X-rays. The exposure changes the charge distribution in the selenium to produce an electrostatic image stored on the drum. A probe then scans the electrostatic image to produce a voltage that is subsequently sent to an analog-to-digital converter (ADC), which digitizes the signal and sends the digital data stream to a computer for digital processing. The image is then displayed for viewing by the radiologist.

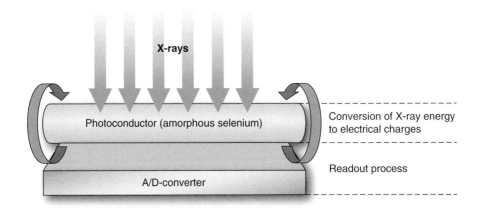

FIGURE 5-2. A dedicated digital radiography imaging system that is based on selenium drum technology.
Source: *Korner, et al. (2007). Advances in digital radiography: Physical principles and system overview. Radiographics, 27, 675–686. Reproduced by kind permission of RSNA*

The quality of the selenium drum image has been shown to be superior to that of both FS radiography and CR imaging (Kloft et al., 2005; Neitzel et al., 1994; Ramli et al., 2005; Veldkamp et al., 2006).

Flat-Panel DR: System Components

A flat-panel DR imaging system (detectors and associated technical components) is illustrated in Figure 5-3. It is clearly apparent that there are several components coupled to the flat-panel detector. As shown in the diagram, the flat-panel digital detector is a single unit (a thin flat-panel device) that contains not only the flat-panel X-ray detection array but also the associated electronics. These include the pre-amplifiers, switching control, central logic circuits, ADCs, and internal memory. It is important to note that X-ray detection and digitization of the X-ray signal take place within the flat-panel detector. There is no need to take the flat-panel detector to a separate unit for signal readout as is a characteristic feature in CR. The different types of flat-panel detectors, imaging principles, and technology will be described in detail later in the chapter.

As can be seen in Figure 5-3, the host computer acts as an interface between the flat-panel detector and the X-ray machine (X-ray tube, generator, and control panel) and other system components such as the image display device, network communication, and the image storage device. The host computer plays an important role in controlling X-ray production and signal readout from the flat-panel detector (Yorkston, 2004). In addition, the host computer applies the appropriate image processing "to perform image correction and optimization for display" (Yorkston, 2003).

Other system components such as the image display, image storage, and network communication are responsible for several tasks. The computer output image is first displayed on a monitor for viewing, image postprocessing, and interpretation by a radiologist. The image storage provides a repository for all images obtained from the flat-panel detector that are acceptable by the radiologist, and these are appropriately archived. Finally, the network component provides the opportunity to distribute the images to interested parties located anywhere in the world.

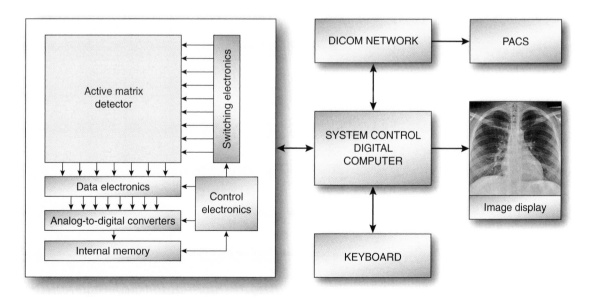

FIGURE 5-3. A schematic representation of a flat-panel digital radiographic imaging system. The flat-panel detector contains all essential X-ray detection elements and electronics for image capture and retrieval respectively.
Source: *Delmar, Cengage Learning*

Types of Flat–Panel Detectors

The use of flat-panel digital detectors in X-ray imaging is referred to as direct radiography (Korner et al., 2007; Lanca & Silva, 2009). Currently, there are two categories of flat panel digital radiography detectors, namely, indirect detectors and direct detectors based on the type of X-ray absorber used (Figure 5-4). While indirect detectors use a phosphor, direct detectors use a photoconductor, as is clearly illustrated in Figure 5-4. With the above in mind, Yorkston (2003) points out that "the rationale for this nomenclature is that the systems that use phosphors convert X-ray energy into electrical change through an intermediate stage of light photons, while those that use photoconductors convert the X-ray energy directly into electrical charge without the intermediate stage." In this respect, therefore, the terms indirect conversion and direct conversion have been used synonymously to refer to indirect detectors and direct detectors respectively.

Indirect Digital Detectors: Technical Components

As illustrated in Figure 5-4, there are two types of indirect digital detectors (Figure 5-4A) the charge-coupled device (CCD) digital detector and the flat-panel thin film transistor (TFT) digital detector (Figure 5-4B). The most conspicuous difference

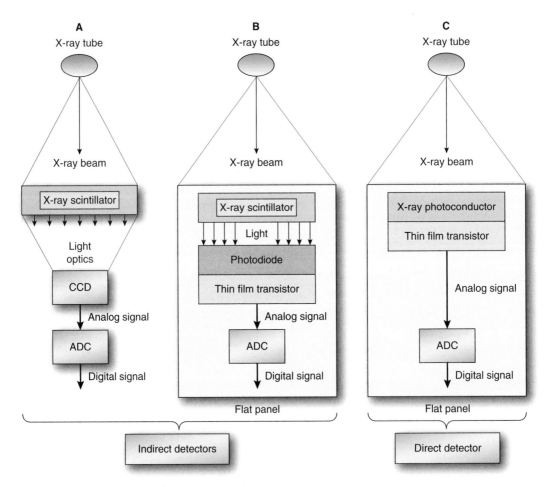

FIGURE 5-4. Two categories of flat–panel digital radiography detectors, indirect detectors (A and B) and direct detectors (C). The CCD detector is not generally considered a flat–panel detector.
Source: *Delmar, Cengage Learning*

between these two types of detectors is the technical component used to convert light into electrical signals.

• *CCD Digital Detectors*

The CCD digital detector is based on an indirect conversion process and uses a CCD chip to convert light to electrical charge. The CCD digital detector is not classified as a flat-panel digital detector; however, because it is a system that is available commercially, it is included in this chapter.

The main technical components of a CCD-based digital radiography detector are shown in Figure 5-5, including an X-ray absorber, light optics, and the CCD, which is a sensor (chip) for capturing the light. The CCD is also an electrical charge

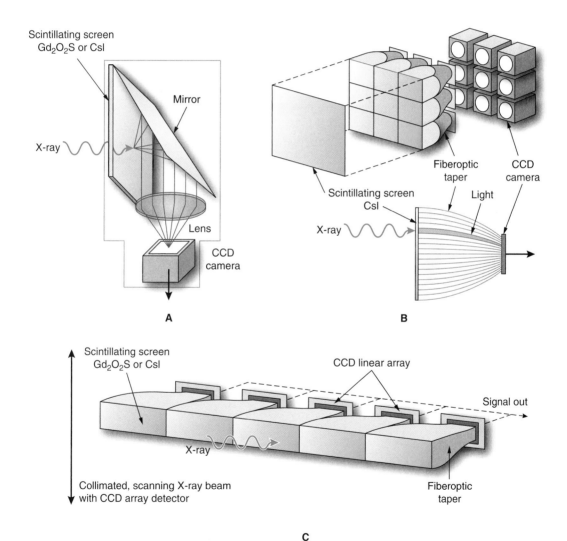

FIGURE 5-5. Three types of CCD digital detector systems. A lens coupled system is shown in A; a fiber–optic coupled system and a fiber–optic scanning array CCD system is shown in B and C respectively.
Source: *Samei, E. et al. (2004). AAPM/RSNA Tutorial on Equipment Selection: PACS Equipment Overview: General Guidelines for Purchasing and Acceptance Testing of PACS Equipment. RadioGraphics, 24, 313–334. Reproduced by kind permission of RSNA*

readout device. An important point to note about Figure 5-5A is that only one chip is shown; however, a CCD digital detector consists of several CCDs in order to increase the size of the detection area. Additionally, there are three other noteworthy components: the scintillation screen (detects X-rays and converts them into light); the light collection optics; and an array of CCDs, also referred to as the CCD camera. While the CCD detector shown in Figure 5-5A is a fiberoptic-coupled CCD system, other systems may use a lens-coupled CCD (Figure 5-5B) or a fiberoptic-coupled scanning array as shown in Figure 5-5C (Samei et al., 2004).

- **Indirect Flat-Panel TFT Digital Detectors**

An indirect flat-panel digital detector is based on an indirect conversion process and uses several physical components to convert X-rays into light that is subsequently converted into electrical charges. These components include an **X-ray scintillator** (X-ray conversion layer), followed by an **amorphous silicon (a-Si) photodiode** flat-panel layer, with a **thin-film transistor (TFT)** array for readout of the electrical charges by the photodiode array. The organization of these components is illustrated in Figure 5-6.

The X-ray scintillator layer used in the indirect flat-panel digital detector is usually either **cesium iodide (CsI)** or gradolinium oxysulfide (Gd_2O_2S).

These phosphors are not new to X-ray imaging for they have been used in X-ray image intensifiers (CsI) and in rare-earth intensifying screens (Gd_2O_2S). An interesting design fabrication of these phosphors is the manner in which they are deposited into the a-Si photodiode array. CsI crystals are deposited in a needle-like fashion (structured phosphor) and run in the direction of the X-ray beam, while Gd_2O_2S crystals are deposited as powdered particles (turbid phosphor). The former is sometimes referred to as a structured scintillator and the latter as an unstructured scintillator. In addition, powdered phosphors produce lateral spreading of light, which destroys the spatial resolution of the image; whereas structured phosphors like the CsI needles reduce the lateral dispersion of light, thus improving the spatial resolution of the image. This effect is clearly illustrated in Figure 5-7.

Following the X-ray scintillator (X-ray detection medium) is an a-Si photodiode flat-panel array. This component is made by a process referred to as "plasma-enhanced chemical vapor deposition" in which "layers of a-Si are deposited onto a thin glass substrate (typically ~0.7 mm) ..." (Yorkston, 2003). The purpose of the a-Si photodiode layer is to convert the light from the X-ray detection scintillator into electrical charges. Adjacent to the a-Si photodiode layer is a thin-film transistor (TFT) array, as well as storage capacitors and associated

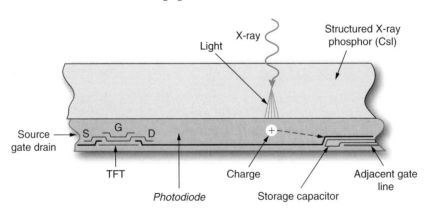

FIGURE 5-6. The main system components of an a–Si photodiode TFT indirect flat-panel digital detector.
Source: Samei, E. et al. (2004). AAPM/RSNA Tutorial on Equipment Selection: PACS Equipment Overview: General Guidelines for Purchasing and Acceptance Testing of PACS Equipment. RadioGraphics, 24, 313–334. Reproduced by kind permission of RSNA

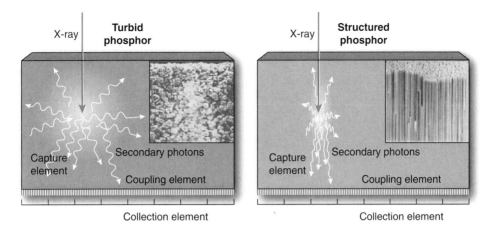

FIGURE 5-7. The amount of light scattering in a turbid (powdered) and structured phosphor indirect flat-panel digital detector. The structured phosphor "needle-like" design reduces the lateral spread of light which serves to improve the spatial resolution of the image
Source: *Samei E. Performance of digital radiographic detectors: Factors affecting sharpness and noise. In E. Samei & M. J. Flynn (Eds.). (2003)* Advances in Digital Radiography: RSNA Categorical Course in Diagnostic Radiology Physics *(pp. 49–61). Reproduced by kind permission of RSNA*

electronics (Figure 5-6). The purpose of the capacitor is to collect and store the electrical charge produced in the a-Si photodiode array. In this regard, the flat-panel described above is also referred to as an indirect conversion TFT digital detector. The flat-panel design will be described later in the chapter.

Direct Digital Detectors: Technical Components

A cross-sectional diagram of a direct flat-panel TFT digital detector is shown in Figure 5-8. This detector consists of several components such as a source

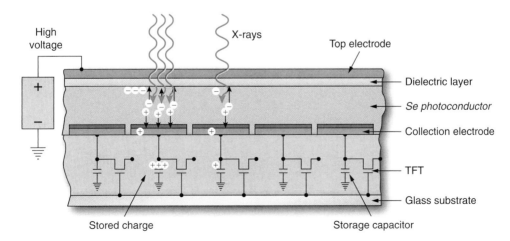

FIGURE 5-8. The main system components of an a–Se TFT direct flat-panel digital detector.
Source: *Samei, E. et al. (2004). AAPM/RSNA Tutorial on Equipment Selection: PACS Equipment Overview: General Guidelines for Purchasing and Acceptance Testing of PACS Equipment.* RadioGraphics, 24, 313–334. *Reproduced by kind permission of RSNA*

of high voltage, top electrode, dielectric layer, photoconductor, collection electrode, TFT, storage capacitor, and the glass substrate. It is not within the scope of this book to describe the details of each of these components; however, the basics of the photoconductor will be highlighted.

The photoconductor is usually amorphous selenium (a-Se), although other photoconductors such as lead oxide, lead iodide, thallium bromide, and gadolinium compounds can be used (Korner et al., 2007). The use of a-Se, however, has become commonplace simply because of "its excellent X-ray detection properties and a very high spatial resolution" (Kotter & Langer, 2002). The photoconductor detects X-ray photons from the patient and converts them directly into electrical charges. The TFT and associated electronics (capacitors for example) collect and store the changes for subsequent readout.

The operational principles of indirect and direct flat-panel TFT digital detectors will be described later in this chapter. The next section of this chapter deals with the design (or construction framework) of the flat-panel TFT digital detector.

Design Characteristics of Flat-Panel Detectors

Configuration of the Flat-Panel

The flat-panel TFT digital detector is designed as a matrix of detector elements, each of which can be regarded as a pixel and constructed as shown in Figure 5-9. This design principle is referred to as large area integrated circuit (Rowlands & Yorkston, 2000).

The matrix, also referred to as an active matrix array, consists of rows and columns that play a role in addressing and readout of the signal from each pixel. As seen in Figure 5-9, each pixel contains a TFT (switch), a storage capacitor, and a sensing area, referred to as the sensing/storage element (Yorkston, 2004). The sensing area will detect the light from the CsI scintillator in the indirect flat-panel TFT detector, or in the case of a direct flat-panel TFT detector, X-ray photons passing through the patient. In particular, the sensing/storage element of an indirect flat-panel TFT detector is the photodiode (photosensitive storage element), while it is the storage capacitor (capacitive storage element) in the direct flat-panel TFT detector that uses the a-Se photoconductor (Yorkston, 2004).

In addition to the matrix of pixels, there are other electronic components that are included in the flat-panel detector (gateline or data line). These include switching electronics to activate each row of pixels and electronic amplifiers and associated electronic devices (multiplexer) for signal readout from each column of pixels. The electronic (analog) signal is subsequently sent to the analog-to-digital converter (ADC) for digitization. The ADC is also included in the flat-panel detector. Finally, the digital data stream is sent to a computer for digital image processing.

Dimensions of the Detector and its Components

As noted earlier, the flat-panel TFT digital detector consists of a matrix of pixels (individual elements). Since there are different sizes of body parts to be imaged, different sizes of detectors are commercially available for clinical imaging. Typical detector dimensions, for example, include 43 cm × 43 cm, 30 cm × 40 cm, and 18 cm × 18 cm.

The matrix size also varies depending on the size of the detector. Typical matrix sizes include 1760 × 2140, 2000 × 2500, 2736 × 2736, 2560 × 3072, 2688 × 2688, and 3121 × 3121 (Korner et al., 2007).

The pixel size and spacing (i.e., pixel pitch, the distance from the midpoint of one pixel to the midpoint of the adjacent pixel) determine the spatial resolution of the image. The number of pixels can be obtained by multiplying the dimensions of the matrix size. For example, the number of pixels in a 2688 × 2688 matrix is 7,225,344 pixels. In general, pixel sizes in current detectors can be 139 μm, 143 μm, 160 μm, 162 μm, 167 μm, and 200 μm (Korner et al., 2007).

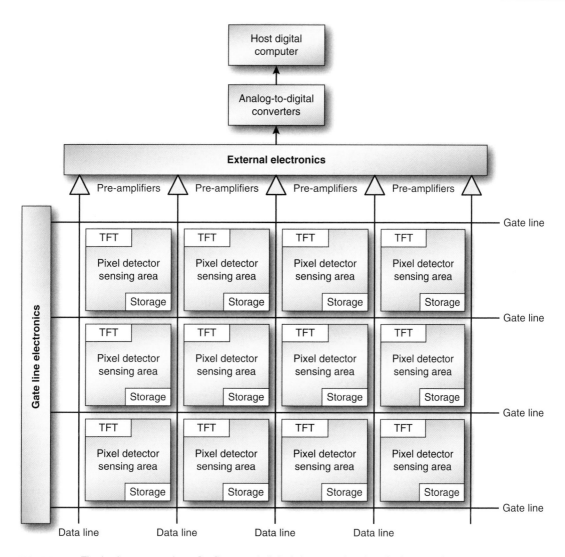

FIGURE 5-9. The basic construction of a flat-panel digital detector showing the layout of the major system components. The flat panel detector captures radiation from the patient and converts it into an electrical signal, which is subsequently digitized by the analog-to-digital converters. The digital data are sent to the host computer for image processing.
Source: *Delmar, Cengage Learning*

The Fill Factor of the Pixel

An important feature of the pixel in the flat-panel TFT digital detector active matrix array is the fill factor, as shown in Figure 5-10. A pixel contains generally three components: the TFT, the capacitor, and the sensing area. The sensing area of the pixel receives the data from the layer above it that captures X-rays that are converted to light (indirect flat-panel detectors) or electrical charges (direct flat-panel detectors). The fill factor, then, is defined as the ratio of sensing area of the pixel to the area of the pixel itself (Bushberg et al., 2004;

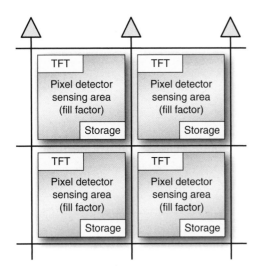

FIGURE 5-10. The sensing area of a single pixel of a flat-panel digital detector is referred to as the fill factor. Source: *Delmar, Cengage Learning*

Kotter & Lauger 2002; Yorkston 2004), and can be expressed as

$$\text{Fill Factor} = \frac{\text{Sensing area of the pixel}}{\text{Area of the pixel}}$$

The fill factor is also expressed as a percentage, where a fill factor of 80% means that 20% of the pixel area is occupied by the detector electronics with 80% representing the sensing area.

The fill factor affects both the spatial resolution (detail) and contrast resolution (signal-to-noise ratio) characteristics of the detector (Bushong et al., 2009). Detectors with high fill factors (large sensing areas) will provide better spatial and contrast resolution than detectors with low fill factors (small sensing area).

Principles of Operation

The principles of operation of digital detectors based on CCD and flat-panel technologies are complex and demand a good understanding of the physics of scintillation phosphors, photoconductors, and semiconductors, as well as electronics. Since this is not a physics or electronics textbook, it is not within the scope here to describe the physics

or electronics in any detail. In addition, some of the technical aspects of these detectors are proprietary and are not disclosed to the public; therefore, only a generalized description of how these detectors work will be presented.

The topics described in this section will focus on how the CCD detectors and flat-panel detectors work (from exposure of the detector to readout of the electrical charges that create a latent image), exposure latitude of flat-panel digital detectors, exposure indicators, and image processing.

CCD Digital Detectors

Figure 5-5 shows the various design structures of the CCD digital detector. These are indirect conversion detectors using the CCD to collect light from the scintillator. The CCD silicon chip is made up of millions of discrete pixels forming a matrix array of pixels. Light from the scintillator falls upon each pixel to produce electron-hole pairs (charges) in direct proportion to the amount of light falling upon them.

During readout, the system electronics provide a systematic collection of changes on each chip in a manner referred to as a "bucket brigade" (Yester, 2004). The charge from each pixel in a row is transferred to the next row and subsequently down all the columns to the final readout row. The charge pattern from the readout row of pixels is sent to the ADC for digitization. The digital data stream is then sent to a computer for processing to produce a digital image.

One of the limitations of the CCD digital detector is related to the light optics (lenses, mirrors, and fiber-optics; Figure 5-5) used to couple the X-ray scintillator to the CCD silicon chip. Specifically, the optical system reduces the output image from the scintillator phosphor to the size of the CCD array. This minification, or demagnification, reduces the image quality (Kotter & Langer, 2002; Yorkston, 2004) by producing, for example, a reduced signal-to-noise ratio (Korner et al., 2007). In this respect, efforts have been made to design other CCD detectors to deal with image quality degradation in CCD detectors that have a small area (Figure 5-5). More studies are needed to assess the objective imaging performance of these detectors (Korner et al., 2007).

Flat-Panel TFT Digital Detectors

As described earlier in the chapter, there are two types of flat-panel TFT digital detectors for use in radiographic imaging, the indirect flat-panel TFT detector (Figure 5-6) and the direct flat-panel TFT detector (Figure 5-8). While indirect detectors use a light-sensitive photodiode (to capture light from the scintillator phosphor such as CsI) to produce electrical charges, the direct detectors use an a-Se photoconductor to convert X-rays directly into electrical charges.

The physics of the interaction of X-rays with scintillators, photodiodes, and photoconductors (a-Se, which is also a semiconductor [Wolbarst, 1993]) will not be described in this book. Such description can be found in any good radiologic physics textbook. Additionally, a radiologic physics course for technologists should address the basic physics of how X-rays interact with these materials.

One important physical concept that is essential to understanding the rationale for the use of specific X-ray scintillators and a-Se in digital detectors is that of X-ray attenuation or absorption. Recall from physics that X-ray attenuation depends on several factors, such as the atomic number (Z), density, and thickness of the attenuating materials. As noted earlier, X-ray scintillators are CsI and Gd_2O_2S for indirect flat-panel TFT detectors and a-Se for direct flat-panel TFT detectors.

A conspicuous feature of these detectors is that they are commonly used in radiography, fluoroscopy, and angiography that are based on the use of the Brems, or continuous X-ray, spectrum. This spectrum ensures that a wide range of voltages (say from 50 kVp to 140 kVp) can be used for the varying types of body parts imaged in the three modalities mentioned above. In addition, flat-panel detectors are used in digital mammography (Chapter 7) where a dedicated X-ray tube is used to produce a specific spectrum (discrete or characteristic spectrum) in which the range of energies is optimized to image the breast. Recall that mammographic kV can range from 26 kV to 32 kV (Bushberg et al., 2004).

Additionally, the Z for CsI is about 54 (Z for Cs = 55; Z for I = 53) and the thickness of the CsI scintillator layer is about 600 μm. These characteristics make this type of detector suitable for radiography, fluoroscopy, and angiography. For mammographic imaging, a thinner layer of CsI, about 150 μm, combined with the mammographic X-ray spectrum, is an essential requirement for optimum imaging (Spahn, 2005).

For a-Se digital detectors, apart from the k-edge characteristic that plays an important role in X-ray absorption (see any radiographic physics textbook), a thickness of about 250 μm is required for mammography, while about 1000 μm thickness is essential for radiographic and angiographic pixel imaging (Spahn, 2005).

Two processes—the detection and conversion of X-rays into electrical charges and subsequent readout of the charges—characterize the operating principles of flat-panel digital detectors and will now be described.

Indirect flat-panel TFT digital detectors (Figure 5-6) utilize a scintillator layer such as CsI to first convert X-ray photons into light photons. These light photons strike the a-Si photodiode layer, which converts them into electrical charges. For direct flat-panel digital detectors, X-ray photons fall upon the a-Se photoconductor layered on top of a matrix of a-Si TFT array (Figure 5-8). In this detector, an electric field is created between the top electrode and the TFT elements. As X-rays strike the a-Se, electrical charges are created and the electric field causes them to move towards the TFT elements, where they are collected and stored. These two processes are illustrated in Figure 5-11 for both indirect and direct detectors. In both cases, the distribution of the charges in the matrix array of pixels represents the so-called "latent" image. It is at this point that all charges must be read out. This is accomplished by what is referred to as the readout electronics.

The flat-panel TFT digital detector uses complex and sophisticated electronic circuitry to read out the electrical charges produced and stored in the matrix array. This is a very systematic process, also referred to as an active matrix readout (Kotter & Langer, 2002), in which pixels are read out row by row.

The general readout process is illustrated in Figure 5-12, which shows a small portion of the flat-panel detector matrix array, a 3 × 3 pixel region.

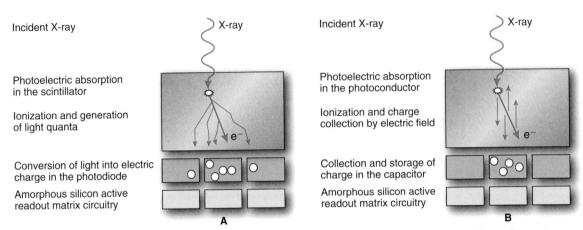

Incident X-ray

Photoelectric absorption in the scintillator

Ionization and generation of light quanta

Conversion of light into electric charge in the photodiode

Amorphous silicon active readout matrix circuitry

A

Incident X-ray

Photoelectric absorption in the photoconductor

Ionization and charge collection by electric field

Collection and storage of charge in the capacitor

Amorphous silicon active readout matrix circuitry

B

FIGURE 5-11. The processes of detection and conversion of X-ray photons into electrical signals (charges) in indirect (A) and direct (B) flat-panel digital detectors.
Source: *Spahn, M. (2005). Flat detectors and their clinical applications. European Journal of Radiology, 15, 1934–1947. Reproduced with kind permission of Springer Science and Business Media*

The essential components shown are switch lines, data lines, control voltage, and external electronics. It is clearly apparent in Figure 5-12 that "all the control contacts of the pixel switching elements along a horizontal line are connected to the same horizontal readout control line and all the signal readout connections of the pixels along a vertical column are connected to the same vertical data output line" (Yorkston, 2004).

Before the flat-panel detector can be used for an X-ray examination, it must be prepared. This preparation is referred to as initialization. The basic principles of operation of the flat-panel are best described by Yorkston (2003), (see Figure 5-12) as follows:

> "Once the array has been put into a suitable 'initialized' state, all switching elements are held in an 'off' state by the appropriate control voltage (−5V in this example) (Figure 5-12 left). The x-ray exposure is made, and the pixels now contain the image information in the sensing/storage element. This image information is then read out one line at a time by changing the control line voltage (to +10V in this example) such that all pixels along a single row become connected to their

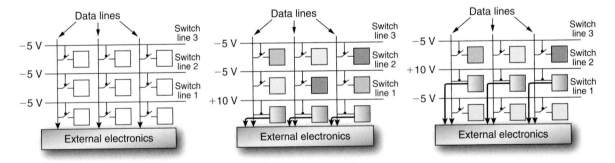

FIGURE 5-12. Schematic diagram of a generic flat-panel array readout scheme. Left: The array is in an initialized state ready for X-ray exposure. Center: The X-ray exposure has been made, and switching line 1 is being read out. Right: Switching line 2 is being read out.
Source: *Yorkston J. Digital radiography technology. In E. Samei & M. J. Flynn (Eds.). (2003) Advances in Digital Radiography: RSNA Categorical Course in Diagnostic Radiology Physics (pp. 23-36). Reproduced by kind permission of RSNA*

corresponding data line (Figure 5-12 center). The signal charge from this row of pixels is transferred along the data lines to the external electronics, where it is amplified, digitized, and stored. The controlling voltage for this line is then returned to the 'disconnect' value (−5V), and the next line is connected by switching its control line voltage to +10V (Figure 5-12 right). This process is repeated for each line of the detector"

For the flat-panel TFT digital detectors used in fluoroscopy, the readout process and readout electronics are somewhat different to the detectors used for radiographic applications. While radiography produces static images, fluoroscopy produces dynamic images to demonstrate motion. Digital fluoroscopy will be described in Chapter 5.

Exposure Latitude

The **exposure latitude** in radiographic imaging is a concept that examines the response of the image receptor (screen-film detector or digital detector) to the radiation falling upon it. Exposure latitude for computed radiography detectors (photostimulable phosphor imaging plate) was described in Chapter 3.

The exposure latitude for various screen-film detectors, CR, and flat-panel digital detectors (DR) is illustrated in Figure 5-13. Essentially, the exposure latitude for digital detectors (CR and DR detectors) is much wider (0.1 – 1000 µGy) compared to the screen-film receptors shown. The major advantage of such wide dynamic range is that the detector can respond to different levels of exposure (low to high) and still provide an image that appears acceptable to

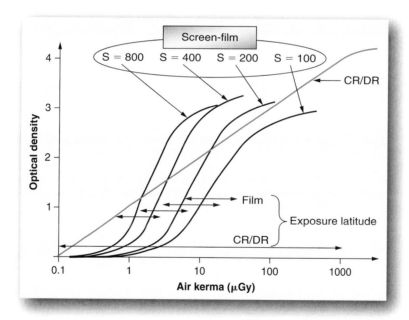

FIGURE 5-13. Response of film to variations in radiation exposure is nonlinear. Contrast enhancement and radiographic speed are based on the characteristics of the intensifying screen (phosphor) and the design of the light–sensitive silver halide emulsion to respond to chemical processing. A selection of screen–film speeds can be chosen to achieve appropriate optical density for a given dose (SNR). CR and DR exhibit a linear response over 10,000 in exposure latitude to allow the user to achieve an SNR sufficient to enable a reliable diagnosis.
Source: *Seibert, J. A. (2006). Computed radiography/Digital radiography: Adult, In D. P. Frush & W. Huda (Eds.), From Invisible to Visible–The Science and Practice of X-Ray Imaging and Radiation Dose Optimization: RSNA Categorical Course in Diagnostic Radiology Physics (pp 57–71). Figure and legend reproduced by kind permission of RSNA*

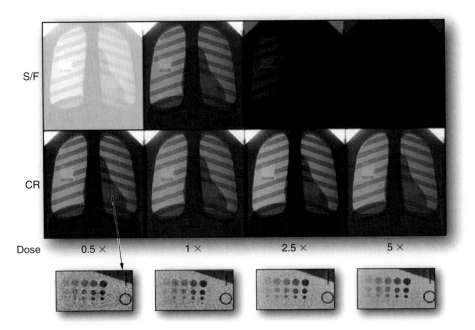

FIGURE 5-14. CR and DR devices can compensate for a wide exposure range by using histogram, analysis methods corresponding to specific patient anatomy. This permits the signal amplification needed to render a visible image. In this example a 10-fold range in incident exposure for CR is illustrated with a phantom image. Underexposure results in an image with low SNR and poor contrast sensitivity as shown by the contrast-detail phantoms on the bottom row. Overexposures give higher SNR with better contrast sensitivity but also higher dose. Of concern is the wide range of exposures that can easily go undetected without substantially increasing SNR. Screen-film (S/F) response (top row) provides direct feedback.
Source: *Seibert JA. Computed radiography/Digital radiography: Adult, In Frush DP and Huda W (Eds), From Invisible to Visible-The Science and Practice of X-Ray Imaging and Radiation Dose Optimization: RSNA Categorical Course in Diagnostic Radiology Physics, pp. 57-71, 2006. Figure and legend reproduced by kind permission of RSNA*

the observer, as is clearly illustrated in Figure 5-14. However, a significant disadvantage of this digital detector response is that while higher doses provide excellent image quality, the patient's radiation dose increases. Since operators and observers tend to favor excellent image quality, operators may use a higher exposure than is normally required for a particular examination. This situation is referred to as "exposure creep," or simply "dose creep" (Seibert 2006; Willis, 2006).

Exposure Indicator

The exposure indicator (EI) or exposure index as it is sometimes referred to, is a useful tool to address the problem of "exposure creep." The

exposure indicators for CR systems were explained in Chapter 3. In review, the EI is a numerical value usually displayed on the digital image to indicate the exposure to the digital detector. Therefore, the EI provides a visual cue as to the amount of exposure used for a particular examination and whether the exposure falls within the guidelines suggested by the manufacturer. A representative sample of EIs for both CR and flat-panel digital detectors is provided in Table 5-1. As is clearly seen in the table, there is a lack of standardization of EIs, and this can create problems in the intelligent use of EIs in a clinical environment (Willis, 2006). As mentioned in previous chapters, currently, the American Association of Physicists in Medicine (AAPM) and the International Electrotechnical Committee (IEC)

TABLE 5-1. Different exposure indicators and values and their associated receptor radiation exposure.

Type of System and Manufacturer	Symbol	Exposure		
		0.5 mR (5 μGy)	1.0 mR (10 μGy)	2.0 mR (20 μGy)
Fuji CR (ST plates)	S	400	200	100
Kodak CR (GP plates)	EI	1700	2000	2300
Agfa CR (speed class = 200)	lgM	2.0	2.3	2.6
Canon DR (brightness = 16, contrast = 10)	REX	50	100	200
IDC DR (S_T = 200)	f#	−1	0	1
Philips DR	EI	200	100	50
Siemens DR	EI	500	1000	2000

Source: Willis C. Computed radiography/Digital radiography: Pediatric. In Frush DP and Huda W (Eds.) *From Invisible to Visible-The Science and Practice of X-Ray Imaging and Radiation Dose Optimization: RSNA Categorical Course in Diagnostic Radiology Physics*, pp. 57-71, 2006. Figure and legend reproduced by kind permission of RSNA
(Note: Agfa HealthCare, Ridgefield, NJ; Canon, Lake Success, NY; Eastman Kodak, Rochester, NY; FujiFilm Medical Systems, Stamford, Conn; Imaging Dynamics Co (IDC), Calgary, Alberta, Canada; Philips Medical Systems, Bothel, Wash; and Siemens Medical Solutions, Malvern, PA.)

are working together to standardize the EI for digital radiographic imaging systems (see Appendix A).

The value of the EI can be affected by several factors, such as collimation, patient positioning, centering, image processing, and so on. Additionally, Schaefer-Prokop and Neitzel (2006) note that "different combinations of patient body constitutions and exposure can result in the same detected signal. Variation in the EI may occur because of varying imaging content (eg. a chest radiograph with or without pneumonia) even if the same exposure settings were used and patient entrance exposures are identical. This means that the EI in digital systems can be used only as a surrogate for dose management; EI does not represent an equivalent for patient entrance exposure."

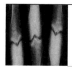

Image Processing: Optimizing the Display of the Image

The fundamental principles of digital image processing were described in Chapter 2 and specific image processing techniques used in CR imaging systems were discussed in Chapter 3. Essentially, the same image processing algorithms used in

CR are used in flat-panel digital imaging systems (Andriole, 2006).

The purpose of image processing in systems using flat-panel digital detectors is twofold:

1. To provide corrections to the raw digital data obtained from the detector. This will reduce artifacts in image postprocessing and will be described subsequently.

2. To optimize the display of the image that is presented to the radiologist for diagnostic interpretation. This means that contrast and sharpness are enhanced while noise is reduced.

Both 1 and 2 above are clearly demonstrated in Figure 5-15, which illustrates how the raw image can be optimized to provide images that have good contrast (a), smoothness (b), and sharpness (c).

Image Processing Stages

There are two image processing stages that are used to accomplish the two tasks listed above; the image pre-processing stage and the image post-processing stage, as illustrated in Figure 5-16. The raw digital data from the detector has low image contrast simply because of the wide exposure latitude of the digital detector. Therefore the raw digital data is first subject to pre-processing and presented as

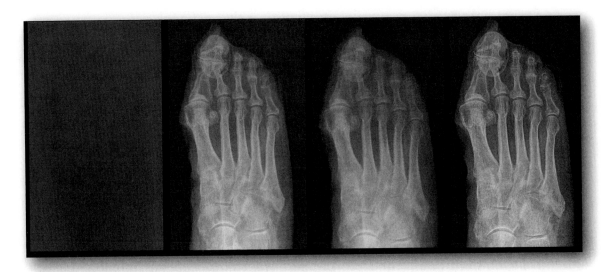

FIGURE 5-15. Optimization of the image display quality by digital image processing.
Source: *Korner et al. (2007). Advances in digital radiography: Physical principles and system overview. Radiographics, 27, 675–686. Reproduced by kind permission of RSNA*

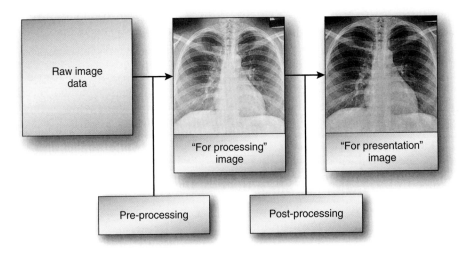

FIGURE 5-16. The framework for processing raw digital data for image display and viewing by an observer.
Source: *Delmar, Cengage Learning*

a DICOM "for processing" image. This image then undergoes digital image post processing, and the resultant post-processed image is labeled a "for presentation" image (Krugh, 2007; Seibert, 2006). While pre-processing operations deal with applying corrections to the raw data, post-processing operations address the appearance of the image displayed on a monitor for viewing and interpretation by a radiologist.

Pre-processing techniques are intended to correct the raw data collected from bad detector elements that create problems in the proper functioning of the detector. The image obtained initially from the detector, referred to as a flat-field image, contains artifacts due to the bad detector elements. Examples of these artifacts are shown in Figure 5-17A, and include those due to dead or bad pixels, bad columns of pixels, and the "seam

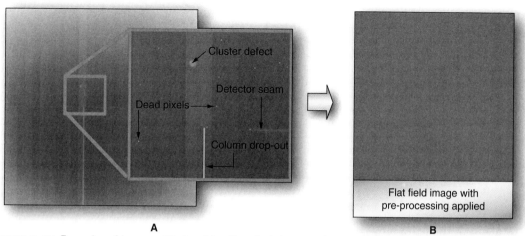

FIGURE 5-17. Examples of image artifacts arising from bad detector elements (A) and flat–field image after corrections applied (B).
Source: *Kerry Krugh, PhD, Medical Physicist, The Toledo Hospital, Toledo, Ohio*

where sub-panels are filled together" (Krugh, 2007). These artifacts can be corrected by a pre-processing technique referred to as flat-fielding (Seibert, 2006), shown in Figure 5-17B. This correction process is popularly referred to as system calibration, and it is an essential requirement to ensure detector performance integrity. The column artifact arising from a bad column of pixels indeed provides a rationale for ongoing calibration of the digital imaging system.

The purpose of post-processing is shown in Figure 5-16, where the "for processing" image is converted into the "for presentation" image that has better contrast. The poor contrast of the "for processing" image in Figure 5-16 is due to the wide exposure latitude of the digital detector. This image is subsequently subject to image post-processing and presented with improved contrast (Figure 5-16) to suit the viewing needs of the radiologist. As shown in Figure 5-18, the wide exposure latitude (linear

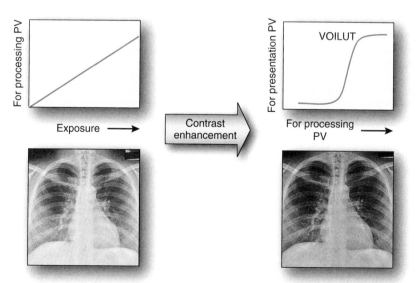

FIGURE 5-18. The fundamental process of producing an image of optimum image contrast
Source: *Kerry Krugh, PhD, Medical Physicist, The Toledo Hospital, Toledo, Ohio*

response) is converted into the well-known characteristic curve (nonlinear response) to produce an image with improved contrast (contrast enhancement). This is the "for presentation" DICOM image (Clunie, 2003; Krugh, 2007).

There are several steps in image processing to get from the "for processing" image to the "for presentation" image. These steps were described in Chapter 2 and then again in Chapter 3 for CR systems. In review, the steps include "exposure recognition and segmentation of the pertinent pre-processed image data. These two steps find the image data by using image processing algorithms and histogram analysis to identify the minimal and maximal useful values according to the histogram-specific shape generated by the anatomy. This usually requires the user to choose the correct examination-specific processing algorithm" (Seibert, 2006).

The next step involves scaling the histogram based on the exposure falling on the detector. If the exposure is too low (underexposure), for example, the raw data is adjusted to generate an image that looks pleasing to the observer. Clunie (2003) labels this image as the DICOM "for processing" image.

The third step in image processing is contrast enhancement, where the adjusted or scaled raw data values are mapped to the "for presentation" values to display an image with optimum contrast and brightness (Figure 5-18). The displayed image can be post-processed further to enhance image detail or sharpness and to reduce image noise, using the spatial frequencies (high and low frequencies contained in the image). While the high frequencies contain fine details of the image, low frequencies contain the contrast information in the image. By using a high-pass filter, low frequencies are suppressed and the image details are enhanced and the image appears sharper. This is an edge enhancement algorithm. Too much edge enhancement, however, produces image noise and creates the "halo" effect. This was clearly shown in Figure 3-23.

In a similar manner, a low-pass filter can be used to suppress the high frequencies to smooth (blur) the image. Such smoothing operations can help the radiologist to make a diagnosis, since they serve to reduce the noise present in the image. These algorithms were described in Chapters 2 and 3.

Image Display Optimization

Just as exposure technique factors (mAs and kV) should be optimized to meet the requirements of the ALARA (as low as reasonably achievable) philosophy, image display should be optimized so that the best possible image is available to the radiologist for diagnostic interpretation (Korner, 2007; Seibert, 2006).

There are several factors that affect the display of an image on the monitor and it is not within the scope of this book to describe these in any detail. The interested student should refer to the work of the AAPM Task Group 18 (2006) for a comprehensive coverage of image display. It is important, however, that the technologist is aware that the following play a role in image display optimization (Krugh, 2007):

(a) Image post-processing operations

(b) Technologist workstation (also referred to as the image acquisition workstation) problems

(c) Communication of the image from the technologist workstation to the PACS workstation (radiologist workstation)

The effective use of image post-processing is a fairly complex process. Image processing is not intended to correct poor images due to routine errors that are made during image acquisition. If a technologist has to post-process every single image to improve its quality, this may be a sign that indicates a problem with the imaging system. Furthermore, different anatomical regions should be processed with their respective algorithms. For example, a chest image should not be processed with a shoulder algorithm, even though this may have a positive impact on the image displayed on the technologist workstation. In addition, there should be what Krugh (2007) refers to as "processing optimization rules":

"1. Avoid having technologists manipulate processing on a case-by-case basis – creates inconsistency in image appearance.

2. Ensure modified processing parameters work on a variety of cases including various patient sizes.

3. Evaluate processing parameter modifications on whatever the radiologist reads from (i.e., not the acquisition workstation)."

Problems arising as a result of image post-processing may also be related to the differences in the acquisition workstation and the higher-quality PACS workstation used by the radiologist. These workstations may have different display resolution and luminance characteristics, for example. In addition, the acquisition workstation may not be calibrated to a standard called the DICOM Grayscale Standard Display Function (GSDF), whereas the PACS radiologist workstation is always calibrated to that standard.

Finally, it is important that the DICOM format "for presentation," such as the presentation look-up table (LUT) and image rotation used at the acquisition workstation, "are correctly transferred to the PACS and are used by the PACS for image display" (Sheppard, 2004) to ensure system integrity.

Optimization of the image displayed on monitors for viewing by both technologists and radiologists requires a good working knowledge of not only image processing but also display workstation (acquisition and PACS) principles and technology.

 ## Imaging Performance Characteristics

The imaging performance of a detector generally refers to the "ability of the detector to produce a high-quality X-ray image" (Yorkson, 2004). Several authors such as Korner et al. (2007), Seibert (2006), Spahn (2005), Yorkston (2004), Samei (2003), and Kotter and Langer (2002) have identified and described in detail a wide range of characteristics affecting image quality. These include spatial resolution (sharpness), modulation transfer function (MTF), dynamic range, detective quantum efficiency (DQE), image lag, ghosting, and artifacts created by a host of factors, such as dead pixels. A complete description of these characteristics is beyond the scope of this chapter, however, it is noteworthy to describe the essential elements of the most important ones. These are identified by Spahn (2005), and Korner et al. (2007) as the spatial resolution, dynamic range, MTF, DQE, and image lag. Each of these will be reviewed briefly, leaving out the underlying physics and mathematics.

Spatial Resolution

Spatial resolution is the ability of the imaging system to resolve fine details present in an object. It also refers to the sharpness of the image. For digital imaging systems, the spatial resolution depends on the size of the pixels in the matrix. Smaller pixels will produce images with better spatial resolution compared with larger pixels.

Measuring the spatial resolution is a complicated process that involves at least three methods. These include imaging a bar test pattern, a sharp-edged object, or a narrow slit (Yorkston, 2004). While the image of the bar test pattern is easy to interpret visually for the sharpness of the lines (Figure 5-19), the latter two are more complicated. For the edged object and the narrow slit, an edge-spread function (ESF) and a line-spread function (LSF) have to be obtained, respectively. The LSF is shown in Figure 5-20 for four digital radiography detectors. The narrower the LSF, the better the spatial resolution. The spatial resolution is best with the a-Se detector and the structured CsI a-Si TFT detector produces better spatial resolution (narrower LSF) than the turbid Gd_2O_2S or CsI digital detector. The three methods listed above can be used to produce yet another function called the modulation transfer function (MTF).

Modulation Transfer Function

The modulation transfer function (MTF) is a complex mathematical function that measures the ability of the detector to transfer its spatial resolution characteristics to the image. Bushong (2009) notes that the MTF can simply be expressed as a ratio of the image to the object, and an MTF of 1 represents a perfect detector. How is this MTF obtained?

Consider a patient's abdomen, which consists of both fine and coarse objects. These objects can be represented as spatial frequencies (line pairs/mm = lp/mm), where fine and coarse objects generate high and low spatial frequencies respectively. While the high spatial frequencies represent fine detail or sharpness, the low spatial frequencies represent object contrast information. The image would contain both sharpness and contrast (intensity grayscale values). The MTF is a graph of the contrast plotted as

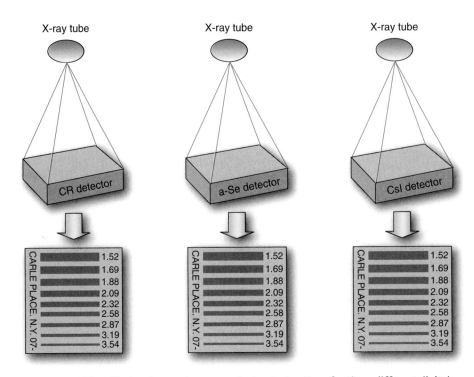

FIGURE 5-19. The effect on image sharpness of a bar test pattern for three different digital radiography detector systems.
Source: *Images of the test pattern provided by the kind courtesy of John Yorkston PhD, Senior Research Scientist, Clinical Applications Research, Carestream Health Inc. Rochester, NY*

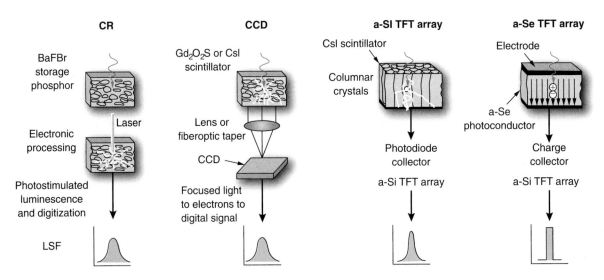

FIGURE 5-20. The line spread function (LSF) for four different digital detector systems.
Source: *Seibert, J. A. (2006). Computed radiography/Digital radiography: Adult, In D. P. Frush & W. Huda (Eds.), From Invisible to Visible–The Science and Practice of X-Ray Imaging and Radiation Dose Optimization: RSNA Categorical Course in Diagnostic Radiology Physics (pp. 57–71). Figure and legend reproduced by kind permission of RSNA*

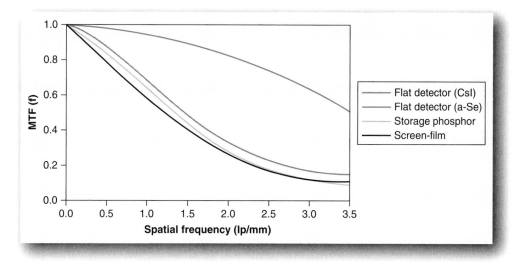

FIGURE 5-21. The MTFs for four image receptors, three digital detectors, and one screen–film system. Source: *Spahn, M. (2005). Flat detectors and their clinical applications. European Journal of Radiology, 15, 1934–1947. Reproduced with kind permission of Springer Science and Business Media*

a function of spatial frequency. As noted earlier, an MTF of 1 represents a perfect transfer of spatial and contrast information.

The MTFs for various detectors (digital and screen-film) are illustrated in Figure 5-21. It is clear that as the spatial frequency increases, the MTF decreases. A higher MTF value at a higher spatial frequency means that the detector provides better spatial resolution than lower MTF values at low frequencies. Furthermore, a higher MTF value at lower spatial frequencies means that the detector provides better contrast resolution.

All digital imaging systems have what is referred to as the limiting resolution, which is the spatial frequency limit that is obtained at an MTF value of 0.1. A system that has a higher spatial frequency at an MTF of 0.1 will show better spatial resolution than a system that has a lower spatial frequency at an MTF of 0.1.

Dynamic Range

The dynamic range of a digital detector is the response of the detector to different levels of radiation exposure. As described earlier, the digital detector responds to a wider range of exposure compared with film-screen image receptors. This is one of the most obvious differences that allow the digital detector to respond to both underexposure and overexposure without the need for repeat exposures. It is important, however, to ensure that technologists use these detectors wisely in order to avoid exposure creep.

Detective Quantum Efficiency

The detective quantum efficiency (DQE) is yet another performance characteristic of digital detectors, described in Chapter 3 for CR. Essentially, the DQE deals with "the efficiency of a detector to convert the x-radiation signal at its entrance window into useful image signal" (Spahn, 2005). The DQE measurement is quite complicated and is obtained from other physical quantities such as the MTF, noise power spectrum (NPS), the incident X-ray flux, X-ray photon energy, and the spatial frequency (f) (Spahn, 2005; Yorkston, 2004).

The DQE provides information about the signal-to-noise ratio (SNR). In imaging, the goal is to obtain good contrast information in the image. This is, in general the signal, and the detector must provide the maximum signal possible. However, noise is also present in the signal due to a few photons striking the detector (quantum noise), as well as system

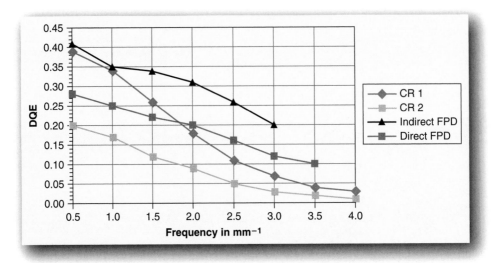

FIGURE 5-22. The DQE for four different digital detectors as a function of spatial frequency. Source: *Korner et al. (2007). Advances in digital radiography: Physical principles and system overview. Radiographics, 27, 675–686. Reproduced by kind permission of RSNA*

noise (electronic noise). These two parameters put together create the SNR concept. In imaging applications, since contrast resolution (the ability to resolve small differences in tissue contrast) is mandatory for diagnostic interpretation, it is important to have a high SNR. This means that the signal is high and the noise is low.

The DQE can be expressed as follows:

$$DQE = \frac{SNR_{out}^2}{SNR_{in}^2}$$

A perfect digital detector would have a DQE of 1. Examples of the DQE values for detectors used in clinical practice are shown in Figure 5-22. It is clearly apparent that the indirect conversion CsI a-Si TFT flat-panel detectors offer the highest DQE at low frequencies. As the spatial frequencies increase, the DQE decreases rapidly (Spahn, 2005; Siebert, 2006).

A very important point about the DQE that the technologist should pay careful attention to is quoted from expert medical physicist Dr. Anthony Seibert, PhD as follows:

"A DR system with higher DQE, however, does not necessarily translate into a system with *superior image quality or lower dose. For instance, a slot-scan digital system can achieve comparable image quality for chest imaging with a lower dose compared to a flat-panel large-area detector, despite having a lower intrinsic DQE(f). Besides intrinsic detector efficiency, other considerations affecting patient dose and image quality include effective X-ray energy, beam uniformity, wide-latitude response, spatial and temporal sampling, grid use, examination-specific image processing, image display quality, monitor calibration, viewing conditions, radiologist capability (alertness, experience), and working environment. The difference between a diagnostic and non-diagnostic image often has a cause other than the detector itself" (Seibert, 2006).*

As mentioned earlier, the DQE also depends on the photon energy (kV). Under controlled conditions it has been shown that the quantum efficiencies (based on the X-ray absorption properties of the detector converter materials) at 70 kV is about 67% for a-Se and 77% for CsI phosphor. At 120 kV, efficiencies are 37% for a-Se and 52% for CsI. In lower kV applications such as mammography, a-Se performs better than CsI and has a higher DQE (Sphan, 2005).

Image Lag

An important imaging performance characteristic of a flat-panel detector that has an impact on clinical practice is that of image lag (Spahn, 2005; Yorkston, 2004). Image lag, also referred to as "memory effect" (Spahn, 2005), refers to the persistence of the image, that is, charge is still being produced after the radiation beam from the X-ray tube has been turned off. The reason for this is that the "charge has been trapped in the metastable band-gap states in the a-Si and a-Se material during exposure and is only released slowly over time" (Yorkston, 2004). Image lag times vary and are shortest for flat-panel digital detectors based on indirect conversion (Spahn, 2005).

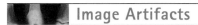 ## Image Artifacts

Flat-panel digital detectors are complex devices and pose numerous challenges in the manufacturing process. Flaws in the various components that make up the panel can lead to image artifacts. Flaws include dust, scratches, chemical reactions among the various materials that the detector is made of, and defective pixels (Yorkston, 2004). Image artifacts can also arise from vibrations or poor performance of the electronics, as well as scattered radiation grids. Examples of some of these artifacts are shown in Figure 5-17.

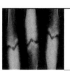 ## Other Applications of Flat-Panel Digital Detectors

Flat-panel digital detectors are used not only in general static radiography examinations in the main department but also in other imaging applications. Flat-panel detectors can be used in portable radiography applications and in applications involving fluoroscopy. Fluoroscopic applications include gastrointestinal tract fluoroscopy, angiography, portable fluoroscopy, and dedicated systems that have now become available for cardiology.

As flat-panel detector techniques improve, they will become increasingly commonplace in the imaging environment and may replace other digital imaging systems such as CR systems. Already, they are becoming more and more popular and are replacing the image intensifier tube used in fluoroscopy. Therefore, the technologist must make every effort to have a good understanding of this technology. This chapter offers one small step in this direction.

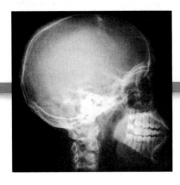

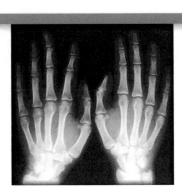

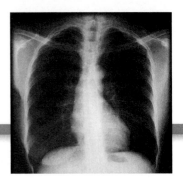

REVIEW QUESTIONS

1. What are the limitations of computed radiography?
2. Define the term "flat-panel digital radiography."
3. Draw a diagram of a generic flat-panel digital radiography imaging system and label the main components.
4. State the purpose of each of the components identified in Question 3.
5. Briefly compare and contrast two types of flat-panel detectors (FPDs) systems.
6. Draw a diagram of an indirect FPD, label its components, and describe each component and its function.
7. Draw a diagram of a direct FPD, label its components, and describe each component and its function.
8. What is meant by the term "fill factor" of a pixel in an FPD system?
9. Explain how a CCD detector works.
10. Explain the detection and conversion of X-rays into electrical charges in an FPD.
11. Explain how charges are read out in an FPD.
12. What is the purpose of an exposure in FPD imaging systems?
13. What is the purpose of image processing in FPD imaging systems?
14. List several image postprocessing operations used in FPD imaging systems and state the purpose of each of them.
15. What are the three factors that play a role in optimizing the FPD image-for-image display?
16. List three of Kerry Krugh's "processing optimization rules" for FPD imaging systems.

17. What are the characteristics affecting image quality in FPD imaging systems?
18. What is meant by image lag in an FPD?
19. List several sources of artifacts in FPD imaging systems.

REFERENCES

Andriole, K. (2006). Image acquisition. In K. J. Dryer, D. S. Hirschorn, J. H. Thrall, A. Metha (Eds.), *PACS A Guide to the Digital Revolution* (pp. 189–227). New York: Springer Science and Business Media Inc.

Antonuk, L. E., Yorkston, J., Huang, W., Siewerdsen, J. H., Boudry, J. M., el-Mohri, Y., & Marx, M. V. (1995). A real time flat-panel amorphous silicon digital X-ray imager. *Radiographics, 15,* 993–1000.

Bushberg, J. T., Seibert, J. A., Leidholdt, E. M., & Boone, J. M. (2004). *The Essential Physics of Medical Imaging* (2nd ed.). Philadelphia: Lippincott Williams and Wilkins.

Bushong, S. (2009) *Radiologic Science for Technologists.* (9th ed.). St Louis: Elsevier-Mosby.

Chotas, H. G., Dobbins, J. T., III, & Ravin, C. E. (1999). Principles of digital radiography with large-area electronically-readable detectors: A review of the basics. *Radiology, 210,* 595–599.

Clunie, D. A. (2003). DICOM implemenmtations for digital radiography. In E. Samei & M. J. (Eds.), *Categorical Course in Diagnostic radiology Physics-Advances in Digital Radiography* (pp. 163–172). Oak Brook, Ill: RSNA.

Gransfors, P. R., & Aufrichtig, R. (2000). DQE(f) of an amorphous silicon flat-panel x-ray detector: Detector parameter influences and measurement methodology. *Proceedings of SPIE, 3977,* 2–13.

Hammerstrom, K. et al. (2006) Recognition and prevention of computed radiography image artifacts. *Journal of Digital Imaging, 19*(3), 1–15.

Korner, M., Weber, C. H., Wirth, S., Pfeifer, Klaus-Jürgen, Reiser, M. F., & Treitl, M. (2007). Advances in digital radiography: Physical principles and system overview. *Radiographics, 27,* 675–686.

Krugh, K. (2007). Personal communications. Medical Physicist, The Toledo Hospital, Toledo, Ohio.

Lanca, L., & Silva, A. (2009). Digital radiography detectors: A technical overview. *Radiography, 15*(1), 23–35.

Neitzel, U., Maack, I., & Günther-Kohfahl, S. (1994). Image quality of a digital chest radiography system based on s selenium detector. *Medical Physics, 21,* 509–516.

Samei, E., Seibert, J. A., Andriole, K., Badano, A., Crawford, J., Reiner, B., Flynn, M. J., & Chang, P. (2004). General guidelines for purchasing and acceptance testing of PACS equipment. *Radiographics, 24,* 313–334.

Samei, E. (2003). Performance of digital radiographic detectors: Factors affecting sharpness and noise. In E. Samei & M. Flynn (Eds.), *Advances in Digital Radiography. RSNA Categorical Course in Diagnostic Radiology Physics* (pp. 49–61). Oak Brook, Ill: RSNA.

Schaefer-Propkop, C., & Neitzel, U. (2006). Computed radiography/Digital radiography: Radiologist perspective on controlling dose and study quality. In D. P. Frush & W. Huda (Eds.), *From Invisible to Visible-The Science and Practice of X-ray Imaging and radiation Dose Optimization: RSNA Categorical Course in Diagnostic Radiology Physics* (pp. 85–98). Oak Brook, Ill: RSNA.

Seibert, J. A. (2006). Computed radiography/Digital radiography: Adult. In D. P. Frush & W. Huda (Eds.), *From Invisible to Visible-The Science and Practice of X-ray Imaging and radiation Dose Optimization: RSNA Categorical Course in Diagnostic Radiology Physics* (pp. 57–71). Oak Brook, Ill: RSNA.

Spahn, M. (2005). Flat detectors and their clinical applications. *European Journal of Radiology, 15*, 1934–147.

Willis, C. E. (2006). Computed radiography/Digital radiography: Pediatric. In D. P. Frush & W. Huda (Eds.), *From Invisible to Visible-The Science and Practice of X-ray Imaging and radiation Dose Optimization: RSNA Categorical Course in Diagnostic Radiology Physics* (pp. 78–83). Oak Brook, Ill: RSNA.

Yorkston, J. (2004). Flat-panel DR detectors for radiography and fluoroscopy. In L. Goldman & M. V. Yester (Eds.), *Specifications, Performance, and Quality Assurance of Radiographic and Fluoroscopic Systems in the Digital Era* (pp. 177–229). AAPM Monograph 30. College Park: MD.

Yorkston, J. (2003). Digital radiographic technology. In E. Samei & M. Flynn (Eds.), *Advances in Digital Radiography. RSNA Categorical Course in Diagnostic Radiology Physics* (pp. 23–36). Oak Brook, Ill. RSNA.

CHAPTER 6

Digital Fluoroscopy

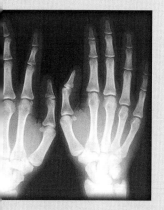

OBJECTIVES

Upon completion of this chapter, the student should be able to:

1. Describe the major components of conventional fluoroscopy and explain how the system works.

2. Describe the major characteristic imaging features of a digital fluoroscopic system using image intensifiers and video camera technology.

3. State the limitations of image intensifier-based digital fluoroscopy.

4. Describe the equipment configuration of a digital fluoroscopy imaging system using flat-panel detectors.

5. Identify the types of flat-panel detectors used in digital fluoroscopy.

6. Describe the major characteristics of flat-panel detectors used in digital fluoroscopy.

7. Outline the operating principles of flat-panel digital fluoroscopy imaging.

8. Explain the advantages of flat-panel digital fluoroscopy.

9. State what is meant by connectivity of flat-panel digital fluoroscopy and PACS.

10. State the purpose of digital image post processing in digital fluoroscopy.

11. Explain the effect of each of the following image postprocessing operations on the fluoroscopy image:

    • Grayscale image manipulation

    • Last-image hold

    • Temporal frame averaging

    • Edge enhancement

12. Describe briefly the nature of digital subtraction angiography (DSA).

KEY TERMS

Closed–circuit television chain

Contrast ratio

Conventional fluoroscopy

Digital fluoroscopy systems with flat-panel detectors (FPDs)

Digital subtraction angiography (DSA)

Dynamic FPDs

Energy subtraction

Frame rate

Grayscale–image manipulation

Host computer

Image intensification

Image intensifier artifacts

Image intensifier tube

Image intensifier-based digital fluoroscopy

Last–image hold (LIH)

Magnification

Matrix size

Pulsed fluoroscopy

Temporal frame averaging

Temporal subtraction

Video camera

Introduction

In Chapters 3 and 5, the technical characteristics (equipment components and features) of digital radiographic imaging systems; namely, computed radiography (CR) and flat-panel digital radiography (DR) were described in detail. While these systems produce static or stationary images, fluoroscopy is an imaging modality that produces dynamic or moving images, displayed in real time. The purpose of fluoroscopy is to study not only anatomical structures but also, more importantly, the motion of organs and the movement of contrast media in blood vessels and organs with the goal of obtaining functional information.

The introduction of fluoroscopy dates back to 1896, soon after the discovery of X-rays in 1895, when Thomas Edison developed the first fluoroscope (Bushong, 2009), which allowed for the observation of moving images such as the beating heart in real time. Through the years, fluoroscopy has developed into a sophisticated imaging system as new technologies have emerged to improve its imaging system characteristics. For example, the image intensifier tube was developed to solve the image quality problems imposed by the fluoroscopic screen of the early fluoroscopes. A brief timeline of the introduction of several technologies for fluoroscopic imaging is shown in Figure 6-1, which illustrates how fluoroscopy has evolved from analog imaging systems to digital imaging systems that use flat-panel digital detectors.

The purpose of this chapter is to review the principles and technology of conventional fluoroscopy and describe the unique features that characterize digital fluoroscopy. These features include the conversion of analog data from the image receptor (image intensifier) and/or the flat-panel digital detectors into digital data. The digital data is subsequently processed by a computer to produce digital fluoroscopic images.

Conventional Fluoroscopy Principles: A Review

The term conventional fluoroscopy refers to the use of an image intensifier coupled to a video camera that converts the image from the output screen of the image intensifier into a video signal (analog data). This signal is sent to a television monitor where images are displayed at frame rates of at least 30 frames per second (fps) to provide the effect of motion (Bushberg et al., 2004; Bushong, 2009, Holmes et al., 2004). This section of the chapter will review the physical principles and major technical components of a conventional fluoroscopic imaging system and its associated image quality characteristics.

Imaging Principles and Technical Components

A typical conventional fluoroscopic imaging chain is shown in Figure 6-2. The major technical components include the X-ray tube and generator,

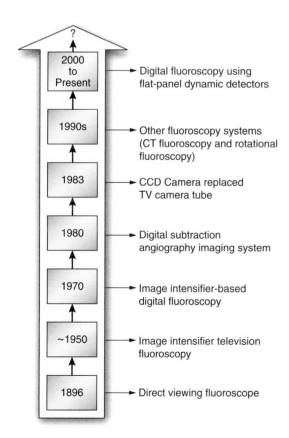

FIGURE 6-1. A brief timeline of the introduction of different technologies for fluoroscopic imaging.
Source: *Delmar, Cengage Learning*

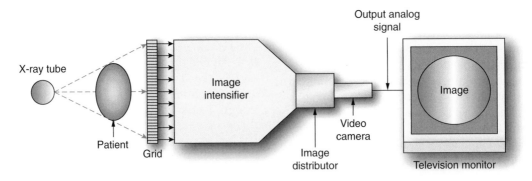

FIGURE 6-2. The technical components of a typical conventional fluoroscopic imaging chain.
Source: *Delmar, Cengage Learning*

spot film device, image intensifier tube, optical image distributor, photospot camera, and video camera coupled to an X-ray television display monitor.

While the X-ray tube and generator provide the appropriate X-ray beam for both fluoroscopy and radiography, the image intensifier converts X-rays into light that is captured by the video camera. The output video signal from the video camera goes to the television display monitor to create fluoroscopic images. Single static images can be recorded by using the spot-film device (in which case, the system must switch from fluoroscopic exposure technique factors to radiographic factors) and/or the photospot film camera. These two methods are becoming obsolete with the transition to digital fluoroscopy, since they both use film for recording images.

Another important element of a conventional fluoroscopic imaging system is closed-circuit X-ray television. This system couples the video camera to the television monitor by means of a coaxial cable and control electronics. It is important to note that the video camera can be either a television "pick-up" tube or a charge-coupled device (CCD). In modern fluoroscopic systems using image intensifiers, the CCD has replaced the television camera tube.

• *X-Ray Tube and Generator*

The X-ray tube used in fluoroscopy must be capable of producing X-rays either continuously or in short bursts or pulses (**pulsed fluoroscopy**). While the former allows for real time image display (30 fps at 33 ms), the overall goal of the latter is to reduce patient dose, especially in pediatric fluoroscopy. In pulsed systems, pulses are as short as 3–10 ms/image (Schueler, 2000). Furthermore, pulsed fluoroscopy requires the use of a grid-controlled X-ray tube, and the dose can be reduced by as much as 90% compared to non-pulsed fluoroscopy (Seeram, 2001). Additionally, since the pulses are very short (3–10 ms), there is less blurring of moving structures.

Modern conventional fluoroscopy imaging units use a high frequency generator to ensure efficient production of X-rays. In addition, fluoroscopic exposure techniques utilize low mA and high kV exposure factors. For example, mA values from 1–3 mA and kV values from 65–120 kV are not uncommon. For recording images using the cassette-loaded spot film device, radiographic factors are used. This means that the imaging system generator must be capable of switching from fluoroscopic mode to radiographic mode. In the latter mode, the tube current is increased to higher mA values.

• *The Image Intensifier Tube*

The image intensifier tube has been developed to replace the conventional fluorescent screen of the early fluoroscopes. An early fluoroscope is graphically illustrated in Figure 6-3. The screen was made of zinc cadmium sulfide (ZnCdS) and emitted a yellow-green light when

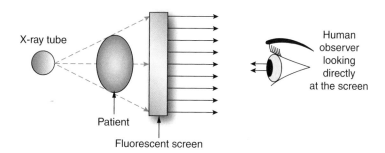

FIGURE 6-3. The fluoroscope was the first system for the direct observation of moving structures in the patient's body. The images are produced on a fluorescent screen that emits light when struck by X-rays. Source: *Delmar, Cengage Learning*

struck by X-rays. A major problem with this screen was that the image lacked detail, contrast, and brightness. Geometric factors, rod vision, and the low brightness levels of the screen limited detail perception. Efforts to solve these problems only resulted in greater dose to patients. Additionally, early fluoroscopy had to be performed in the dark using red goggles for the purpose of dark adaptation. The above problems have been solved with the image intensifier through a process referred to as image intensification.

Image intensification refers to the brightening of the fluoroscopic image using the image intensifier. The structure of the image intensifier tube is shown in Figure 6-4. These include the input screen, photocathode, electrostatic lens, and an output screen, all enclosed in an evacuated glass envelope.

The input screen is coated with a phosphor that converts X-ray photons to light photons. The state-of-the-art phosphor is cesium iodide (CsI). The CsI phosphor absorbs twice as much radiation as ZnCdS and is packed in a needle-like fashion (structured phosphor, as described and illustrated in Chapter 5) to reduce the lateral spread of light in an effort to improve the spatial resolution compared to powdered CsI phosphors. The diameter of the input screen is variable; however, diameters ranging from 13 cm to 30 cm are not uncommon. Larger diameter image intensifiers (36 cm–57 cm)

have become available for imaging larger anatomical regions such as the abdomen.

The light from the input screen (phosphor) strikes the photocathode, which is made of antimony cesium (SbCs) and which emits photoelectrons. At an energy of 60 keV, one X-ray photon at the input screen will result in about 200 photoelectrons being emitted at the photocathode (Wang & Blackburn, 2000). Multialkali photocathodes with a combination of potassium, sodium, and cesium will emit about three times more photoelectrons than SbCs photocathodes, making these image intensifiers much more efficient that single alkali photocathodes.

The electrostatic lens, or electron optics as it is often referred to, consists of a series of electrodes that accelerate and focus the photoelectrons from the photocathode to the output screen. This requires a voltage of about 25 to 30 kV applied between the photocathode and the output screen.

The output screen is coated with a ZnCdS phosphor that converts the photoelectrons into light. The diameter of the output screen is about one-tenth the diameter of the input screen. Due to the acceleration of the photoelectrons and the small size of the output screen, the image at the output screen is extremely bright. This increase in brightness is conveniently referred to as brightness gain (BG). BG can be obtained using the following relationship:

BG = Minification Gain (MG) × Flux Gain (FG)

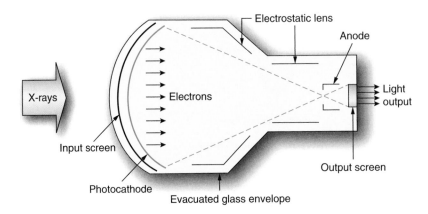

FIGURE 6-4. The major components of an image intensifier tube.
Source: *Delmar, Cengage Learning*

The MG is a ratio expressed as follows:

$$MG = \left[\frac{\text{Diameter of the input screen}}{\text{Diameter of the output screen}}\right]^2$$

The FG is also a ratio expressed as follows:

$$FG = \frac{\text{Number of light photons at the output screen}}{\text{Number of light photons at the input screen}}$$

The brightness gain concept has been replaced by another method used to measure the intensification of the image intensifier tube. This is the conversion factor (CF), which measures the light gain at the output screen using the following relationship:

$$CF = \frac{\text{Luminance of the output screen}}{\text{Exposure rate at the input screen}}$$

The unit of luminance (light brightness) is the candela/square meter (Cd/m^2), and the unit is milliroentgens/second (mR/sec) for the exposure rate. Bushong (2004) reports that while the brightness gain can range from 5000–30,000, the conversion factor for image intensifiers can range from 50–300. A higher conversion factor implies that the intensifier is much more efficient than one with a lower conversion factor.

- *Image Intensifier Tube Housing*

The image intensifier glass envelope is enclosed in a metal housing that not only provides mechanical support for the glass envelope but also shields the intensifier against magnetic fields. Since the housing is lined with lead, it also shields from any radiation scattered within the glass envelope.

- *Optical Image Distributor*

The position of the optical distributor is shown in Figure 6-2. The purpose of the image distributor is to split the total light (100%) from the output screen between the video camera and the photospot film camera. Using a system of lenses and a beam-splitting mirror, 10% of the light goes to the video camera and 90% of the light goes to the photospot film camera.

Magnification Fluoroscopy

Magnification of the image in conventional fluoroscopy is an important feature of the image intensifier. The purpose of magnification fluoroscopy is to enhance the image in order to facilitate diagnostic interpretation.

Magnification fluoroscopy is only possible with multifield image intensifiers. These include the popular dual-field and the triple-field intensifiers that use a technique referred to as electron optical magnification (Seeram, 2001). This technique changes the voltage on specific electrodes of the electrostatic lens system in the image intensifier tube, causing the electron beam crossover point to increase its distance from the output screen. A dual-field intensifier (25 cm/17 cm) can operate in the full-field mode (25 cm) and in the magnification mode (17 cm). When the magnification mode is used, the X-ray beam is automatically collimated to fall upon the central portion of the input screen to cover a diameter of 17 cm. A triple-field intensifier (25 cm/17 cm/12 cm) can operate in two magnification modes, 17 cm and 12 cm modes. The 12 cm mode provides greater magnification than the 17 cm mode.

Magnification provides increased spatial resolution, but at the expense of increased dose to the patient. In general, the increase is about 2.2 times that used in the full-field mode of operation. For example, the exposure rate for a 25 cm mode is about 30 μR/sec, while it is 60 μR/sec, and 120 μR/sec for the 17 cm and 12 cm modes respectively (Wang & Blackburn, 2000). The approximate dose can be computed by using the ratio of the two fields as follows:

$$\text{Dose} = \frac{(\text{Full-field diameter})^2}{(\text{Magnification mode})^2}$$

For example, the dose increase when going from a 25 cm mode of operation to a magnification mode of 12 cm is about 4.3 times ($25^2/12^2 = 4.3$).

Image Quality Characteristics

There are at least three image quality parameters of the image intensifier that are worthy of review in this chapter. These are spatial resolution, contrast ratio, and noise. In addition, image intensifiers do exhibit a few artifacts, such as image lag, vignetting, pincushion distortion, and "S" distortion, as well as veiling glare (Bushberg et al., 2004; Bushong, 2009; Holmes, 2004; Wang & Blackburn, 2000). Each of these will now be highlighted briefly.

- ### Spatial Resolution

  The spatial resolution of an image intensifier refers to its ability to resolve fine details in an object (patient). Since the input screen is convex with respect to the X-ray tube (see Figure 6-4), the spatial resolution is much better at the center of the input screen compared to the screen's periphery. The spatial resolution for a CsI

image intensifier operating in the 25 cm mode, 4 line pairs/mm (l p/mm), and it is 6l p/mm in the 10 cm mode. This means that 0.125 mm objects can be visualized for the 4l p/mm, and 0.08 mm-sized objects can be seen when the resolution is 6l p/mm (Bushong, 2009).

- ### Contrast Ratio

  The contrast ratio of an image intensifier tube is the ratio of the image brightness at the periphery to that at the center of the output screen. A typical contrast ratio is about 20:1, but this can range from 10:1 to 30:1 and 15:1 to 35:1, depending on where it is measured (Wang & Blackburn, 2000).

- ### Noise

  Conventional fluoroscopy with an image intensifier operates in the low mA mode, and therefore the noise level is usually high. To reduce the noise, the mA can be increased, but this results in a proportional increase in patient dose. To reduce this dose, the ZnCdS input phosphor used in the early image intensifier tubes was replaced with CsI input phosphor, since CsI has a higher quantum detection efficiency (QDE) and uses very little radiation dose to produce good quality images that are noise free.

- ### Image Intensifier Artifacts

  Image intensification fluoroscopy can produce several of the **artifacts** mentioned earlier.

Image lag is the continued emission of light from the screen when the radiation beam has been turned off. This is not a serious problem, however, with newer image intensifiers, since the lag time is in the order of about 1 ms (Wang & Blackburn, 2000). Vignetting refers to a loss of brightness at the periphery of the image. This means that the image is sharper and much brighter in the central portion of the screen. The image intensifier may also exhibit veiling glare, an artifact that results when light is scattered in the intensifier tube.

Two other image intensifier artifacts include pincushion distortion and S distortion, as illustrated in Figure 6-5. When a rectangular grid is imaged with an intensifier, pincushion distortion (Figure 6-5A) results due to the fact that the input

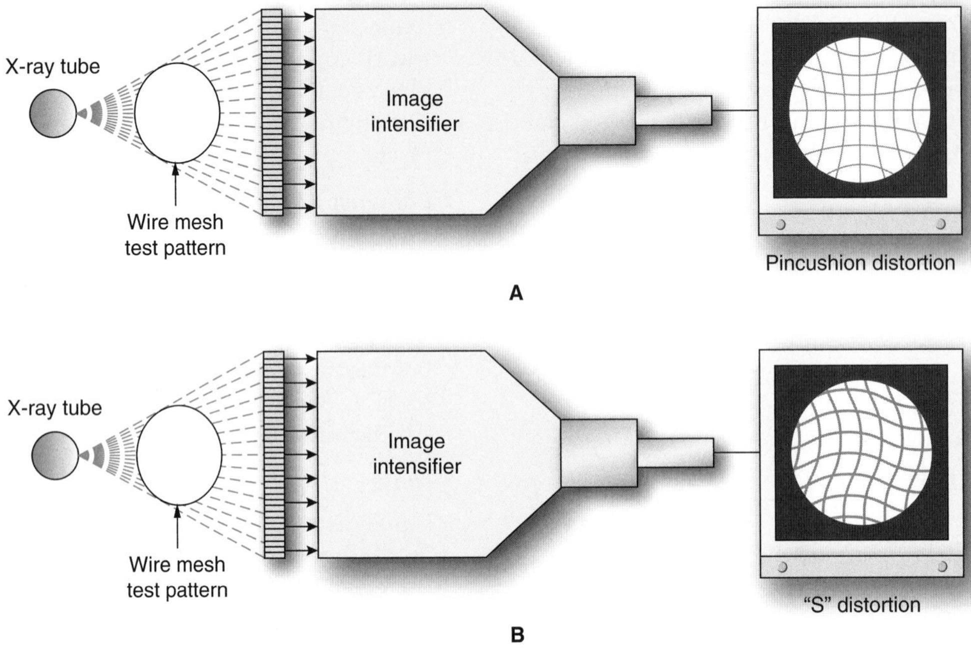

FIGURE 6-5. A graphic illustration of two typical image artifacts characteristic of image intensifier fluoroscopy. While pincushion distortion is seen in A, "S" distortion is shown in B.
Source: *Delmar, Cengage Learning*

screen is curved. On the other hand, S distortion (Figure 6-5B) appears if an electromagnetic field is close to the intensifier. This field will influence the electrons, especially those at the "the perimeter of the image intensifier more so than those nearer the center" (Wang & Blackburn, 2000).

Fluoroscopic Television Chain

The image at the output screen of the image intensifier tube is far too small and too bright to be observed directly by a radiologist. Therefore, a closed-circuit television chain is used to display this image onto a television monitor for proper viewing and interpretation. The technical components of a fluoroscopic television chain are shown in Figure 6-6. These include a video camera and a television monitor coupled by a cable referred to as a coaxial cable.

The video camera can be a television "pick-up" camera tube or a CCD camera, and it is coupled to the image intensifier by means of the image

distributor. The video camera converts the light from the output screen of the image intensifier into an electrical signal (output video signal), which is sent to the television monitor where it is converted into a visible image that can be viewed in real time. Television camera tubes were used in early image intensifier systems but they were replaced by the CCD camera (Yester, 2004), and therefore they will not be described further in this chapter; however, the interested student should refer to any good radiologic physics or equipment textbook for a description of how these tubes work.

The CCD chip (about 100 mm × 100 mm square) is mounted onto a camera head that is coupled to the output screen of the image intensifier tube. The CCD consists of a matrix (1024 × 1024, for example) of pixels that capture the image from the output screen. Each pixel consists of a photosensitive region that produces electrons when struck by light. The electrical charge from each pixel is read-out very systematically using suitable electronics

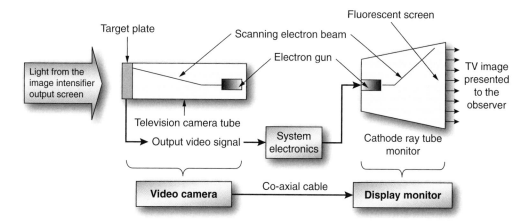

FIGURE 6-6. The technical components of a fluoroscopic television chain. The television camera tube is connected to the television monitor by means of a coaxial cable.
Source: *Delmar, Cengage Learning*

to produce an output video signal that goes to the television monitor to create fluoroscopic images displayed in real time.

The CCD camera is more compact and has a longer life span than television camera tubes. In addition, there is no image lag with the CCD camera and no spatial distortions. Furthermore, the CCD camera has a high dynamic range. As noted by Holmes et al. (2004), the dynamic range is a "ratio of the largest detectable signal to the smallest, corresponding to the brightest and darkest regions of the image. The CCD camera has a significant advantage with a dynamic range of 3000:1 compared with the pick-up tube's linear usable range of approximately 1000:1."

The final component in the fluoroscopic television chain is the television monitor. These monitors can be either of the cathode ray tube (CRT) type or the liquid crystal display (LCD) type. The monitor receives the video signal from the video camera and with suitable electronics uses the signal to create the television image. This image is made up of lines from the scanning process. Scanning can be interlaced or it can be progressive. In the case of **interlaced scanning**, 262.5 odd lines (one TV field) are first scanned, followed by 262.5 even lines (one TV field). These two fields are interlaced to create one TV frame that is made up of 525 lines.

This type of scanning reduces image flickering. At a frequency of 60 Hz (60 cycles/sec), 30 frames per second (60 fields/sec) can be displayed and no flickering is observed. In **progressive scanning**, each line is read sequentially (1, 2, 3, 4, and so on, to 525 lines). Progressive scanning is important in digital fluoroscopy (Bushong, 2009).

 Digital Fluoroscopy with Image Intensifiers

The next developmental stage in the evolution of digital fluoroscopy was the digitization of the output video signal (either from the television camera tube or the CCD camera) and the use of a computer to process the digitized data and subsequently display the image on a television monitor. To accomplish this task, two new components have been added to the conventional fluoroscopic imaging system. These are the analog-to-digital converter (ADC) and a computer. The location of these two components is shown in Figure 6-7. This is known as an image intensifier–based digital fluoroscopy system, and it consists of the X-ray tube and generator, image intensifier, video camera, ADC, computer, digital-to-analog converter (DAC), and the television monitor.

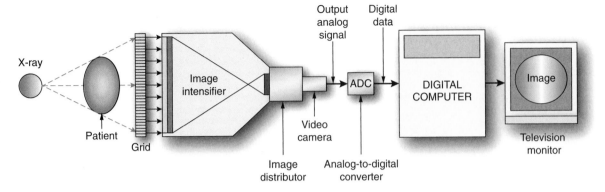

FIGURE 6-7. Two new components have been added to the conventional fluoroscopic imaging system, the analog-to-digital converter (ADC) and a computer, as shown in this figure. This is now known as an **image intensifier-based digital fluoroscopy** system, and it consists of an X-ray tube and generator, the image intensifier, the video camera, the ADC, the computer, a digital-to-analog converter (DAC), and the television monitor.
Source: *Delmar, Cengage Learning*

X-Ray Tube and Generator

The X-ray tube and generator provide the appropriate radiation beam for imaging in digital fluoroscopy. The X-ray tube is a high-capacity tube and is pulsed in operation. The generator is a high-frequency generator and can provide the high mA values used in digital fluoroscopy, as opposed to the low mA values typical of conventional fluoroscopy. As noted by Bushong (2009), the mA is sometimes 100 times higher in digital fluoroscopy. These higher values are especially important in digital angiography. The generator ensures that the X-ray beam is pulsed rather than being produced continuously. The pulsing is referred to as "pulsed-progressive fluoroscopy" (Bushong, 2009). Another important point emphasized by Bushong (2009) is that "during digital fluoroscopy, the X-ray tube operates in the radiographic mode."

Video Camera

As noted earlier in this chapter, the video camera used in fluoroscopy can be either a television camera tube or a CCD camera. While the first-generation systems use television tubes, second-generation systems use CCD cameras. If a television camera tube is used, it must have a higher signal-to-noise ratio (SNR) than tubes used in conventional fluoroscopy. While the SNR for conventional fluoroscopy systems is about 200:1, it is 1000:1 for digital fluoroscopy with image intensifiers (Bushong, 2009).

Television camera tubes should also have low image lag.

The CCD camera, described earlier in this chapter, is now used in digital fluoroscopy systems using image intensifiers (Yester, 2004). It is important to note, however, that the CCD camera has extremely high sensitivity and low readout noise level. Images can also be acquired at 60/sec compared with 30/sec for television tubes.

Analog-to-Digital Converter

The analog-to-digital converter (ADC) is an integral component in digital imaging technologies. In digital fluoroscopy, the ADC receives the output video signal (analog signal) from the video camera. Since a computer is used, the analog signal must be converted into digital data for computer processing. The process of digitizing the analog signal requires dividing it (the signal) into a number of parts. This is referred to as sampling (Chapter 2). The unit of the parts is the bit (contraction for binary digit). A bit can be a 1 or it can be a 0. A 2-bit ADC will divide a signal into 4 (2^2) parts. Similarly, a 10-bit ADC will divide the signal into 1024 (2^{10}) parts. The higher the number of bits, the more accurate is the ADC.

Computer System

At the heart of a digital fluoroscopy imaging system is a **host computer**, a minicomputer system capable of receiving dynamic digital data from the

ADC and processing it quickly for image display and subsequent storage. It is not within the scope of this chapter to describe the details of the computer system; however, the following points are noteworthy:

- The computer operates on the data it receives from the ADC in a matrix format. This means that the digital image is a matrix of pixels, and for digital fluoroscopy, matrix sizes of 512 × 512 and 1024 × 1024 are typical (Pooley et al., 2001).

- Each pixel in the image contains the atomic number and mass density characteristic of the tissue, and a single number for the pixel represents this information.

- The matrix of numbers is transformed into a gray scale image, as illustrated in Figure 6-8. The image can be characterized by the term "bit depth," which describes the number of shades of gray that a single pixel in the matrix (image) can assume. For example, in a 3-bit depth image, each pixel can have 8 (2^3) shades of gray; an 8-bit depth image will provide 256 (2^8) shades of gray for each pixel.

- The spatial resolution for a digital fluoroscopic image depends on the pixel size. As the matrix size increases for the same field-of-view (FOV), the pixel size decreases and the image appears sharper.

- Images displayed on the television monitor can be post-processed using a number of different image-processing operations. These include last-image hold, grayscale image manipulation, and edge enhancement (Pooley et al., 2001). Such processing is a function of the computer, and it is intended to alter the image to enhance diagnostic interpretation as detailed in previous chapters.

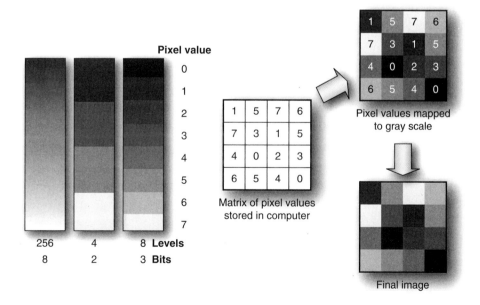

FIGURE 6-8. Formation of a displayed image from a 4 × 4 matrix of pixel values (stored as a series of binary numbers). A 3-bit binary system is used, which can encode up to eight (2^3) different values (0–7 in decimal). The eight values are assigned to eight shades of gray between white and black. The gray level assigned to a pixel value will be displayed at that pixel location in the matrix. Likewise, an 8-bit image may have a maximum of 256 different pixel values and 256 different shades of gray

Source: *Pooley, R. A., McKinney, M. I., & Miller, D. A. (2001). Digital fluoroscopy. Radiographics, 21, 521–534. Figure and legend reproduced by permission of RSNA and the authors*

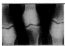

Digital Fluoroscopy with Flat-Panel Detectors

Recently, digital fluoroscopy systems with an image intensifier and video camera (both television camera tubes and CCD cameras) in the imaging chain have been replaced with digital fluoroscopy systems with flat-panel detectors (FPDs). Digital fluoroscopy with FPDs has become commonplace in angiography, and a few systems are currently being used for gastrointestinal tract fluoroscopy (at the time of writing this chapter). This section will therefore focus on the fundamental principles guiding the performance of FPDs in digital fluoroscopy.

Limitations of Image Intensifier Technology

Image intensifier tube technology poses several problems when used for fluoroscopic imaging. These problems were identified earlier in this chapter and include vignetting, image lag, and pincushion and S distortions. Additionally, light and electron scattering within the tube degrades the image contrast (veiling glare) and image magnification results in increased dose to the patient.

Equipment Configuration

The overall equipment configuration of an FPD digital fluoroscopy imaging system (real-time imaging) is shown in Figure 6-9, which clearly demonstrates that the most significant difference between this system and the image intensifier-based system shown in Figure 6-7 is the presence of the FPD. FPDs used in radiographic imaging (Chapter 5) produce static images and are therefore referred to as static FPDs. One significant and important technical characteristic of an FPD for fluoroscopy is that it must be capable of producing dynamic images that can be displayed and viewed in real time. For this reason, these detectors are sometimes referred to as dynamic FPDs.

The components shown in Figure 6-9 include the X-ray tube, patient, grid, dynamic FPD, host computer, and the television display monitor. The next subsection of this chapter will highlight the basics of the dynamic FPD.

Types of Dynamic FPDs

Two types of dynamic FPDs are currently available for digital fluoroscopy, namely, the CsI a-Si TFT indirect digital detector and the a-Se TFT direct digital detector. In general these detectors are similar in design to the static FPDs used for radiographic imaging (Granfors et al., 2003; Hunt et al., 2004) described in Chapter 5. There are a few significant differences, however, and they will be reviewed subsequently.

Various medical imaging vendors utilize different dynamic FPDs in their digital fluoroscopy systems. For example, General Electric (GE) Healthcare, Philips Medical Systems, Luminos, and Siemens Medical Solutions use the CsI a-Si indirect FPDs; Toshiba Medical Systems and Shimadzu use the

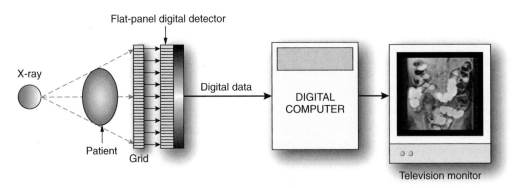

FIGURE 6-9. The overall equipment of a digital fluoroscopy imaging system using flat-panel digital detectors. The detector is also referred to as a dynamic flat-panel detector since it provides images in real time. Source: *Delmar, Cengage Learning*

a-Se direct FPDs, specifically the GE Innova 4100™ and the Siemens AXIOM®.

Characteristics of Dynamic FPDs

The characteristics worthy of consideration in this chapter are the dimensions of the detector, matrix sizes, pixel considerations, and the zoom feature. Typical dimensions of these detectors vary, however: 31 cm × 31 cm, 35 cm × 35 cm, 30 cm × 40 cm, and 41 cm × 41 cm are commonplace. Recently, 43 cm × 43 cm dynamic FPD has become available for both digital fluoroscopy and digital radiography (Gans, 2007).

Matrix sizes vary as well, depending on the physical dimensions of the detector. Generally, larger detectors have larger matrix sizes, and typical sizes include 1024 × 1024, 2304 × 2304, and 2048 × 2048.

For digital fluoroscopy detectors, the pixel size is larger than the pixel size used in digital radiography detectors. In some systems it is possible to "adjust the pixel size by binning four pixels into one larger pixel. Such dual-use systems have pixels small enough to be adequate for radiography (e.g., 100 to 150 μm), but the pixels can be binned to provide a detector useful for fluoroscopy (e.g., 200 to 300 μm)" (Bushberg et al., 2004).

An example of a dual-use system is the Siemens AXIOM® Luminos dRF imaging system, which can be used for both digital fluoroscopy and digital radiography.

Another characteristic feature of the dynamic FPD is that it offers "zoom" modes, enabling the operator to zoom into the survey image and examine details of smaller structures (Mioni & Franssen, 2004).

Operating Principles

There are other significant differences between FPDs for digital radiography and dynamic real time fluoroscopy, most notably the "complexity of the readout electronics" (Yorkston, 2004). Such complexity is beyond the scope of this book; however, the interested reader should refer to the paper by Lai et al. (2005) on this subject. One primary consideration is that the electronics must facilitate high frame rates and fast data transfer rates. Frames rates of 15 to 30 fps or greater are possible

at readout speeds of 30 to 50 msec (Holmes et al., 2004; Lai et al., 2005; Yorkston, 2004).

Additionally, dynamic FPDs can operate in at least two readout modes, the frame rate (fps) in continuous X-ray mode and the fps in the pulsed X-ray mode. For example, the ANRAD dynamic FPD can provide 7.5 fps and 30 fps and 7.5 fps (<72 ms) and 30 fps (<11 ms) in the full-panel continuous and pulsed X-ray modes respectively. In the zoom (23 cm × 23 cm) readout mode, it can provide 30 fps and 60 fps in the continuous X-ray mode and 30 fps (<8 ms) and 60 fps (<4 ms) in the pulsed X-ray mode (ANRAD Corporation, 2004).

In general, the operational elements of a dynamic FPD involve three sequences that result in a single image that must be completed in at least 33 ms for fluoroscopy. These elements include initialization, integration, and readout (Lai et al., 2005). While initialization prepares the detector electronics for X-ray exposure, integration and readout are intended to collect the detector (analog) signal for subsequent digitization and image display. It is interesting to note that a light-emitting diode (LED) array located below the detector produces a "refresh" light to erase images after every frame to get rid of image ghosting (Sivananthan et al., 2004). According to Yorkston (2004), image ghosting "is generally identified as a change in sensitivity of the X-ray converter after exposure to X-rays. Consequently, in contrast to image lag, it is only observed in images taken with further exposure."

Advantages

Compared to image intensifier-based digital fluoroscopy, dynamic FPD fluoroscopy offers several advantages. These include "high low-contrast resolution; high DQE across all dose levels, particularly for a CsI a-Si based flat detector, high dynamic range covering all dose levels from fluoroscopy to digital subtraction angiography (DSA)" (Spahn, 2004). Furthermore, artifacts such as pincushion distortion and veiling glare that are present with image intensifier-based system do not occur with dynamic FPDs.

Dynamic FPDs also make use of scattered radiation grids that can be removed when imaging children (since the use of grids during the examination will increase the dose to the patient). It is vital to

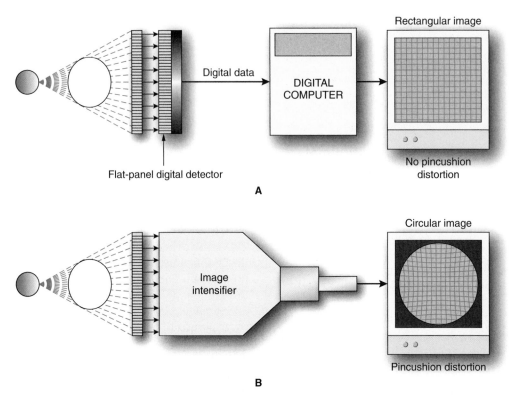

FIGURE 6-10. The image display format when using a flat-panel digital fluoroscopy imaging system is rectangular (A), whereas it is circular for an image intensifier-based fluoroscopy system (B). The rectangular format matches the display format of the television monitor. Note that the pixels in B are distorted, especially at the periphery of the image, while the pixels in the A are not distorted.
Source: *Delmar, Cengage Learning*

note that during its use the grid lines are oriented diagonally to the detector matrix to eliminate any aliasing artifacts (Brennan et al., in press).

Another notable advantage is clearly illustrated in Figure 6-10. The image display with an FPD system is clearly rectangular, whereas it is circular for intensifier-based systems. This format makes efficient use of the rectangular display offered by television monitors.

Finally, digital fluoroscopy using FPDs is much more compact in design, and this feature enables excellent access to the patient during the examination.

Connectivity

Digital fluoroscopy imaging systems can be configured with the DICOM standards to ensure connectivity and integration with picture archiving and communication systems (PACS) and information systems such as the radiology information system (RIS) and the hospital information system (HIS). For example, the DICOM "Query/Retrieve" service classes can provide direct access to archived images (in PACS) for display at the radiologist workstation.

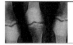 ## Digital Image Postprocessing

All digital imaging modalities, including digital fluoroscopy, make use of various types of image postprocessing algorithms (software), essentially to manipulate the image presented to the observer in order to enhance diagnostic interpretation (Seeram & Seeram, 2008). Digital fluoroscopy can be applied to both gastrointestinal (GI) tract imaging and DSA, and the image post-processing operations are specific to each application. For example, while grayscale image manipulation is common to GI fluoroscopy, road mapping is an operation commonly used in DSA. DSA will be described briefly later in this chapter.

Image post-processing operations specifically for digital fluoroscopy have been reviewed by Pooley et al. (2001). These operations include grayscale image manipulation, temporal frame averaging, last-image hold, and edge enhancement. Each of these will be described briefly.

Grayscale–Image Manipulation

Grayscale-image manipulation was described in detail in Chapter 2. In review, the purpose of grayscale-image manipulation is to change the contrast and brightness of an image displayed on the monitor in order to facilitate diagnostic interpretation.

Recall that a digital image is made up of a matrix of pixels in which each pixel is assigned a number and each number corresponds to a gray shade. An 8-bit image, for example, will consist of 256 (2^8) pixels ranging from 0 to 255 on the grayscale. This image will also consist of 256 shades of gray, where low numbers are dark and higher numbers are bright. The range of the numbers is defined as the window width (WW) and the center of the range is defined as the window level (WL). The WW changes the image contrast and the WL changes the brightness of the image. Figure 6-11 demonstrates the effect of the WW (a) and the WL (b) on image contrast and brightness, respectively.

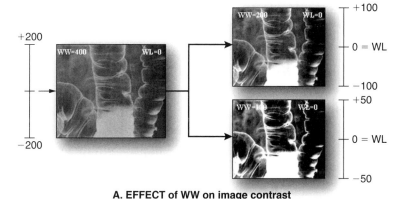

A. EFFECT of WW on image contrast

B. EFFECT of WL on image brightness

FIGURE 6-11. The effect of changing the window–width (WW) and window–level (WL) settings on the grayscale appearance of the image.
Source: *Delmar, Cengage Learning*

Last-Image Hold

Last-image hold (LIH) is an image-processing technique used to reduce the radiation dose to the patient. Figure 6-12 illustrates the concept of LIH. When the X-ray beam is turned on, images are obtained. The LIH operation displays the last frame continuously when the X-ray beam is turned off. The process repeats itself when the beam is turned on once again.

Temporal Frame Averaging

The purpose of temporal frame averaging is to reduce the noise present in an image "by continuously displaying an image that is created by averaging the current frame with one or more previous frames of digital fluoroscopic image data" (Pooley et al., 2001), as shown in Figure 6-13. In this figure, averaging five frames will reduce the noise by about 44%; however, as more and more frames are averaged, image lag results.

Edge Enhancement

Edge enhancement is an image-sharpening post-processing operation (Chapter 2). Several image-sharpening algorithms are currently available (Seeram & Seeram, 2008) including the unsharp masking operation shown in Figure 6-14. In this operation, a blurred image (b) of the original image (a) is first obtained, followed by subtraction of the blurred image from the original image. The subtraction process produces a new image (c) that is subsequently added to the original image to produce the final image, referred to as the edge-enhanced image (d).

Proprietary Post-processing Techniques

It is understandable that different vendors will have post-processing algorithms specific to their equipment, and students and technologists alike will experience this when they work with different vendor equipment. While it is not necessary to describe all of these proprietary algorithms, it is noteworthy to mention one example as an illustration.

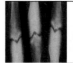

Digital Subtraction Angiography: A Brief Overview

As noted earlier in the chapter, dynamic FPD detectors were first used in angiography, rather than in GI tract fluoroscopy. Dynamic FPDs have replaced image intensifier/video camera technology

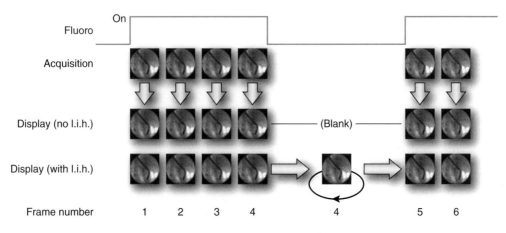

FIGURE 6-12. The technique of last image hold (LIH) in which the last frame acquired during the fluoroscopic sequence of frames obtained when the X-ray beam is "on" is displayed continuously. This technique is essentially intended to reduce the radiation dose to the patient.
Source: Pooley, R. A., McKinney, M. I., & Miller, D. A. (2001). Digital fluoroscopy. Radiographics, 21, 521–534. Reproduced by permission of RSNA and the authors

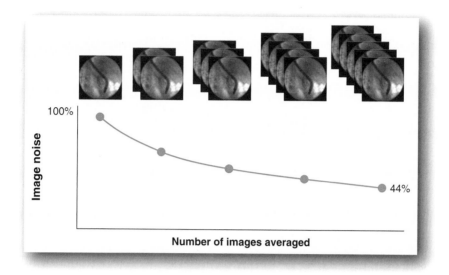

FIGURE 6-13. Temporal frame averaging during digital fluoroscopy is one technique that can be used to reduce image noise.
Source: *Pooley, R. A., McKinney, M. I., & Miller, D. A. (2001). Digital fluoroscopy. Radiographics, 21, 521–534. Reproduced by permission of RSNA and the authors*

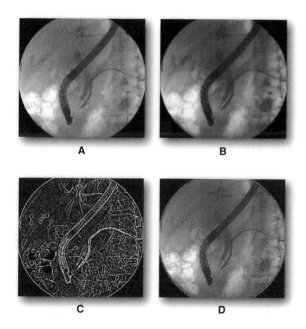

FIGURE 6-14. The edge–enhancement image–processing operation involves creating a blurred image (B) and then digitally subtracting it from the original image (a) to obtain the image (C). Image (C) is added to image (A) to produce the edge–enhanced image (D).
Source: *Pooley, R. A., McKinney, M. I., & Miller, D. A. (2001). Digital fluoroscopy. Radiographics, 21, 521–534. Reproduced by permission of RSNA and the authors*

in angiographic imaging. Since contrast material is used in angiography, and pre-contrast images are digitally subtracted from post-contrast images during the procedure, the imaging process is referred to a digital subtraction angiography (DSA). There are two methods of DSA, temporal subtraction and energy subtraction, which are described briefly here.

Temporal Subtraction

Temporal subtraction involves the digital subtraction of images in time. In general, a pre-contrast image referred to as a mask image is first obtained and post-contrast images are then digitally subtracted from the mask image. This method of subtraction is illustrated in Figure 6-15. Six post-contrast images (frames) are used in the subtraction sequence to provide images of only the contrast-filled vessels. All other overlying anatomical structures are removed.

Energy Subtraction

The energy subtraction operation is based on subtraction of images taken at different kVs. "Images are recorded based on subtraction of

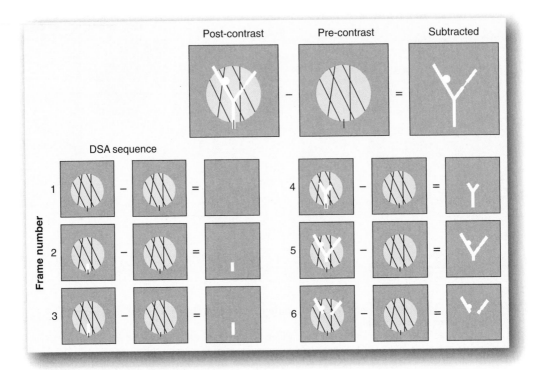

FIGURE 6-15. DSA. A precontrast mask image (which shows a distracting background structure and the tip of the catheter) is subtracted from a postcontrast image obtained at the same location (which shows contrast material–filled vessels). The result is an image of only the contrast material–filled vessels. During the actual imaging sequence, the subtraction process may begin slightly prior to contrast material injection, with each frame capturing a different phase of injection. The sequence of subtracted frames can then be reviewed in cine mode or as still frames. The unsubtracted original digital fluoroscopic images are generally not reviewed. Source: Pooley, R. A., McKinney, M. I., & Miller, D. A. (2001). Digital fluoroscopy. *Radiographics, 21,* 521–534. Reproduced by permission of RSNA and the authors

energies slightly above and slightly below the k-absorption edge of the contrast material used for the examination" (Seeram, 2001). For a further description of temporal and energy subtraction techniques, the student should refer to Bushong (2004).

New Techniques

DSA has advanced from film-based imaging using image intensifier/video camera technology to imaging with dynamic FPDs. Recently, several innovations in angiography have been described on several manufacturers' Web sites and various angiography journals. For example, the *AXIOM Innovation in Intervention* magazine of Siemens Medical Solutions describes several new developments in DSA. One such new technique is 3-dimensional (3D) reconstruction using FPDs that rotate about the patient for at least 180°, and the data collected is reconstructed in a manner similar to that used in computed tomography (CT). Other techniques include stent and vessel assessment. The interested student should refer to any good angiographic imaging textbook for further details of these techniques.

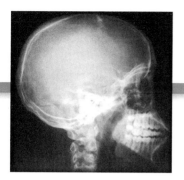
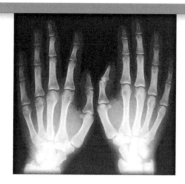
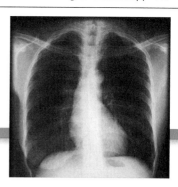

REVIEW QUESTIONS

1. Draw a diagram of a conventional fluoroscopy imaging system, label the components, and explain the contribution of each component to the imaging process.

2. What major components of an image intensifier-based digital imaging system are responsible for digitizing analog data collected from the video camera?

3. Draw a diagram of an image intensifier tube, label its components, and explain how the intensifier tube works.

4. What are the main components of a closed-circuit X-ray television chain?

5. List the shortcomings of an image intensifier-based digital fluoroscopy imaging system.

6. Explain how the dose increases when magnification is used in image intensifier-based fluoroscopy imaging systems.

7. Briefly explain how pulsed-fluoroscopy reduces the dose to the patient.

8. Draw a diagram of an FPD fluoroscopy imaging system and label its components.

9. What types of FPDs are used in digital fluoroscopy?

10. What is one of the most significant differences between an FPD used for digital radiography and one used for digital fluoroscopy?

11. List the advantages of FPD digital fluoroscopy.

12. List several digital image post-processing techniques, and state the purpose of each of them.

13. What is the difference between temporal subtraction and energy subtraction as used in digital subtraction angiography (DSA)?

REFERENCES

Anrad Corporation. (2006). *The FPD14 Digital Detector, a-Se digital flat-panel detector for real time applications.* Product Literature. Quebec, Canada.

AXIOM Luminos dRF. (March, 2007). *AXIOM Innovation in Intervention, 4,* 36–41.

Brennan, P., McKentee, M., Seeram, E. et al. (in press). *Digital Diagnostic Imaging.* Oxford: Blackwell Publishing.

Bushberg, J. T. et al. (2004). *The Essential Physics of Medical Imaging.* (2nd ed.). Philadelphia: Lippincott Williams and Wilkins.

Bushong, S. (2009). *Radiologic Science for Technologists.* (9th ed.) St Louis: Elsevier-Mosby.

Gaus, N. (2007). Editorial. *AXIOM Innovation in Intervention.* No. 4, March, 1.

Granfors, P. A., Aufrichtig, R., & Possin, G. E. et al. (2003). Performance of a $41 \times 41 cm^2$ amorphous silicon flat-panel detector designed for angiographic and R&F imaging applications. *Medical Physics, 30*(10), 2715–2726.

Holmes, D. R., Laskey, W. K., et al. (2004). Flat-panel detectors in the cardiac catheterization laboratory: Revolution or evolution-What are the issues? *Catheterization and Cardiovascular Interventions, 63,* 324–330.

Hunt, D. C., Tousignant, O., & Rowlands, J. A. (2004). Evaluation of the imaging properties of an amorphous selenium-based flat-panel detector for digital fluoroscopy. *Medical Physics, 31*(5), 1166–1175.

Lai, J., Safavian, N. et al. (2005). Active pixel TFT arrays for digital fluoroscopy in a-Si:H technology. *Materials Research Society Symposium Proceedings, 862,* 635–640.

Mioni, D. & Franssen, B. (2004). A large-area flat-detector interventional X-ray imaging system. *Medicamundi, 43,* 19–21.

Pooley, R. A., McKinney, M. I., & Miller, D. A. (2001). Digital fluoroscopy. *Radiographics, 21,* 521–534.

Seeram, E. (2001). *Rad Tech Guide to Equipment Operation and Maintenance,* Malden: Blackwell Science.

Seeram, E. & Seeram, D. (2008). Image postprocessing in digital radiology: A Primer for technologists. *Journal of Medical Imaging and Radiation Sciences, 39*(1), 23–43.

Sivananthan, M. U., Moore, J., Pepper, C. B. et al. (2005). A flat-detector cardiac cath lab system in clinical practice. *Medicamundi, 48*(1), 4–12.

Spahn, M. (2005). Flat detectors and their clinical applications. *European Journal of Radiology, 15,* 1934–147.

Wang, J., & Blackburn, T. J. (2000). X-ray image intensifiers for fluoroscopy. *Radiographics, 20,* 1471–1477.

Yester, M. V. (2004). CCD digital radiographic detectors. In L. Goldman & M. V. Yester (Eds.), *Specifications, Performance, and Quality Assurance of Radiographic and Fluoroscopic Systems in the Digital Era* (pp. 177–229). AAPM Monograph 30. College Park, MD.

Yorkston, J. (2004). Flat-panel DR detectors for radiography and fluoroscopy. In L. Goldman & M. V. Yester (Eds.), *Specifications, Performance, and Quality Assurance of Radiographic and Fluoroscopic Systems in the Digital Era* (pp. 177–229). AAPM Monograph 30. College Park, MD.

Yorkston, J. (2003). Digital radiographic technology. In E. Samei & M. Flynn M (Eds.), *Advances in Digital Radiography. RSNA Categorical Course in Diagnostic Radiology Physics* (pp. 23–26). Oak Brook, Ill: RSNA.

CHAPTER 7

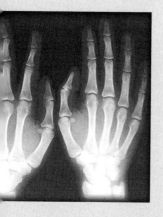

Digital Mammography

OBJECTIVES

Upon completion of this chapter, the student should be able to:

1. State the limitations of screen film mammography.

2. Describe briefly what is meant by digital mammography.

3. List the advantages of digital mammography.

4. Describe the technical requirements for digital mammography.

5. Outline the major characteristics of four types of digital detector systems used in digital mammography.

6. State the purpose of digital image processing in digital mammography.

7. List several specific digital image processing operations for use in digital mammography.

8. Outline the characteristic features of computer aided diagnosis, digital tomosynthesis, and contrast-enhanced digital mammography.

KEY TERMS

Clinical trials
Computer-aided detection and diagnosis (CAD)
CR digital mammography
Digital tomosynthesis
Flat panel a–Se detector

Flat panel a–Si detector
Image processing algorithm
Mammography
Screen–film mammography (SFM)

Introduction

Mammography is defined as radiography of the breast, and it is a prime example of soft tissue radiography, since the breast is composed of soft tissues such as adipose (fat), fibrous, and glandular tissue. Mammography was developed as a dedicated imaging technique to detect breast cancer that has become prevalent among women in North America. The imaging technique is dedicated because it uses equipment designed especially to produce an X-ray beam that will allow for maximum X-ray absorption by the soft tissues, microcalcifications, and thin fibers so that they can be shown on radiographic film with excellent spatial resolution or detail. Mammography must be able to show the contrast between a lesion that is located in the breast and the normal anatomy that is around that lesion. This imaging technique is referred to as screen–film mammography (SFM).

Screen–Film Mammography: A Review of the Basics

It is not within the scope of this chapter to describe the physics and technical details of SFM, and therefore the interested reader should refer to any good radiologic physics textbook (such as Bushberg, Seibert, Leidholdt, & Boone, 2004; Bushong, 2009; Huda & Slone, 2002) for comprehensive coverage of these topics.

The Imaging Process

The basic process of SFM is shown in Figure 7-1. A dedicated X-ray tube produces a special X-ray beam (soft X-rays) that passes through the breast to fall upon the mammography cassette. This cassette contains the intensifying screen and the film that has been made for use in mammographic imaging. X-rays cause the screen to emit light and a latent image is formed on the film. The film is processed using a chemical processor to render the latent image visible. This film image is then displayed on a lightview box for interpretation by a radiologist, who makes a diagnosis of the patient's medical condition. In this entire process, the film acts as the acquisition device, the display medium, and the storage medium, since it is placed in an envelope and housed in a room for long-term storage and archiving.

SFM has been successful for decades since it offers several advantages (Mahesh, 2004); most notably, it provides not only high image

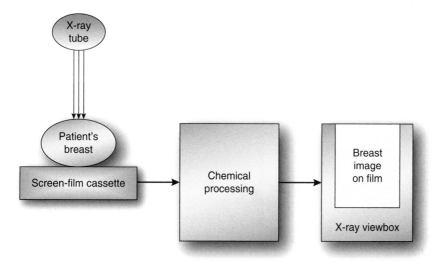

FIGURE 7-1. The major components of a SFM imaging system. The radiation passes through the patient's breast to create a latent image on the film. The film is processed using chemical solutions to render the latent image visible. The image in then displayed on a light box (viewbox) for viewing and interpretation by a radiologist.
Source: *Delmar, Cengage Learning*

contrast but also high spatial resolution of about 15–20 line pairs/mm limiting resolution, which is needed to detect specks of calcium hydroxyapatite (microcalcifications) with diameters of around 0.01 mm (100 μm) (Huda & Slone, 2002).

Limitations of SFM

Although it possesses the above advantages, SFM also has several drawbacks. First, it has a limited dynamic range (narrow exposure latitude) of the film. This is illustrated in Figure 7-2. The film will only respond to a narrow range of exposures and therefore the technologist must be extremely careful in selection of the optimum exposure factors to provide the best image contrast. Such contrast falls on the slope of the characteristic curve (the H and D, or Hurter-Driffield, curve). Second, the display characteristics of film, such as its brightness and contrast, are fixed once the film

is developed in the chemical processor. If the radiologist needs a lighter or darker film or if the image contrast needs to be changed, then the technologist must perform the exam using a different set exposure technique factors to demonstrate these required characteristics. This strategy increases the radiation dose to the patient. Third, the film serves three roles: acquisition, display, and storage, as mentioned above.

Over the years, SFM progressed along with significant developments in the field, such as technical and clinical improvements and regulatory approval. One such significant technical development/improvement is digital mammography, designed to overcome the limitations of SFM.

 ## What is Digital Mammography?

Digital mammography (DM) is radiography of the breast using a digital detector coupled to a computer that makes use of digital image processing techniques to enhance the visibility of detail and contrast of the image and therefore to improve the detectability of breast lesions. The major components of a DM imaging system and imaging steps are clearly illustrated in Figure 7-3.

In DM, a digital detector replaces the screen-film image receptor used in conventional film-screen mammography. X-rays passing through the breast fall upon the digital detector to produce a latent image that is subsequently processed by a computer.

The development of DM dates back to more than a decade ago. In September 1991, the National Cancer Institute was advised by a group of well-known breast imaging experts to develop the technique of DM (Pisano, 2000). Today, several research groups and manufacturers are actively engaged in developing DM into a useful clinical imaging tool. Manufacturers who are actively engaged in DM development include Fischer Imaging (SenoScan System), Fuji Medical Systems (Computed Radiography (CR) Mammography System), General Electric Medical Systems (Senograph 2000 D System), and Trex Medical (Trex

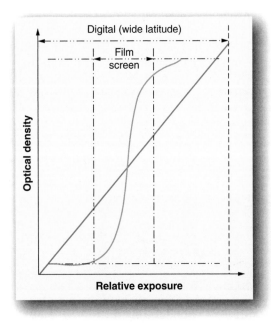

FIGURE 7-2. The exposure latitude (dynamic range) of SFM is very narrow compared to the wide latitude of DM. Source: *Mahesh, M. (2004). Digital Mammography-Physics Tutorial for Residents.* Radiographics, 24, 1747–1760. *Reproduced by permission*

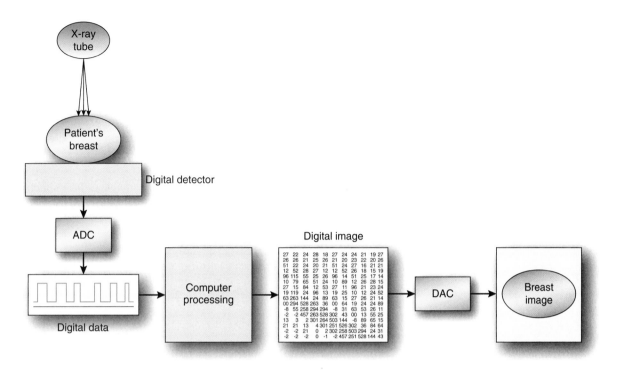

FIGURE 7-3. The major components of a DM imaging system. The basic steps in producing the image are clearly illustrated. Source: *Delmar, Cengage Learning*

Digital Mammography System). These manufacturers have developed several DM imaging systems, each based on a different set of technical principles.

In 2000, the Food and Drug Administration (FDA) approved the first DM unit after much research dedicated to improving its technical performance as well as clinical trials (Pisano, Yaffe, & Kuzmiak, 2004). Today, the FDA has approved two more DM systems. The only DM system that has not been approved by the FDA is the Fuji Computed Radiography (CR) mammography system, even though this system is being used in Japan and in Europe as well (Pisano & Yaffe, 2005).

Advantages of DM

Digital mammography uses a digital detector and computer processing to generate images, as opposed to the chemical processing of film characteristic of SFM. Because of this, DM offers the following advantages over SFM:

- The digital detector offers a wider dynamic range. As seen in Figure 7-2, the dynamic range for SFM is about 40:1, while it is 1000:1 for DM
- Greater contrast resolution, especially for dense breast tissue
- Use of digital image post-processing operations to enhance image quality
- The ability to communicate with a picture archiving and communication system (PACS)
- Computer-aided detection and diagnosis (CAD)
- Digital tomosynthesis
- Contrast-enhanced DM

Digital image post-processing, CAD, telemammography, digital tomosynthesis, and contrast-enhanced DM will be described briefly later.

Technical Requirements for DM

Digital mammography involves at least five fundamental steps, as shown in Figure 7-4. These include data acquisition, analog-to-digital conversion (ADC), digital image processing, image display, image storage, archiving, and communications via the PACS. Once in the PACS, images and text data can be sent to remote locations via communication networks.

Data Acquisition

Data acquisition is the first step in producing a DM image. The data acquisition system consists of the X-ray tube and generator systems coupled to the digital detector imaging system. X-rays pass through the breast and fall upon the digital detector to create an electronic signal that must subsequently be digitized for input into a computer. Currently, there are four types of digital detector systems used for DM: flat-panel phosphor, charge-coupled device (CCD), flat-panel amorphous selenium (a-Se), and a CR DM system (Mahesh, 2004; Pisano & Yaffe, 2005). Each of these will be described briefly later in this chapter.

Detectors for DM must be capable of providing a spatial resolution of at least 10 lp/mm to improve lesion detectability and must have an image area of at least 24 cm × 30 cm in order to capture the entire breast. Additionally, since the pixel size affects the spatial resolution, pixels must be spaced about

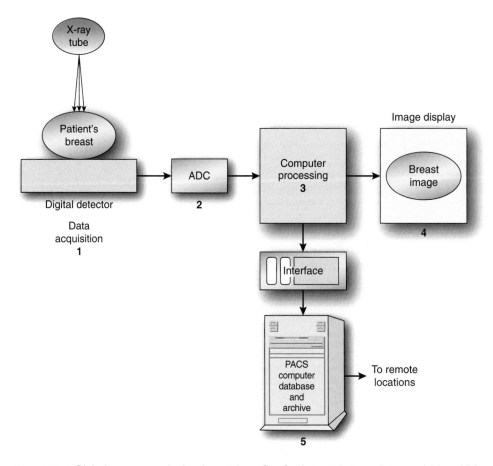

FIGURE 7-4. Digital mammography involves at least five fundamental steps: data acquisition, ADC, digital image processing, image display, image storage, archiving, and communications via the PACS. Source: *Delmar, Cengage Learning*

25 μm (0.025 mm) apart. For a large detector, a 9600 × 12,000 matrix size is a fundamental requirement (James, 2004). In addition, as noted by James (2004), "for good image quality, a high intensity signal is required with low-intensity noise (a good Signal-to-Noise Ratio [SNR])." Recall that the SNR describes the information quality in the image.

Another measure of the detector's performance in DM is the detective quantum efficiency (DQE). This is how well the DM imaging system can efficiently transfer the input SNR (at the detector) to the output SNR (image displayed on the monitor) so that it is useful to the observer in making a diagnosis. The DQE is expressed as follows:

$$DQE = SNR_{out}^2/SNR_{in}^2$$

In a perfect imaging system, the DQE would be equal to one (100%). The DQE for F-S mammography system is about 45% (Pisano, Yaffe, & Kuzmiak, 2004). The reader will have to refer to the various manufacturers for the DQE of their DM systems.

Analog-to-Digital Conversion

The digital detectors convert X-ray photons to an electronic signal (analog signal) that must first be digitized for input into a computer. DM systems require ADCs with very high digitization capability. DM systems may use 12–14-bit ADCs. A 14-bit ADC can divide an electronic signal into 16,384 (2^{14}) discrete parts. This is rated as excellent digitization and will enable images to be displayed with excellent grayscale resolution (James, 2004).

Digital Image Processing

The computer is central to a DM imaging system. The computer generates a digital mammographic image, using the digital data it receives from the ADC, using a defined set of image processing algorithms. (It is not within the scope of this text to describe these algorithms.) In addition, a number of post-processing operations are available to enhance images to suit the viewing needs of the observer. These operations include windowing, measurement and annotation tools, and various sophisticated digital post-processing techniques, such as frequency processing for enhancing the

sharpness of an image. These will be discussed later in the chapter.

Image Display

The digital output from the computer must be converted back into an analog signal so that it can be displayed on a monitor workstation (soft-copy image) that has a display resolution of at least 5 megapixels (Mahesh, 2004). Image display also takes into consideration the luminance and contrast resolution of the display monitors.

Two types of display technologies for DM are in use today, the cathode-ray tube (CRT) and the liquid crystal display (LCD). Recently, Samei (2005) has described the technological and psychophysical factors for these types of displays. The psychophysical factors (contrast resolution and noise) play a role in image interpretation. It is interesting to note that "optimal display of mammograms is achieved by taking these factors into consideration and by using time-efficient, intuitive, and reader-specific user interfaces" (Samei, 2005).

Digital mammography computer display monitors should also be located in rooms that have ambient light of less than 5 lux^2. Various studies have evaluated the performance of radiologists on soft-copy images; the results of these studies indicate that "the lower luminance and contrast resolution of soft copy systems, compared with those printed on film displays, do not significantly affect the interpretation performance of radiologists" (Samei, 2005). Since it is not within the scope of this chapter to describe the details of image display, the interested reader should refer to the works of Pisano, Yafee, and Kuzmiak (2004); Pisano and Yaffe (2005); and James (2004).

PACS Integration

Picture archiving and communication systems are now commonplace in hospitals, and the next consideration for DM is to send all the digitally acquired images to the PACS. As described in previous chapters, the PACS is characterized by several components working together to achieving a common goal, including image storage, archiving, and communications. Of course, the DM acquisition components are connected to the PACS,

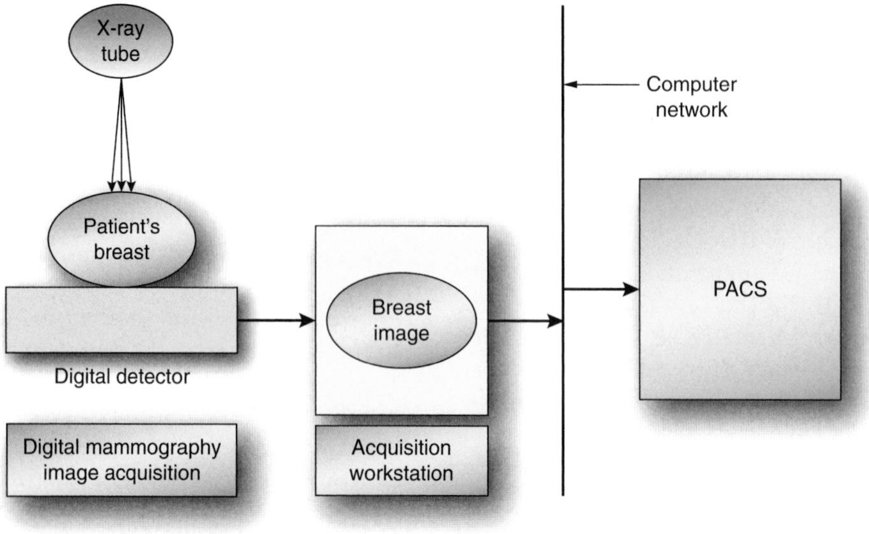

FIGURE 7-5. The DM image acquisition system and the acquisition workstation are connected to the PACS via computer networks and an interface (not shown) that facilitate the communication of images to the PACS.
Source: *Delmar, Cengage Learning*

as shown in Figure 7-5. The purpose of the PACS is to improve the management efficiency of the large amount of DM images, including storage, retrieval, and communication of images.

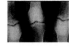

Types of Digital Detector Systems for DM

As noted earlier in the chapter, there are four different types of DM systems available commercially based on the digital detector structure and function as shown in Figure 7-6. These include Type 1 digital detectors such as the flat-panel scintillator/amorphous silicon (a-Si) System; Type 2 digital detectors such as the CCD system; Type 3 digital detectors such as the CR DM system; and Type 4 digital detectors such as the flat-panel a-Se system. These systems are manufactured by General Electric Medical Systems, Fisher Medical Imaging, Fuji Medical Systems, and Lorad/Hologic, respectively. Recall that the FDA currently approved three of these four systems at the time of writing this chapter.

The overall basic principles of these detectors were described in Chapter 1 and elaborated on in

Chapters 3 and 4. In this chapter, the following brief principles of how each works are relevant and noteworthy:

Flat-Panel Scintillator/Amorphous Silicon (a-Si) DM System

The basic structure of the flat-panel a-Si detector system is shown in Figure 7-6 and is labeled Type 1. As can be seen, the detector consists of three major components, a scintillator, photodiodes, a thin film transistor (TFT) array, and a glass support. This detector system is sometimes referred to as an indirect conversion system by some authors (Smith, 2005), only because the detector first converts the X-ray photons falling upon it into light photons. Subsequently, the light is converted into electricity by the photodiodes.

The scintillator is made up of cesium iodide (CsI) activated by thallium. The CsI phosphor is deposited on top of the a-Si TFT array in a needle-like fashion (to reduce lateral dispersion of light in order to improve image detail) and converts X-rays into light. The light falls upon the a-Si TFT array, which is constructed as a matrix of photodiodes and is subsequently converted into electrical signals. These

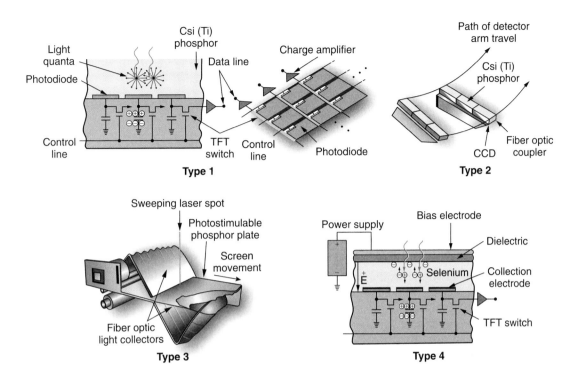

FIGURE 7-6. The four different types of digital detectors used in DM systems. Type 1 is the flat-panel scintillator/a-Si digital detector. Type 2 is CCD digital detector. Type 3 is the CR imaging plate digital detector. Type 4 is the flat-panel a-Se digital detector.
Source: *Pisano, E. D., & Yaffe, M. J. (2005). Digital Mammography. Radiology, 234, 353–362. Reproduced by permission of RSNA*

signals are sent to a digitizer and are converted into digital data for input into a computer. The computer performs the appropriate digital processing to produce a digital image of the breast. An example of this type of DM system based on this type of digital detector is the Senographe 2000D manufactured by General Electric Medical Systems.

Charge-coupled Device DM System

The charge-coupled device (CCD) DM detector is illustrated in Figure 7-6, labeled Type 2. The main structural components include a thallium-activated CsI scintillator phosphor similar to the one described above, deposited upon a matrix of CCDs. This system is also referred to as an indirect conversion system by some authors (Samei, 2005), simply because X-rays are first converted into light and not directly into electricity. In addition, the CsI phosphor is coupled

to the CCD array via a fiberoptical system that directs the light from the CsI to the CCD array.

The CCD array is arranged as a matrix of pixels that are sensitive to the light from the CsI phosphor. The CCD system converts the light into electrical signals that are read out in a very systematic way and sent to the digitizer, which generates digital data for input into a computer for processing. The result of computer processing is a digital image of the breast.

This system is somewhat different to the system described above. A fan beam from the X-ray tube falls upon the detector, which "has a long, narrow, rectangular shape, with dimensions of approximately 1 × 24 cm. The X-ray beam is collimated into a narrow slot to match this format" (Pisano & Yaffe, 2005). For this reason, this system is also referred to as a slot-scanning DM system and it "has a distinct advantage over the area detectors in that it is very compact and therefore the detector assembly costs less. Also the system has excellent scatter rejection due to the small breast volume exposed at any time. The need for a grid does not arise in these systems, thereby reducing the overall breast dose. However, these systems need powerful X-ray tubes and generators and elaborate signal readout and image reconstruction. Also, relative to other mammography systems, the system requires longer breast compression" (Mahesh, 2004). An example of this type of DM system based on this type of digital detector is the SenoScan manufactured by Fischer Medical Imaging in Denver, Colorado.

Computed Radiography DM System

Computed radiography was introduced around 1981 by Fuji Medical Systems and has found widespread applications in general radiographic imaging. Fuji, however, has extended its use to mammographic imaging. As noted earlier, this is the only DM system that has not been approved by the FDA; however, since it is being used in Europe and Japan its essential elements will be described here.

The basis for CR is photostimulable luminescence. This means that when photostimulable phosphors such as barium flurohalides (barium fluorobromide, for example) are exposed to X-rays, electrons are raised to a higher energy state and are stored as a latent image. To render this latent image visible, the phosphor is exposed to a laser light and the electrons return to their original state. In doing so, light is emitted and subsequently converted into electrical signals that are digitized for computer processing to produce a CR image. As described in earlier chapters, the phosphor is deposited on a special support called the imaging plate (IP) that can be placed in a cassette and looks similar to a film-screen cassette; however, the IP replaces the film, and it can be used again and again for several hundred exposures.

The typical CR digital mammography system is illustrated in Figure 7-7. There are three steps. First, the IP is exposed to X-rays to produce a latent image. The IP is then taken to the CR image reader, or processor, as it is often referred to. A laser beam scans the IP in a systematic fashion (to render the latent image visible) as illustrated in Figure 7-6, labeled Type 3, and the light emitted as a result of laser scanning is collected by a light guide and sent to a digital processor, which produces a CR digital image. In step three, the IP is exposed to a high intensity light, which erases the plate, thereby making it ready for another exposure.

As noted by Pisano and Yaffe (2005), the "potential advantages of this technology are the small detector element size, the fact that the plates can be used in any mammography unit, the ease of having multiple plate sizes, and the relatively low cost. Potential weaknesses are loss of spatial resolution due to scattering of the laser light during readout, which can cause adjacent areas of the phosphor to discharge; the difficulty of correcting flat-field corrections; the need to spend technologist time on processing and printing of images; and the addition of noise associated with low collection efficiency of emitted light."

Flat–Panel Amorphous Selenium (a–Se) DM System

Yet another type of DM system commercially available for clinical use is one that is based on the flat-panel a-Se detector system shown in Figure 7-6, labeled Type 4. It is clearly apparent that the major difference between this system and the others mentioned above is that the components of this system allow for a direct conversion of X-rays to electrical signals, eliminating the light conversion process. Some authors refer to these DM systems as direct conversion systems.

The detector system consists of a thin layer of a photoconductor, a-Se, deposited onto a readout layer of electronics. This layer (laid down upon a glass support) is similar to the phosphor flat-panel system described above; however, "the photodiodes are replaced by a set of simple electrode pads to collect the charge" (Pisano & Yaffe, 2005). When X-rays fall upon the a-Se layer, an electric charge is released and readout using an electric field. The electrical signal generated is then digitized and computer processed to produce a digital image of the breast. An example of this type of DM system based on the a-Se flat-panel digital detector is the Lorad Selenia DM system manufactured by Hologic, Inc., Bedford, MA.

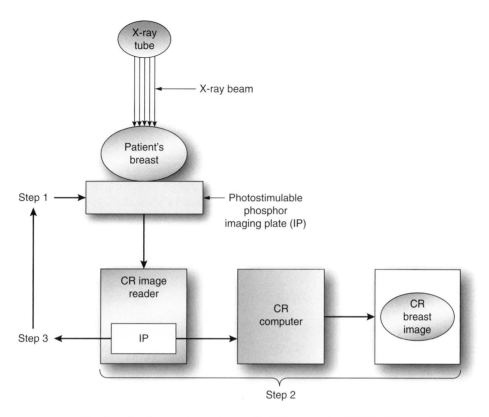

FIGURE 7-7. The three fundamental steps in a typical CR system for DM. The IP is considered the digital detector in a CR imaging system.
Source: *Delmar, Cengage Learning*

Digital Image Post-Processing Techniques

The basic concepts of digital image processing were described in Chapter 2. In this section, digital image post-processing techniques specific to DM will be presented. Once the image is displayed on a monitor for viewing, the observer can now apply digital image post-processing techniques (Seeram & Seeram, 2008). James (2004) points out that "image processing is designed to optimize the quality of the output, but it should be remembered that sub-optimal image processing and display has the potential to result in image degradation and misdiagnosis."

In Chapter 2, digital image processing techniques were described in detail. These techniques, or

operations as they are often referred to, can be classified into three types: point-processing operations, such as grayscale processing (windowing, image subtraction, and temporal averaging); local processing operations (such as spatial filtering, edge enhancement, and smoothing); and global operations such as the Fourier transform (FT). These processing algorithms can also be applied to DM; however, there are processing operations that are specific to DM.

Specific Image-Processing Algorithms for DM

There are several image-processing algorithms developed specifically for use in DM systems, and, more importantly, manufacturers have developed algorithms specific to their systems; several individuals

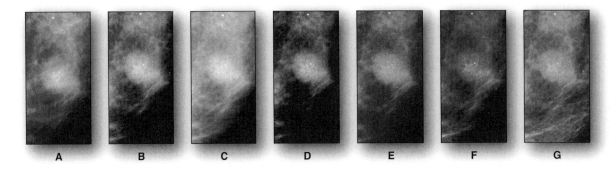

FIGURE 7-8. The visual effects of seven digital image processing algorithms for use in DM (A) cyst on mammogram; processes with M1W1 (B); H1W (C); MM1W (D); CLAHE (E); unsharpe masking (F); and peripheral equalization (G). Source: *Pisano, E., Cole, E., Hemminger, B., Yafee, M., Aylward, S., Maidment, A., et al. (2000). Image Processing Algorithms for Digital Mammography: A Pictorial Essay.* Radiographics, 20, 1479–1491. Reproduced by permission of RSNA

have also developed others independently. Pisano, Yafee, and Kuzmiak (2004), for example, have described seven of these algorithms. These include manual intensity windowing (MIW), histogram-based intensity windowing (HIW), mixture-model intensity windowing (HMIW), contrast-limited adaptive histogram equalization (CLAHE), unsharp masking, peripheral equalization, and Trex processing. The visual effects of these algorithms are illustrated in Figure 7-8.

While it is not within the scope of this chapter to describe the details of each of these, Pisano, Cole, Hemminger, Yaffe, Aylward, and Maidment (2000) provide a comprehensive summary description of each as follows:

"Manual intensity windowing can produce digital mammograms very similar to standard screen-film mammograms but is limited by its operator dependence. Histogram-based intensity windowing improves the conspicuity of the lesion edge, but there is a loss of detail outside the dense parts of the image. Mixture-model intensity windowing enhances the visibility of lesion borders against the fatty background, but the mixed parenchymal densities abutting the lesion may be lost. Contrast-limited adaptive histogram equalization can also provide subtle edge information but might degrade performance in the screening setting by enhancing the visibility of nuisance information. Unsharp masking enhances the

sharpness of the borders of mass lesions, but this algorithm may make even an indistinct mass appear more circumscribed. Peripheral equalization displays lesion details well and preserves the peripheral information in the surrounding breast, but there may be a flattening of the image contrast in the nonperipheral portions of the image. Trex processing allows visualization of both lesion detail and breast edge information but reduces image contrast."

Future Applications of DM

There are several applications of DM that have been described in the literature and which are intended to assist in not only the detection of breast cancer but also to enhance the diagnostic interpretation skills of the radiologist. These include computer-aided detection and diagnosis, digital tomosynthesis, and contrast-enhanced DM (James, 2004; Mahesh, 2004; Pisano & Yaffe, 2005).

Computer–Aided Detection and Diagnosis

In computer–aided detection and diagnosis (CAD), computer software is used as a tool to provide additional information to the radiologist and other related individuals in order to make a diagnosis. In other words, the computer output is regarded as a "second opinion." The purpose of

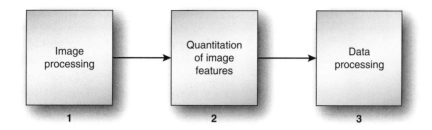

FIGURE 7-9. Three major components of a CAD system for DM: image processing, quantitation of image features, and data processing.
Source: *Delmar, Cengage Learning*

CAD is to improve diagnostic accuracy as well as to improve the consistency of image interpretation using the computer results as a guide.

CAD systems are essentially based on two approaches: those that use location of lesions by using the computer to search for abnormal patterns and those that quantify the image features of normal and/or abnormal patterns (Erickson & Bartholmai, 2002; Lemke, 2005). CAD has been applied to screening and diagnostic mammography, chest radiography, chest CT, cardiovascular systems, neuroradiology, virtual colonography, pediatric radiology, and to the musculoskeletal system.

There are three major technical components of a CAD system: image processing, quantitation of image features, and data processing, as shown in Figure 7-9. It is not within the scope of this chapter to describe these in any detail; however, the following points are noteworthy.

Image Processing

The computer uses image-processing algorithms for enhancement and extraction of lesions. This process allows the computer (not the human) to pick up initial lesions and suspicious patterns. To perform this task, a number of processing operations have been used, such as filtering baser, Fourier analysis, artificial neural networks, wavelet transform, etc., to enhance and extract lesions.

Quantitation of Image Features

Quantitation involves at least three steps to distinguish between lesions and normal anatomical structures. The first step in quantifying features in the image is to select size, contrast, and shape of candidates. The second step uses image features that have been used by radiologists for years, because diagnostic accuracy is generally high and reliable. Quantitation finds unique features that can be readily distinguished reliably between a lesion and other normal anatomical structures.

Data Processing

The third component of CAD systems is data processing. Data processing uses techniques such as rule-based methods and other approaches such as discriminant analysis, artificial neural networks, and the decision-tree method to distinguish between normal and abnormal patterns based on features obtained in quantitation (Erickson & Bartholmai, 2002; Lemke, 2005). These methods are beyond the scope of this text, and will not be described here.

Commercial Systems

Two CAD systems commercially available for use in Radiology are the R2 "Image Checker," R2 Technology from R2 Technology, Inc., Los Altos, California; and the CADx "Second Look," CADx Medical Systems, Quebec, Canada.

Digital Tomosynthesis

Digital tomosynthesis is a technique that uses the principles of conventional tomography to produce tomographic images that are intended to enhance the conspicuity of lesions by blurring out structures above and below the layer of interest. The basic principles of digital tomosynthesis are

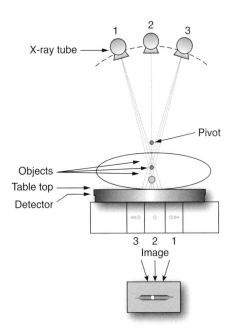

FIGURE 7-10. The basic principles of digital tomosynthesis
Source: *Pisano, E. D. & Yaffe, M. J. (2005). Digital Mammography. Radiology, 234, 353–362. Reproduced by permission of RSNA*

without superimposition. This is accomplished by the image reconstruction process as shown in Figure 7-11b in which images obtained in separate planes are added to produce the final image of the objects of interest. Note that the diamond image is sharp and the oval image is also sharp and free of superimposition.

For a more detailed account of digital tomosynthesis the interested reader should refer to the book by Pisano, Yaffe, and Kuzmiak (2004).

Contrast–Enhanced DM

Digital mammography can be used in visualizing angiogenesis (appearance of new vasculature in a tumor) by using an iodinated contrast medium. This technique has been described by Pisano and Yaffe (2005), who point out that after obtaining a mask (scout) image of the breast, several iodinated contrast images (contrast medium-enhanced) are recorded. Using computer processing, the mask image

illustrated in Figure 7-10. As can be seen, the X-ray tube moves through various angles (three in this case) while the detector is stationary. In this manner, several images are recorded and stored. Subsequent image reconstruction and image processing by the computer renders the objects located at different planes in the patient clearly visible on the image.

The imaging technique for breast tomosynthesis is further elaborated in Figure 7-11, which shows two methods of acquiring data, namely the step-and-shoot method (Figure 7-11a) and the continuous exposure method (Figure 7-11b). In both methods the X-ray tube travels in an arc during the exposure to acquire data while the image detector remains stationary (in some systems the detector may be moving as well). As clearly illustrated in Figure 7-11a, there are two objects that are of interest in the imaging process, the diamond- and oval-shaped objects, which are located at different levels in the breast. These objects are superimposed on the image as shown in Figure 7-11b. The next step is to render each of the objects clearly visible

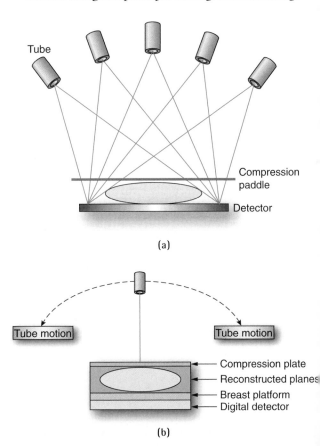

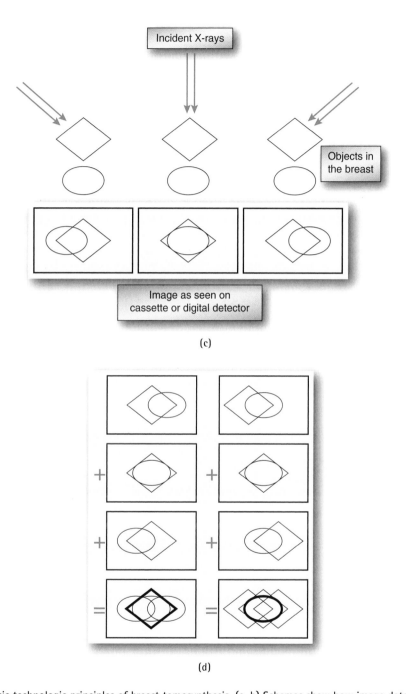

(c)

(d)

FIGURE 7-11. Basic technologic principles of breast tomosynthesis. (a, b) Schemas show how image data are acquired from various angles as the X-ray tube moves in an arc. Either the step-and-shoot method (a) or the continuous exposure method (b) may be used, and the detector may be moving or stationary during image acquisition. The 3D-image data are subsequently reconstructed as conventional mammographic projections (craniocaudal, mediolateral oblique, and mediolateral views). (c, d) Diagrams show how different 3D image data acquired from different angles (c) are reconstructed to provide separate depiction of two overlapping structures located in different planes (d).
Source: *Park, J. M., Franken, E. A., Garg, M., et al. (2007). Breast Tomosynthesis: Present Considerations and Future Applications. Radiographics, 27, S231–S240. Figure and legend reproduced by permission of RSNA and the authors*

is subtracted from the contrast medium-enhanced images to produce another set of images "showing the conspicuity of the uptake of iodine in the vicinity of the lesion" (Pisano & Yaffe, 2005).

DM Clinical Trials

In order to compare the clinical usefulness of a new technique with existing techniques, it is essential to conduct clinical trials. In this regard, several studies have been conducted and the results have been summarized by Pisano and Yaffe (2005); Mahesh (2004); and James (2004). In general, the results of these clinical trials indicate that "there is insufficient evidence to permit conclusions about the superiority of DM compared to F-S Mammography in screening for breast cancer" (Mahesh, 2004).

More recently, however (October 2005), the results of a large clinical trial called the Digital Mammographic Imaging Screening Trial (DMIST) were reported. The goal of this study was to compare the diagnostic performance of DM with F-S mammography for breast cancer screening. This study examined 49,528 asymptomatic women who presented for breast cancer screening in the United States and Canada. Although the methodology will not be reported here, it is interesting to note that the results of this study showed that "the overall diagnostic accuracy of digital and film mammography as a means of screening for breast cancer is similar, but digital mammography is more accurate in women under the age of 50 years, women with radiographically dense breasts, and premenopausal or perimenopausal women" (Pisano, Gatsonis, Hendrick, Yaffe, Baum, & Acharyya, 2005).

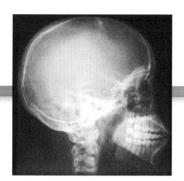

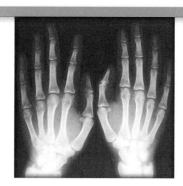

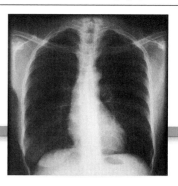

REVIEW QUESTIONS

1. List the limitations of screen-film mammography.
2. Explain what is meant by digital mammography.
3. List the advantages of digital mammography.
4. Draw a diagram of a digital mammography imaging system, label its components, and explain the purpose of each component.
5. List four types of digital detectors used for mammography.
6. Explain how the CsI a-Si TFT detector works.
7. What are the differences between a CCD detector and a CR detector used for digital mammography?
8. Explain how the a-Se digital detector for mammography works.
9. What is the purpose of image post-processing in digital mammography?
10. List several image post-processing operations currently used in digital mammography.
11. What is CAD? Explain how it works.
12. What is digital tomosynthesis? What is its primary purpose in digital mammography?

REFERENCES

Bushong, S. (2009). *Radiologic Science* (8th ed.). St Louis, MO: Mosby Inc.

Bushberg, J., Seibert, A., Leidholdt, E. Jr., & Boone, J. (2004). *The Essential Physics of Medical Imaging.* (2nd ed.). Philadelphia, PA: Lippincott Williams & Wilkins.

Erickson, B. & Bartholmai, B. (2002). Computer-Aided Detection and Diagnosis at the Start of the Third Millennium. *Journal of Digital Imaging, 15,* 59–68.

Huda, W., & Slone R. (2002). *Review of Radiologic Physics.* (2nd ed.). Philadelphia, PA: Lippincott Williams & Wilkins.

James, J. J. (2004). The Current Status of Digital Mammography. *Clinical Radiology, 59,* 1–10.

Lemke, H. (Ed.). (2005). Computer Aided Diagnosis. *British Journal of Radiology, 78,* Special Issue.

Mahesh, M. (2004). Digital Mammography-Physics Tutorial for Residents. *Radiographics, 24,* 1747–1760.

Park, J. M., Franken, E. A., Garg, M., Fajardo, L. L., & Niklason, L. T. (2007). Breast Tomosynthesis: Present Considerations and Future Applications. *Radiographics, 27,* S231–S240.

Pisano, E. (2000). Current Status of Full-Field Digital Mammography. *Radiology, 214,* 26–28.

Pisano, E., Cole, E., Hemminger, B., Yafee, M., Aylward, S., Maidment, A., et al. (2000). Image Processing Algorithms for Digital Mammography: A Pictorial Essay. *Radiographics, 20,* 1479–1491.

Pisano E. D. and Yaffe M. J. (2005). Digital Mammography. *Radiology, 234,* 353–362.

Pisano, E., Yaffe, M. J., & Kuzmiak, C. M. (2004). *Digital Mammography.* Philadelphia, PA: Lippincott Williams & Wilkins.

Pisano, E., Gatsonis, C., Hendrick, E., Yaffe, M., Baum, J., & Acharyya, S., et al. (2005). Diagnostic Performance of Digital versus Film Mammography for Breast-Cancer Screening. *New England Journal of Medicine, 353,* 1–11.

Samei, E. (2005). Technological and Psychological Considerations for Digital Mammography Displays. *Radiographics, 25,* 491–501.

Seeram, E., & Seeram, D. (2008). Image Postprocessing in Digital Radiology: A Primer for Technologists. *Journal of Medical Imaging and Radiation Sciences, 39*(1), 23–43.

Smith A. (2005). *Fundamentals of Digital Mammography: Physics, Technology, and Practical Considerations,* Bedford, MA: Hologic Inc.

CHAPTER 8

Picture Archiving and Communication Systems

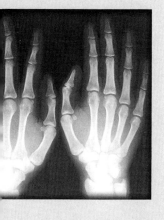

OBJECTIVES

Upon completion of this chapter, the student should be able to:

1. Define the term picture archiving and communication systems (PACS)

2. Trace the historical development of PACS

3. Identify the image acquisition modalities that are connected to the PACS

4. Identify the types of computer networks and describe the elements of each type

5. Explain how images are stored in the PACS

6. State the purpose of image compression in digital imaging

7. Identify and describe briefly two types of compression used in digital imaging

8. Explain briefly what is meant by a display and analysis workstation

9. Identify the basic elements of four types of display workstations available in a PACS environment

10. State the purpose of the RIS/PACS broker and the web server in a PACS environment

11. State what is meant by the term workflow and explain the influence of PACS on the workflow in the imaging department

12. State the purpose of system integration and explain how information systems are integrated with the PACS

13. Explain what is meant by DICOM and explain the bare essentials of DICOM

14. State the problems associated with DICOM and HL-7 and how the IHE has helped to overcome these problems

15. State the meaning of the term "enterprise-wide image distribution"

16. List the basics of four remote-access technological approaches to enterprise-wide image distribution that meet the challenges of effective image distribution

17. Identify several different types of activities that can be accommodated by PACS used in an educational institution

18. Explain briefly the two U.S. Federal Acts that are intended to regulate PACS

19. Discuss the evolving role of the technologist as informaticist

KEY TERMS

Analysis workstation

Application service provider model

Bandwidth

Bridge

Communication protocol

Compression ratio

Computer network

Desktop workstation

Digital Imaging and Communication in Medicine (DICOM)

DICOM conformance statements

DICOM objects

DICOM service class

Digital linear tape (DLT)

Display workstation

Enterprise-wide image distribution

Hardcopy workstation

Health Insurance Portability and Accountability Act (HIPAA)

High-resolution display workstation

Health Level-7 (HL-7)

Image acquisition modalities

Image data set

Image display

Information systems

Information technology (IT)

Integrating the Healthcare Enterprise (IHE)

Integration

Internet

Intranet

Joint photographic experts group (JPEG)

Link

Local area network (LAN)

Long-term storage

Lossless compression

Lossy compression

Medium-resolution display workstation

Nearline storage

Network protocol

Network security

Node

Offline storage

Online storage

PACS administrator

Partnership model

Provider

Query/retrieve

Redundant array of independent disks (RAID)

Random-access memory (RAM)

RIS/PACS broker

Router

Service class provider (SCP)

Service class user (SCU)

Short-term storage

Storage technologies

Turnkey model

Wide area network (WAN)

Workflow

Introduction

The previous chapters described data acquisition modalities for digital radiography and fluoroscopy, as well as digital mammography. These modalities generate a very large number of digital image files. For example, a CR examination consisting of two images with an image size of 2048 × 2048 × 12 will result in 16 MB of data. A digital mammography examination can now generate 160 MB of data. Additionally, the number of images generated in a multislice CT examination can range from 40 to 3000; if the image size is 512 × 512 × 12, then one examination can generate 20 MB of data and up. All digital X-ray imaging modalities, as well as MRI, generate very large amounts of digital images that result in what has been referred to as a "data explosion." Huang (2004) points out that "the number of digital medical images captured per year in the US alone is over pentabytes, that is, 10^{15}, and is increasing rapidly every year."

These data files must be handled in such a manner that they can be easily displayed for viewing and interpretation, stored, and retrieved for retrospective analysis, and be transmitted to remote locations within a health care facility, and to remote institutions, for the general management of the patient's medical condition. In the digital imaging environment, one of the central means of addressing this particular challenge requires the use of a picture archiving and communication systems (PACS). PACS is now an important and significant tool in the digital radiology department (Nagy, 2007) and therefore it is mandatory for technologists to have a firm understanding of the fundamental principles and technologies operating in a PACS environment. This is an essential element for effective and efficient use of the system.

The purpose of this chapter is to present a broad overview of the major components and technologies involved in PACS, as well as to lay the foundations needed for the study of radiology informatics, the application of information technology (IT) to radiology.

PACS: A Definition

What is PACS exactly? Some individuals believe that perhaps it should be called IMACS (image management and communication systems); however, the more popular acronym is PACS.

Mosby's Medical Dictionary (2009) defines PACS as "a network of computers used by radiology departments that replaces film with electronically stored and displayed digital images. It provides archives for storage of multimodality images, integrates images with patient database information, facilitates laser printing of images, and displays both images and patient information at work stations throughout the network. It also allows viewing of images in remote locations."

In a recent article published in *Biomedical Instrumentation and Technology*, McGeary (2009) defines PACS as "a network-based, central server used for interfacing, image storage, and data acquisition of images produced by a myriad of radiology modalities that exist in hospitals today."

These definitions imply that PACS is a digital radiology computer-based system or medical device where images acquired from a patient are

1. Displayed on monitors for viewing and subsequent digital image post-processing
2. Stored and archived in electronic form
3. Transmitted to other locations via computer communication networks

Each of these will be described later in the chapter.

Historical Development

The research leading to the development and implementation of PACS is quite involved and dates back several years. In 1970, for example, Dr Paul Capp introduced the term "digital radiology." Later, in 1980, Heinz Lemke, in Berlin, introduced the notion of digital image communications. From 1982 to 2002, several conferences and meetings were presented, all dealing not only with the feasibility of the technology to accomplish filmless radiology but also the technical elements and economics of full implementation. Today, PACS continue to evolve at a rapid rate, and the technology is becoming more and more commonplace in radiology departments all over the world.

Dr Huang (2004) has categorized PACS into five models based on how they are implemented:

1. The **Home-Grown Model**: This is a PACS developed by the radiology department and hospital using technical components from various manufacturers to suit the needs of the hospital.

2. The **Two-Team Effort Model**: This model is based on collaboration of individuals from both outside and inside the hospital to address PACS specifications and a manufacturer to address implementation issues related to the PACS.

3. *The Turnkey Model:* In this model, the PACS is developed by a manufacturer who sells it to a hospital and accepts full responsibility for implementing the system for use by technologists, radiologists, biomedical engineers, medical physicists, and other related personnel such as information technology (IT) staff.

4. *The Partnership Model:* In this model the manufacturer and the hospital work together to ensure the optimum performance and integrity of the system via training for personnel, upgrading, and general system maintenance.

5. *The Application Service Provider (ASP) Model:* In this model, "a system integrator provides all PACS-related service to a client, which can be the entire hospital or practice group. No IT requirements are required by the client" (Huang, 2004).

Early PACS were based on the use of the UNIX operating system for display and processing workstations. The user interfaces posed several problems for the user, since they were not intuitive. The lack of PACS interfacing to information systems such as radiology information systems (RIS) and hospital information systems (HIS) resulted in workflow problems, such as the delivery of data to specific locations at specific times, a function carried out by technologists in a film-based imaging department.

Today, these problems have been solved; however, PACS are always in a state of evolution for the purpose of improving performance efficiency. For example, the development and refinement of enabling technologies such as communication standards, computer and networking speeds, storage and archival devices, PACS work flow and image management technologies, and PACS/RIS/HIS integration, are ongoing activities. A very recent initiative is Integrating the Health Care Enterprise (IHE). The purpose of IHE is to ensure that all digital imaging systems and information systems from different vendors can communicate with each other using communication standards to integrate all patient clinical information for the purpose of viewing such information collectively. IHE will be described later in this chapter.

Last, but certainly not least, we have seen the evolution of a "PACS administrator," a technologist who should be well-versed in the language of PACS in order to meet the needs of the technologies required for a filmless imaging department. It will be useful for the PACS administrator and all radiologic technologists to be well educated in medical informatics and, in particular, radiology informatics (the application of IT to radiology operations).

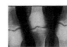

PACS: Major Components and Core Technologies

The major components of PACS and their functional relationships are shown in Figure 8-1. These include digital image acquisition modalities, database/image server, Web server, archive server, short-term and long-term archives, and image-display subsystems, all connected via computer networks, using various gateways and switches. In order to extend their functionality and usefulness, PACS are integrated with RIS and HIS, again through computer communication networks via an RIS-PACS broker and tele-PACS (satellite connection to remote facilities).

Communication and integration of all of these components require the use of communication protocol standards. In this regard, two

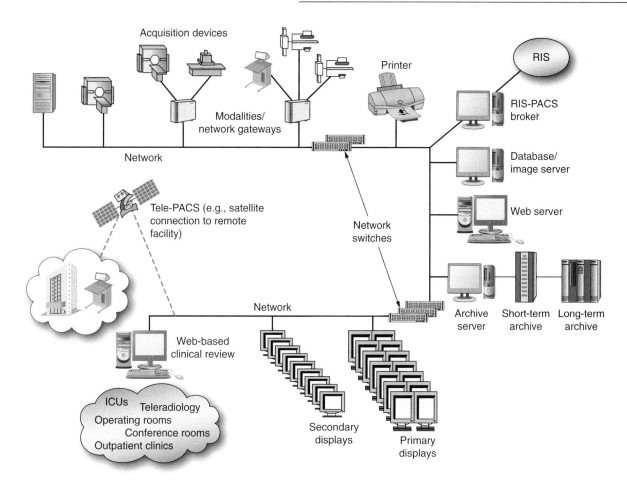

FIGURE 8-1. The major components of PACS and their functional relationships.
Source: Samei, E., Seibert, J. A., Andriole, K., et al. (2004). PACS Equipment Overview. Radiographics 24, 313–334.
Reproduced by permission of RSNA

data standards are now commonplace in a PACS environment:

1. The Digital Imaging and Communication in Medicine (DICOM) standard that essentially addresses the communication of images (image data).

2. Health Level-7 (HL-7) a communication standard configured for information systems, which addresses the communication of textual data, such as patient demographics, admission and discharge transfer, and the type of imaging examinations and radiology reports.

While it is not within the scope of this chapter to elaborate on these two data standards, the bare essentials of DICOM will be highlighted later.

PACS can be classified according to their size and scope. If a PACS is dedicated to a single digital imaging modality such as CR, CT, MRI or US for example, it is usually called a mini-PACS, in which case a single local area network (LAN) is a central feature. This is illustrated in Figure 8-2. On the other hand, PACS can be a large scale system when it includes all the digital imaging modalities that are connected to the digital archive and display workstations and links to a RIS/HIS using either an extended LAN or a wide area network (WAN), as illustrated in Figure 8-1.

Image Acquisition Modalities

To be a part of a PACS, image acquisition modalities must be digital in nature. These include CT, MRI, computed radiography (CR), digital radiography

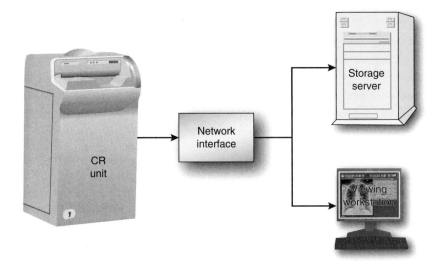

FIGURE 8-2. A mini-PACS, where a single imaging modality (CR) is connected to a storage server and viewing workstations via a local area network.
Source: *Delmar, Cengage Learning*

(DR), Digital fluoroscopy (DF), Digital mammography (DM), film digitizers, nuclear medicine (NM), and ultrasound. Digital image acquisition represents the first point where data and images are entered into a PACS, and, therefore, it is important that such entries are error-free, since "errors generated here can propagate throughout the system, adversely affecting clinical operations" (Andriole, 2002).

Digital image acquisition modalities are of two types: those that are inherently digital, such as CT (Seeram, 2009) and MRI, where the image data is obtained from the scanners at the full spatial resolution and grayscale (bit depth), and those that use frame grabbing. Frame grabbers digitize the analog signals obtained from the image receptor, and images are sent to an image display device such as a cathode ray tube (CRT) monitor for viewing. An example of this is digital fluoroscopy, where the output signal from the charge-coupled device (CCD) is digitized, processed, and sent to the display monitor for image viewing. The frame grabber grabs the same signal and converts it into a digital signal. In this case, image quality is limited to the grayscale resolution of the video signal. Additionally, if the radiology department already has a large number of film images acquired with film-screen cassettes, it may be necessary to convert

these images to digital data. One such device used for this purpose is the film digitizer.

It is not within the scope of this chapter to describe the details of digital image acquisition modalities, including the film digitizer; however, it is important to highlight an important attribute of image acquisition relevant to PACS, namely, image data sets.

Image Data Sets

Image data sets are described in terms of matrix size, inherent spatial resolution, bit depth, number of slices, study sizes, and overall image quality. Clinical image acquisition requirements show huge increases in image data sets that must be handled by the PACS.

Therefore, to be efficient and effective in operating with these data sets and distributing images, there are other issues that must be addressed, such as image compression, which will be described shortly.

Computer Networks

As can be seen in Figure 8-1, the hardware components of PACS and the associated information systems (RIS/HIS) are all connected. These connections are made possible via computer networks.

Essentially, these networks allow information to be transferred and shared among computers and consist of both hardware components and the necessary software to enable the hardware to function. Networking is a complex topic and therefore only the basic concepts will be outlined in this chapter.

First, networks can be discussed in terms of local area networks (LANs) or wide area networks (WANs). The basis for this classification is the distance covered by the network. A LAN for example, connects computers that are separated by short distances such as within a radiology department, a building, or two or more buildings. A WAN, on the other hand, connects computers that are separated by large distances, such as in another state or country. The Internet is a perfect example of a WAN. The network topologies for LANs include bus, star, or ring, as shown in Figure 8-3.

In the bus configuration, computers (nodes) are connected via a single cable, as opposed to the star configuration, where all computers are connected to a central or host computer called a hub. Finally, in the ring topology, a computer is connected to two adjacent computers and all computer connections form a ring.

In general, computers are connected by wires (coaxial cables, optical fiber cables) or wireless connections (radiowave, microwave and satellite links) capable of transferring data at different rates. This data transfer rate of the network is called the bandwidth. The bandwidth will vary depending on the physical connection between computers. The unit of bandwidth is megabits per second (1Mbps = 10^6 bps) or gigabits per second (1Gbps = 10^9 bps).

Information sent through the network is divided into packets of fixed or variable sizes sent via switching devices to the appropriate computer (or other switching devices) on the network. An individual device is referred to as a node, and the connections among nodes are called links. Other hardware components such as bridges and routers play an important role in sending the packets and ensuring that they get to the correct destination computer.

In order for information to be communicated through the network, network protocols are significant to this task. These are communication protocols that must be executed by the hardware and software. One such popular protocol in a PACS environment is the transmission control protocol/Internet protocol (TCP/IP) (actually two protocols, the TCP and the IP). TCP divides the information to be transferred into packets.

Networks often feature a dedicated computer (that is, of course, part of the network) capable of providing various services such as data storage (file server), printing (print server), e-mail (e-mail server), and web access (web server).

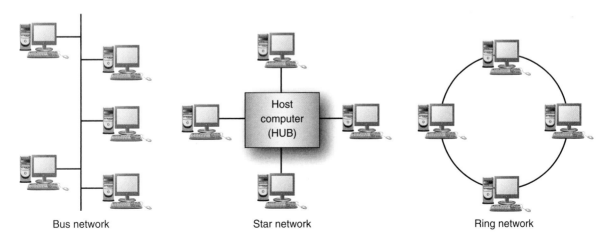

Bus network   Star network   Ring network

FIGURE 8-3. Three network topologies for LANs.
Source: *Delmar, Cengage Learning*

In the case of very large computer networks, LANs can be linked using devices referred to as bridges, the result of which generates an extended LAN. Additionally, routers are used to connect larger and separate networks. The Internet is the largest network of networks. Finally, an intranet is another type of network based on TCP/IP and used within a single organization, such as the radiology department. Another important network concept is long distance telecommunication links. These links are classified according to their data transfer rate, among other things.

The slowest and cheapest link is a telephone modem, with transfer rates of 56 kilobytes/sec (kbps). Others include integrated services digital network (ISDN–128 kbps); digital subscriber line (DSL–up to about 1.5 Mbps); cable modems (500 kbps–10 Mbps); point-to-point links such as T1 (1.544 Mbps) and T3 (44.7 Mbps); and optical carriers (OC) that use optical fibers for data transmission (OC 1 = 51.84 Mbps OC 3 = 155 Mbps) (Bushberg et al., 2004).

The transfer times for images to get to their destination is of vital importance to radiologists, and therefore the type of network technology and bandwidth used is an essential element that must be considered when implementing PACS. The typical maximum image transfer times, bandwidths, and network technologies, are shown in Table 8-1.

One final concept about networks relevant to this module is that of network security. One can understand the need to safeguard confidential information that can be accessed via computer networks by unauthorized individuals.

In a PACS/RIS/HIS environment, network security is paramount. One major security feature is a firewall. This is "a router, a computer, or even a small network containing routes and computers that is used to connect two networks to provide security" (Bushberg et al., 2004). In addition, privacy, authentication, and integrity are vital security concerns surrounding an electronic radiology department. While privacy or confidentiality ensures access only to persons for whom the information is intended, "authentication permits the recipient of information to verify the identity of the sender and permits the sender to verify the identity of the recipient. Integrity means that the received information has not been altered either deliberately or accidentally" (Bushberg et al., 2004). For an extensive coverage of network security for the radiology enterprise, the student should refer to the paper by Eng (2001).

The PACS Main Computer

Images and data acquired from patients are sent via computer networks to the PACS main computer, which is the heart of the system and consists of a "high-end" computer or server. This computer is sometimes referred to as the PACS controller, the database server (Figure 8-1), or the image

TABLE 8-1. Several Computer Network Technologies, their Bandwidths, and associated Times for Transferring Digital Images.

Network Technology	Bandwidth	Transfer Times	
		Chest Radiograph*	Chest CT Scan[†]
Modem	56 kbits/sec	20 min	2 h
T1	1.54 Mbits/sec	43 sec	4.3 min
Ethernet	10 Mbits/sec	6.7 sec	40 sec
Fast Ethernet	100 Mbits/sec	0.7 sec	4 sec
ATM[†]	155 Mbits/sec	0.4 sec	2.6 sec
Gigabit Ethernet	1 Gbit/sec	0.07 sec	0.4 sec

* 8.4 Mbytes
[†] 50 Mbytes
[†] ATM = asynchronous transfer mode

Source: *Samei E., et al. (2004). PACS Equipment Overview–General Guidelines for Purchasing and Acceptance Testing of PACS Equipment.* Radiographics, 24, 313–334. *Reproduced by permission of the RSNA*

server. Images and patient data (demographics, for example) are then sent from the acquisition gateway computer, the HIS and the RIS, to the PACS controller, which has a database server as well as an archive system.

The PACS computer is well equipped with several central processing units that can process data very quickly and has a good deal of internal memory (both random-access memory (RAM) and cache memory) to assist in handling the vast amounts of data that is input into the computer.

Image Storage

The results of computer processing are information and digital images. The images are then sent through the computer network to various computer workstations where they are generally displayed for viewing and stored temporarily and/or permanently for retrospective viewing and analysis.

As noted earlier, the digital images acquired in a total digital radiology department (filmless imaging) are large files with varying matrix sizes. For example, a typical CR image is about a 2048 × 2048 matrix by 2 bytes per pixel, and a CT image is usually a 512 × 512 matrix by 2 bytes per pixel. These two characteristics alone (matrix size and bit depth) place huge demands not only on storage requirements but also on the speed of transmission over the network.

Current storage technologies for PACS include solid-state memory magnetic data carriers (disk and tapes), and optical disks (Dandu, 2008). Each of these data carriers varies in terms of cost, storage capacity, and access time. While RAM and magnetic disks are expensive, optical and magnetic tape storage are inexpensive. Additionally, while the storage capacities for RAM and magnetic disks are limited, storage capacity is large for optical disks and magnetic tapes. For example, while RAM can be in the MB (1000 kbytes) to GB (1000 Mbytes) range, optical disks and magnetic tapes can store image files in the terabyte (TB-1000 Gbytes) to pentabyte (PB) (1PB = 1000 TB) range.

One popular storage technology used in PACS is the redundant array of independent disks (RAID), which can contain several magnetic or optical disks that can perform as a single large disk drive. The result is an automated library system (ALS), or a

"jukebox." RAIDs are used primarily for short-term storage. In addition, robotic technology is now used to manage the movement of storage media to and from the storage shelves and image reader components.

Digital linear tape (DLT) is usually 0.5-inch magnetic tape that is intended for long-term storage of images. Multiple DLT drives can be arranged to create a "jukebox" similar to the RAID situation. It is important to note here that these image storage components can be connected by a sub-network called a storage area network (SAN), a fiberoptic high-speed network (up to about 100 megabits/sec) sometimes referred to a fiber channel. SAN was designed solely for image storage as shown in Figure 8-4.

Storage can be online, nearline, and offline. While online storage cannot be removed and provides immediate access to images (RAM for example) within seconds, nearline storage is removable (RAID for example) with longer image retrieval times. Offline storage on the other hand, refers to storage devices that must be retrieved by an individual and loaded into a drive for access to images. Offline storage is of course cheap and provides the largest storage capacity.

Image Compression

One effective way to manage the size of image files for transmission and storage is that of image compression (Seeram & Seeram, 2008). Image compression is a topic in itself that is quite complex and beyond the scope of this chapter; however, the following basic facts are noteworthy for radiologic technologists:

a. The purpose of compression is to speed up transmission of information (textual data and images) and to reduce storage requirements.

b. Several image compression methods are available, each providing advantages and disadvantages. Compression can be either

- lossless compression, or reversible compression, where no information is lost in the process, as shown in Figure 8-5A

- lossy compression or irreversible compression, where some information is lost in the process, as shown in Figure 8-5B

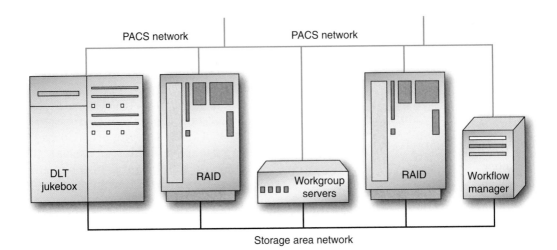

FIGURE 8-4. A dedicated image storage network called a storage area network (SAN) for connecting image storage devices in PACS.
Source: *Delmar, Cengage Learning*

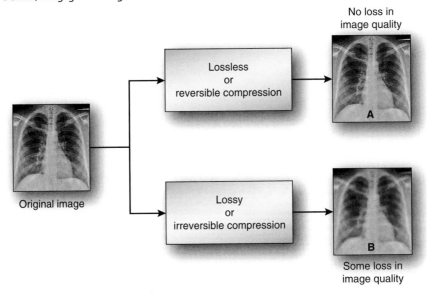

FIGURE 8-5. The visual effect of two image compression methods used in PACS: lossless or reversible compression in which there is no loss in image quality (A), and lossy or irreversible compression in which there is some loss in image quality. Higher compression ratios are possible with the latter.
Source: *Delmar, Cengage Learning*

Joint photographic experts group (JPEG) image compression features both lossy and lossless compression methods. For medical images, JPEG is DICOM's present compression method. Furthermore, JPEG 2000 uses wavelets (wavelet compression) in an effort to decrease the compressed image size and enhance image quality (Mann, 2002; Seeram & Seeram, 2008).

The compression ratio is the element that reduces the size of the image file, and therefore it is a very important variable in studies examining the effects of image compression on image quality.

Huang (2004) provides a brief explanation of compression ratio as follows:

> *"The compression ratio between the original image and the compressed image file is the ratio between computer storage required to save the original image and that of the compressed data. Thus a 4:1 compression on a 512 × x 8 = 2,097,152 bit image, requires only 524,288 bit storage, 25% of the original image storage required. There is another way to describe the degree of compression by using the term bit per pixel (bpp). Thus, if the original image is 8 bpp, a 4:1 compression means the compressed image becomes 2 bpp."*

The size of the compressed image is influenced by the compression ratio (see definition of terms), with lossless compression methods yielding ratios of 2:1 to 3:1 (Huang, 2004), and lossy or irreversible compression having ratios ranging from 10:1 to 50:1 or more (Huang, 2004). It is well known that as the compression ratio increases, less storage space is required and faster transmission speeds are possible, but at the expense of image quality degradation (Chen et al., 2003).

It is also well established that the quality of digital images plays an important role in helping the radiologist to provide an accurate diagnosis. At low compression ratios (8:1 or less), the loss of image quality is such that the image is still "visually acceptable" (Huang, 2004). The obvious concern here is what Erickson (2002) refers to as "compression tolerance," a term he defines as "the maximum compression in which the decompressed image is acceptable for interpretation and aesthetics."

Since lossy compression methods provide high to very high compression ratios compared to lossless methods, and keeping the term "compression tolerance" in mind, Huang (2004) points out that "currently lossy algorithms are not used by radiologists in primary diagnosis, because physicians and radiologists are concerned with the legal consequences of an incorrect diagnosis based on a lossy compressed image." A recent survey of the opinions of expert radiologists in the United States and Canada (Seeram, 2006, 2007), on the use of irreversible compression in clinical practice showed that the opinions are wide and varied. This indicates that there is no consensus of opinion on the use of irreversible compression in primary diagnosis. Opinions are generally positive on the notion of image storage and image transmission advantages of image compression. Finally, almost all radiologists are concerned about the litigation potential of an incorrect diagnosis based on irreversible compressed images.

Display and Analysis Workstations

A display and analysis workstation used in a PACS environment is a computer workstation consisting of hardware and software to facilitate the display of digital images for diagnostic interpretation and for review purposes. The PACS workstation is often referred to as a soft-copy display workstation.

Two types of image display formats are available for these workstations, a portrait display (Figure 8-6A) and a landscape display (Figure 8-6B). While the former displays more pixels in the vertical than horizontal direction, the latter displays more pixels in the horizontal than in the vertical direction.

The generic hardware components of a PACS workstation include a computer system consisting of a central processing unit, RAM, network interface, serial controller, local disk storage, frame buffers, a display controller, and a display device. Display devices can be a cathode-ray tube (CRT) monitor or flat-panel displays. Flat-panel displays have recently become available for PACS and match the display requirements of CRTs; however, they are more expensive than CRTs.

The workstation is an essential component of PACS, since it provides a system-to-user interface. The ultimate goal of a PACS workstation is to provide the radiologist, in particular, with a tool to make a diagnosis and the technologist to assess the overall image quality before the image is sent to the PACS server. Therefore, the workstation must have adequate spatial and contrast resolution, as well as variable brightness and display speeds that facilitate diagnostic interpretation of digital images. It is important to note in this regard that while the viewing task of the radiologist is lesion detection in particular, the viewing task of the technologist is overall image-quality assessment to ensure that the image contains acceptable density and contrast and accurate positioning and is free of artifacts,

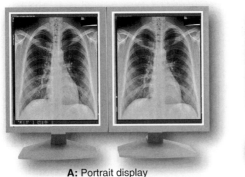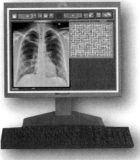

A: Portrait display   **B:** Landscape display

FIGURE 8-6. Two types of image display formats for workstations used in a PACS environment: portrait display (A), and landscape display (B).
Source: *Delmar, Cengage Learning*

all of which will have an impact on the diagnostic interpretation process.

In general, there are at least four types of workstation available in a PACS environment (Hori, 2002):

1. High-resolution display workstations (2.5 K × 2.5 K is not uncommon) used by radiologists for primary diagnosis, since their viewing tasks are fundamentally different to other physicians, medical physicists, and technologists. These are the most expensive of workstations. Higher-resolution monitors (for example, 3 K × 3 K) are now becoming available.

2. Medium-resolution display workstations (1.5 K × 1.0 K is not uncommon) for secondary diagnosis, that is, review function that can be done by radiologists.

3. Desktop workstations for technologists and physicians other than radiologists

4. Hardcopy workstations for image printing. Image printing, however, may eventually become obsolete.

PACS workstations must also be fast enough to retrieve and display images from an archive or an imaging modality to meet the demands of radiologists. For example, it is important to get the workstation to display an image in at least two seconds (Hori, 2002).

Currently, multitasking workstations for PACS can actually let the user perform other tasks, such as interpreting another study, while images are being retrieved. Software for PACS workstations must be intuitive and versatile. Such software facilitates navigation functions, image manipulation functions, and other functions.

A navigation function is one that enables the user of the workstation to find the image or images to be reviewed. Several examples of navigation functions include work list, list all, compare, mark as read, folder display, image icons, consult, next patient (exam), and previous patient (exam), to mention only a few.

Image processing functions (described in Chapter 2) allow users to adjust or manipulate the image to suit their viewing needs. Windowing (grayscale image manipulation) is the most commonly used image-manipulation function. As illustrated in Figure 8-7, the window width (WW = the range of the digital numbers making up the image) and the window level (WL = the center of the range of digital numbers) can be used to alter the image contrast and brightness, respectively. While increasing the WL (for a fixed WW) makes the image darker because more of the lower digital numbers are displayed, decreasing the WL (for a fixed WW) makes the image lighter, since more of the higher digital numbers are displayed (Seeram & Seeram, 2008).

Other image manipulation functions include outlining, boundary detection, region of interest (ROI) cleaning, grayscale invert, undo, pixel statistics, zoom and scroll, various image processing functions (edge enhancement, histogram modification), distance, area, average gray level measurements, and annotation. Equally important are image management functions such as delete, auto delete, print, redirect, scrapbook, and mark for teaching, to mention only a few.

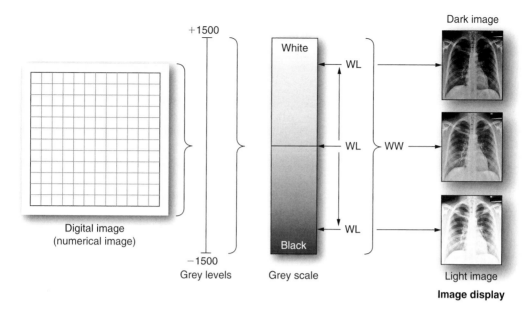

FIGURE 8-7. Windowing can be used to manipulate the image brightness and contrast to suit the needs of the observer.
Source: *Delmar, Cengage Learning*

Since PACS will be a part of the RIS/HIS environment, it is essential that workstations be DICOM compliant. Furthermore, manufacturers should provide a DICOM-conformance statement so that comparisons between devices can be made using the DICOM communication protocol as the basis.

Finally, an important consideration surrounding PACS workstations and their use is that of workstation ergonomics. Ergonomics is the science and art of design that considers not only the physical aspects of the persons using the system but also their mental capabilities in order to reduce unnecessary effort for those using the machine and mistakes that could be made as a result.

Ergonomics considers the design and use of furniture, heat, noise, and lighting in an effort to maximize performance and minimize stress factors such as fatigue and anxiety.

Image Printing

As shown in Figure 8-1, an image printer is part of the components of PACS. Even though the ultimate goal of PACS is a total digital system, some departments may still be printing images to film, for reasons specific to the needs of the department. Today, laser printers are available and they fall into two categories: "wet" printers and "dry" printers. In the early days of PACS development and implementation "wet" printers were common; however, "dry" printers are now commonplace and they have replaced the "wet" printers.

The RIS/PACS Broker

A component of the PACS architecture shown in Figure 8-1 is the RIS/PACS broker. The PACS is concerned primarily with image data, and the RIS deals with textual data such as patient demographics. In order for the PACS and the RIS to communicate with each other, such that patient information for Euclid is linked and associated with Euclid's images, a device is needed that would act as a translator so that communication can be effective and accurate. Such a device is referred to as the "broker," or, more specifically, the RIS-PACS broker. The integration of PACS with information systems (RIS and HIS) will be described subsequently.

The Web Server

The major purpose of the Web Server in PACS is to allow users to access images remotely using Internet browser technology and microcomputers that allow access from within or outside the institution. Several strategies are currently available that provide distribution and display of images throughout the enterprise. These will be described briefly later in this chapter under the heading "Enterprise-Wide Image Distribution."

Workflow in a PACS Environment

In describing radiology operations, the term workflow is often used. This term as noted by Siegel and Reiner (2002), refers to "the movement of patients, images, and information throughout the imaging department and healthcare enterprise." This section will highlight the basic elements of workflow in a PACS environment.

Technologists are all too familiar with workflow in a screen-film radiographic imaging (non-PACS environment) environment, illustrated in Figure 8-8. As shown, there are 59 steps involved from the beginning of the operation (chart is obtained from the radiology clerk) to the end of the operation (review of the report in the chart). In a PACS environment, these steps are reduced to

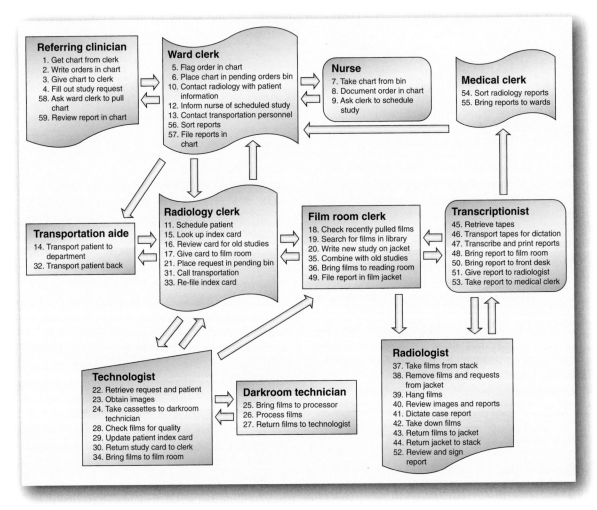

FIGURE 8-8. The workflow in a screen–film radiographic imaging (non–PACS) environment. There are 59 steps involved from the beginning of the operation (chart is obtained from the radiology clerk) to the end of the operation (review of the report in the chart).
Source: *Siegel, E., & Reiner, B. (2002). Work flow redesign: the key to success when using PACS. American Journal of Roentgenology, 178(3), 563–566. Reproduced by permission*

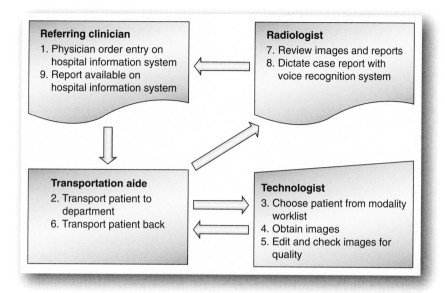

FIGURE 8-9. In a PACS environment, the 59 steps shown in Figure 8-10 are reduced to 9, leading to workflow optimization for digital radiology operations.
Source: *Siegel, E., & Reiner, B. (2002). Work flow redesign: the key to success when using PACS. American Journal of Roentgenology, 178(3), 563-566. Reproduced by permission*

nine, leading to workflow optimization for digital radiology operations, as shown in Figure 8-9.

In a PACS environment, workflow has an impact on clerical personnel, technologists, and radiologists. The ultimate goal of this workflow is to improve patient care and the efficiency of various processes, from patient registration and image acquisition to report generation, archiving, and image/report distribution throughout the health care enterprise. In many cases, there is a need to re-design workflow in a digital radiology department.

It is apparent from the details expressed in Figure 8-9 that, for a logical and smooth flow of images from acquisition to the time they are reported, stored, and distributed, some form of study management is needed. This is accomplished by what is referred to as the folder management function, provided by the PACS software.

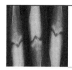

PACS and Information Systems: Integration Overview

While PACS essentially handles images and is usually referred to as an image management

and communication system, it requires other information about a patient (such as the patient demographics, clinical history, previous medical reports, and so forth), in order for the system to be effective and efficient in providing physicians access to all pertinent information during the care and management of the patient. Such information is available from the HIS, RIS, and other information systems that are key components in a digital health care facility. Integration, therefore, serves to combine all the components into a whole system so that they can all communicate with one and other.

A description of PACS is not complete without a discussion of integration of images and information systems. The discussion will focus briefly only on information systems pertinent to digital radiology operations.

Information Systems for Digital Radiology

An information system is a computer-based system that processes data to produce information in a form that can be understood by people using the system in order to solve problems. Several authors, such as Huang (2004), Bushberg et al. (2004), Samei et al. (2004), Dreyer et al. (2002), and Honeyman (1999), have discussed the role of information systems integration in radiology. They have identified at least five separate information systems in an electronic radiology department:

1. PACS
2. RIS
3. HIS
4. Voice-recognition System
5. Electronic teaching/research file system.

Only the RIS and the HIS will be highlighted in this section.

An HIS is a computer-based information system used to gather not only medical information about a patient but also all activities related to the hospital's administration, such as billing, accounting, statistics, personnel, budgets, and materials management, to mention only a few. The major system components for a typical HIS are illustrated in Figure 8-10. The hospital and business component and the hospital operation component are linked, and special software is used to allow the HIS to distribute HL-7 data to other systems external to the HIS.

An RIS is also a computer-based information system that can be a stand-alone system or it can

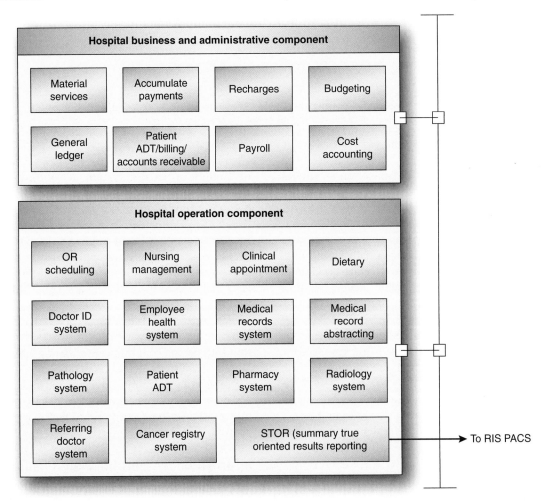

FIGURE 8-10. Major Components of a typical HIS. STOR is a software package (a trade name, other HIS may use a different name) that provides a path for the HIS to distribute HL-7–formatted data to the outside world. Source: *Huang, H. K. (2004). PACS and Imaging Informatics. Wiley–Liss, Hoboken, NJ. Figure and legend reproduced by permission*

be integrated with an HIS. Some of the functions performed by the RIS are:

- patient registration
- Exam scheduling
- Patient tracking
- Film archiving
- Report generation
- Administration and billing
- Documentation
- Inventory control
- Department statistics
- Communication standards.

Systems Integration

The RIS/HIS/PACS must be able to exchange data and information in such a way that it is seamless to technologists, radiologists, and other related personnel in the hospital. The *Oxford Dictionary of Current English* New Edition (1992) states that to integrate means to "combine (parts) into a whole; complete by addition of parts." To perform this task requires a connection, an interface to facilitate communication in order to make up the whole. This interface is a computer program that sets up the rules for communication so that different systems (RIS/HIS/PACS) can exchange data.

As noted by Samei et al. (2004), two types of RIS/HIS integration schemes are available, one that uses a broker and the other that is brokerless and is usually the preferred method. The difference in these two integration schemes is illustrated in Figure 8-11. Systems integration is an ongoing issue in a PACS environment as well as in the digital hospital in general, and currently more research is

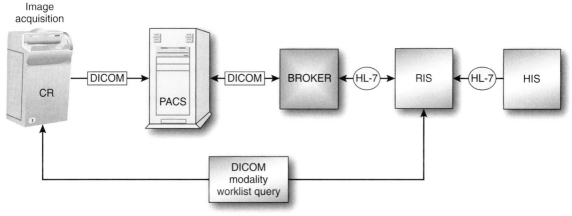

A: Broker technology

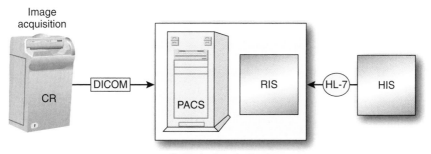

B: Brokerless technology

FIGURE 8-11. Two types of RIS/HIS integration schemes are available, one that uses a broker (A) and the other that is brokerless (B) and is usually the preferred method.
Source: *Delmar, Cengage Learning*

being done by information system vendors and different imaging modality vendors.

Systems integration also requires several elements, all of which play an important role in effective communication among systems. These include a clinical data repository, a data dictionary, mapping, a master patient index, uniform language efforts, and data exchange standards (Hebda, Czar, & Mascara, 2004). Only the last one will be reviewed here.

Integration or Communication Standards for PACS

In order to integrate the two information systems, the RIS and the HIS, several data exchange standards have been developed; however, two standards have become popular and commonplace, especially in the health care enterprise. These are HL-7 and DICOM (Indrajit & Verma, 2007). While HL-7 deals with the flow of textual information between the HIS and the RIS and other information systems, such as nursing information systems (NIS) in the hospital, DICOM deals primarily with the exchange of images in the radiology department and facilitates communication among manufacturer-specific imaging equipment.

In addition, for standards to become commonplace and useful requires the use of some sort of technical framework. Such a framework is that of the IHE (Integrating the Health care Enterprise). Although HL-7 is beyond the scope of this book, DICOM and IHE will be explored briefly.

DICOM: The Bare Essentials

DICOM is complex and its details cannot be described in this chapter. For more comprehensive coverage of DICOM, the student may explore the resources currently available on the Internet. DICOM "specifies a non-proprietary data interchange format and transfer protocol for biomedical images, waveforms, and related information" (Bidgood et al., 1999) and is a "co-operative standard" that enables digital imaging systems to be compatible (Indrajit, 2007).

DICOM was developed in a joint venture between the American College of Radiology (ACR) and the National Electrical Manufacturer's Association (NEMA) that in the early days was referred to as the ACR/NEMA standard 2.0. DICOM is the standard currently used in a PACS environment, simply because it offers

- the specification of a network protocol that runs on top of the Internet standard protocol TCP/IP, allowing DICOM devices to make use of commercial off-the-shelf (COTS) hardware and software;
- the specification of strict requirements on the contents of the image "header" and the form of the pixel data itself for each type of modality, thereby improving interoperability;
- the specification of a conformance mechanism, so that a user can decide whether or not devices are likely to interoperate; and
- an open standard development process that encourages the involvement and consensus of both vendors and users.

What services does DICOM offer for PACS? The answer to this question could be addressed in an entire course on DICOM, since the standard is very large. DICOM is made up of 15 parts, with each part dealing with a specific process. For example, Part 2 deals with conformance issues, Parts 3, 4, and 5 deal with Information Object Definitions, Service Class specifications, and Data Structures and Semantics, respectively, and so on (Whitby, 2007).

DICOM basically specifies

(a) the type of communications referred to as DICOM Service Class

(b) the types of data to be moved around the network and the data format. These are referred to as DICOM Objects (modalities). For example, a DICOM object called CR is a data format for transmitting CR data. Other DICOM objects include CT, MRI, NM, US, and so forth.

DICOM services common to PACS include transfer and storage of images via the network, query and retrieval of images, scheduling of acquisition,

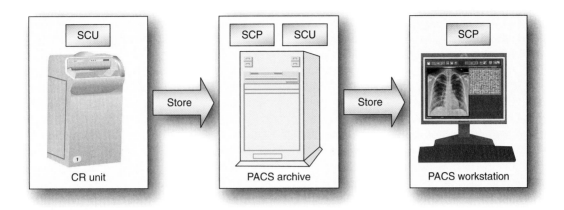

FIGURE 8-12. DICOM communication can involve two devices, one called a *user* and the other a *provider;* hence, the terms *service class user* (SCU) and *service class provider* (SCP). In this basic configuration, a CR unit sends images to a PACS for storage.
Source: *Delmar, Cengage Learning*

completion, notification, image printing, and transferring reports. These services are important to the transfer of image data among various devices in the PACS architecture.

In its most basic configuration, DICOM communication involves two devices, one called a user and the other a provider, hence the terms service class user (SCU), and service class provider (SCP). The Internet provides us with a nice analogue of this type of communication. When you use your computer to access the Internet from anywhere, you are a service user. Your request to access the Internet is answered by your Internet service provider (ISP).

In a simple configuration (Figure 8-12), a CR unit sends images to a PACS for storage. In this case, the PACS is thought of as the provider (SCP), since it provides the storage for the CR images and the CR unit is thought of as the user (SCU), since it uses the storage facility on the PACS; both devices (CR unit and PACS storage) support the DICOM service class-store.

Other configurations exist and can range from several imaging modalities coupled to printers and workstations to a large centralized or a widely distributed PACS architecture.

Other DICOM service classes are available. These include verification, modality work-list

management, performed-procedure step, store, storage commit, print, and query/retrieve. For example, the function query/retrieve can be supported as an SCP and a SCU and can be applied to a number of situations. In a query/retrieve function, an image stored in the PACS archive (SCP) can be sent to a PACS display station (SCU). Another example of query/retrieve function is when the radiologist wants to access the PACS archive and display previous images of a patient on the CT console. These are possible because the modality and the PACS archive support query/retrieve SCU and SCP respectively. In addition, DICOM uses the term "role" to indicate that a device can be either a "user" (SCU) of a service or a "provider" of a service (SCP), as illustrated in Figure 8-12.

Additionally, DICOM specifies information object definitions (IODs) to address what is contained in images (image data and related information) from different imaging modalities. IODs are extremely useful in a PACS environment since images vary in size, acquisition parameters, and textual information.

Another notable element of DICOM is the service object pair (SOP) class, which includes both service class and an IOD. For an MR scanner that sends only MR data to the PACS, for example, the device specifications should show that the service class is store, the role (SCU, SCP) is SCU, and the SOP is MR. Similarly, for a PACS archive that supports DICOM store as a SCU, the device specifications should show that the service class is store, the role (SCU, SCP) is SCP, and the SOP is CT, MR, NM, CR, US, etc.

The last concept to be mentioned here (since this discussion could be extended to an entire course on DICOM) is DICOM conformance statements. These are statements that deal with specific ways of implementation using the services classes, information objects, and communication protocols that are supported. DICOM conformance is a useful specification and implementation strategy.

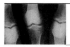

Integrating the Healthcare Enterprise

Problems with DICOM and HL-7

The communication standards DICOM and HL-7 do not address message sequencing and problems that may relate to connectivity of various equipment from different vendors. To solve these problems, Integrating the Healthcare Enterprise (IHE) enters the picture.

IHE Technical Framework

IHE is a standards-based initiative of the Radiological Society of North America (RSNA) and the Healthcare Information and Management System Society (HIMSS). The major role of IHE is to facilitate communications between various computer-based healthcare information systems and imaging modality and PACS vendors through the integrated use of DICOM, which handles mainly image data, and HL-7, which handles textual data exchange. This effort will serve to increase the pace of the digital health care enterprise integration and to remove data redundancy and task repetition by narrowing the information loop between information systems (RIS/HIS, for example) and imaging devices (PACS and image acquisition modalities). It will allow the radiologist, for example, to view relevant patient history, laboratory data, clinical history, and so on, while simultaneously viewing images at the display monitor for diagnostic interpretation.

To accomplish these functions, IHE uses a technical framework built around the following three major components: a data model, actors, and integration profiles. The data model is based on communications standards DICOM and HL-7. Actors are defined by IHE as "information systems or components of information systems that produce, manage, or act on information associated with operational activities in the enterprise" (www.ihe.net). Several actors and their roles are outlined by the IHE and include the patient registration, image acquisition modality, image archive and display systems, image manager, master patient index (MPI), report creator, report manager, print server, post-processing manager, report repository, system scheduler, and order filler.

Integration profiles represent a central feature of IHE specifications. At the time of writing this chapter, there are 12 integration profiles: scheduled work flow, patient information reconciliation, post-processing work flow, charge posting, presentation of grouped procedures, consistent presentation of images, key image notes, simple image and numeric reports, access to radiology information, reporting work flow, evidence documents, and basic security.

The primary function of the IHE integration profiles is to outline the roles of actors in the DICOM and HL-7 environment. For example, the scheduled workflow profile (often viewed as the most important profile) ensures effective communication from the RIS to the imaging modality (via HL-7), which in turn captures the information sent from the RIS using DICOM and subsequently to the PACS, where images from the modality are sent for storage and archiving. The essential point of this example is that if an institution has imaging modalities, PACS, and RIS from different vendors, the IHE scheduled workflow profile ensures that the information exchange (communication) among these different vendor systems is seamless. Additionally, departments purchasing digital imaging equipment, PACS, and RIS systems should ensure that the vendors comply with the IHE profiles.

TABLE 8-2. A comparative overview of health care standards and initiatives relevant to radiology.

Parameter	DICOM	HL-7	IHE
Nomenclature	Digital Imaging and Communications in Medicine	Health Level Seven, Inc.	Integrating the Healthcare Enterprise
Origin	Developed by American College of Radiologists (ACR) and National Electrical Manufacturers Association (NEMA)	Not for profit volunteer organisation headquartered in Ann Arbor MI	Developed by Radiological Society of North America (RSNA) and Healthcare Information Management Systems Society (HIMSS)
Founding Year	1985	1990	1998
Latest Version	DICOM Version 3 (2007)	HL-7 Version 3	Each year new profiles are selected
Role	Provides protocols for integration of image data between imaging, nonimaging modalities, devices and systems	Provides protocols for exchange, management, and integration of varied data in electronic health records	Provides implementation profiles based on existing standards like HL-7 and DICOM
Data	Image information objects and nonimage information objects	Clinical and administrative electronic healthcare data	Functional integration workflow elements
Functional Elements	Protocols, Objects, Services, Service Class, Conformance	Act, Participation, Roles	Actors, Transactions, Integration profiles
Key Area	Image and few nonimage data interoperability	Health record and clinical interoperability	Integration of systems and standards

Source: Indrajit, I. K., & Verma, B. S. (2007). DICOM, HL-7 and IHE. A basic primer on Healthcare standards for radiologists. Indian Journal of Radiology and Imaging, 17, 66-68. Reproduced by permission

A comparative overview of the essential elements of DICOM, HL-7, and IHE is shown in Table 8-2.

Enterprise-Wide Image Distribution

In a PACS environment, it is important to deliver diagnostic reports to referring physicians and specialists in a timely fashion. In the past, physicians relied on the legacy system (a system in which a physician had to go to the radiology department to view films and read reports); however, this classic strategy has been replaced by the remote access concept, or what has been typically referred to as "enterprise-wide image distribution."

There are several approaches to enterprise-wide image distribution that meet the challenges of effective distribution, using four remote access technologies described in Table 8-3 by Samei et al. (2004) These include:

1. Extension of the traditional PACS approach (traditional approach) where images can be sent to all locations in the hospital using the same network, server, and workstation infrastructure.

2. Thin client (web-based) approaches using compressed images. This is a popular strategy.

3. Thin-client approaches using a "just-in-time" data delivery model, that is, instead of compressing the image before transmission, images are delivered only when the user requires them.

4. Compact disk, read-only memory (CD-ROM), where images can be stored and distributed remotely, without the need for computer networks.

TABLE 8-3. Four remote access technologies to enterprise-wide image distribution that meet the challenges of effective distribution.

Technology	Advantages	Disadvantages
PACS Extension	Speed, reliability	Costly, requiring dedicated equipment
Thin Client Web-Based	Relatively low cost, speed, ease of implementation	Possible image quality degradation if compression is applied for speed
Thin Client Just-in-Time	Speed, reliability	Relatively costly, requiring dedicated equipment
CD-ROM*	Low cost, ease of implementation	Slow, low throughput

Source: Samei E. et al. (2004). *PACS Equipment Overview–General Guidelines for Purchasing and Acceptance Testing of PACS Equipment.* Radiographics, 24, 313–334. Reproduced by permission of the RSNA

PACS in an Educational Institution

For the management and care of patients, PACS have been implemented largely in hospitals and clinics where health care and medical information are the primary focus. These systems can also be used for teaching and research purposes.

In an educational environment for medical radiation technologists such as radiological, CT, MRI, ultrasound, and nuclear medicine technologists, as well as radiation therapists, a PACS can prove to be an extremely useful tool for teaching and learning. More importantly, it can serve to prepare students for the interaction with PACS in the hospital.

The architecture of a PACS used for teaching and learning at the British Columbia Institute of Technology (BCIT) Medical Imaging Programs is illustrated in Figure 8-13. The different types of activities that can be accommodated by this system are

1. Students acquire images of phantoms using digital imaging modalities such as CR.

2. These images are assessed for image quality and are then sent to the PACS server and stored for retrospective analysis based on assignments from other courses. For example, in a QC course, the instructor can assign a project whereby the student must access the QC image taken earlier in the laboratory

exercise and evaluate it to meet the needs of the QC assignment.

3. An instructor can access student images for the purposes of assessment of position and techniques requirements covered in a laboratory exercise and/or a theory course assignment.

4. All instructors have access to the PACS server and hence can create teaching files for their respective courses

5. Internet access to the PACS is possible for both instructors and students. Assignments based on images recorded in a laboratory exercise or images discussed in class can now be done at home.

6. Images can be imported form the affiliated hospitals and be housed in the teaching institution's PACS for teaching/learning purposes.

The use of PACS for teaching and learning is an exciting venture and opens up a whole new dimension for both teachers and students.

PACS and Regulatory Approval

PACS is considered a medical device and as such it is subject to federal and other regulations. In the United States, the Food and Drug Administration (FDA) and the Health Insurance Portability and Accountability Act (HIPAA) govern such regulations.

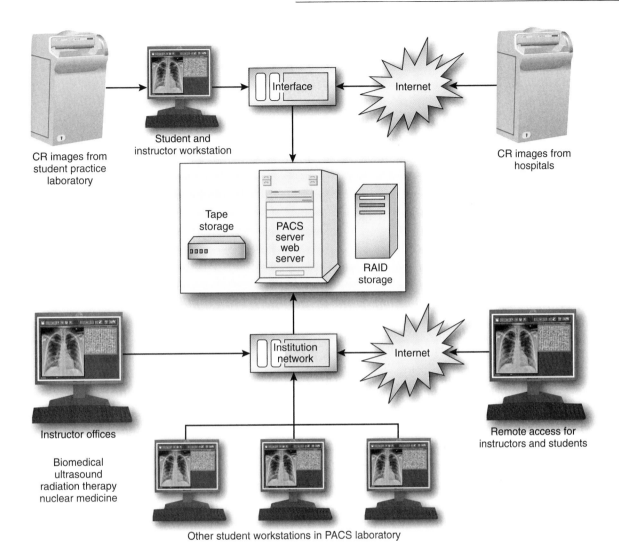

FIGURE 8-13. The framework for a PACS used at the British Columbia Institute of Technology for learning and teaching in several programs in medical imaging, radiation therapy, and biomedical engineering technology.
Source: *Delmar, Cengage Learning*

Food and Drug Administration

The Food and Drug Administration (FDA) notes that medical devices are used for the diagnosis, treatment, and prevention of disease in humans and animals and range from simple devices such as a tongue depressor and a bedpan to more complex devices such as lasers, devices based on micro-chip technology (pacemakers), and radiation emitting devices. Radiation-emitting devices include X-ray equipment, ultrasound, and radiation therapy machines, and so forth.

In the early days of PACS development, FDA approval was not required since PACS was considered accessory equipment to image acquisition modalities. However, with the evolution of more and more sophisticated PACS, the FDA now considers PACS one of the five new classifications for medical image management devices. These are medical devices for image storage, image communications, image digitization, hardcopy images, and PACS.

In summary, PACS are medical devices, and depending on their level of complexity, may require manufacturers to submit a "pre-market approval," or something that the FDA calls a 510 (k), and registration of both the product and the facility (Oosterwijk, 2004).

Health Insurance Portability and Accountability Act

The Health Insurance Portability and Accountability Act (HIPAA) became law in the United States in 1996 in an effort to reform health care by addressing several objectives relating to the protection of the patient's health information, standards for such information, fraud and abuse of such information, and so forth. The act essentially deals with the use and disclosure of such information. Interested readers should refer to the Web site at http://www.hipaaplus.com/abouthippa.htm for further details.

Since PACS stores, archives, and most importantly communicates information with RIS and HIS and to physicians inside and outside the hospital, the HIPPA act is viewed as one intended to protect such information, and essentially places a good deal of importance on the security of electronic data and information. If there is a need to share this information with related parties, then patient permission is required. The interested reader should refer to Oosterwijk (2004) for a more elaborate discussion of HIPPA requirements for PACS.

The Radiologic Technologist as Informaticist: An Evolving Role

The rapid evolution and growth in information systems and technology in health care (RIS/HIS), PAC, and digital imaging modalities (filmless imaging), and notions of enterprise-wide image distribution, ASPs and the IHE, will have an impact on the future role of the technologist in radiology. One such emerging role is that of "informaticist" or "informatician." Both terms have been derived from the popular term "information technology" (IT). IT is defined by the Library of Congress (2002) as

> "the acquisition, processing, storage, and transmission of vocal, pictorial, textual, and numeric information by microelectronics, computers, and telecommunications."

The definition certainly reflects the nature of PACS/RIS/HIS and demonstrates the need for the technologist working in a digital radiology department (filmless imaging) to be IT-literate, that is, to be an informaticist or informatician. Already, we see the technologist assuming the role of "PACS Administrator," a position that demands a good deal of understanding of computer and communication technologies.

PACS Administrator

Digital image acquisition modalities coupled to PACS and enterprise-wide image distribution systems have created the need for personnel trained in IT and computer technology to ensure the integrity of these digital imaging and computer communication systems so as not to comprise patient care and management, image quality, and administrative functions. To address this need, radiology departments have created a new job title, the PACS administrator.

The PACS administrator is usually a senior technologist with some background and interest in computers and IT, or it may be an IT individual from the hospital IT department who provides support to the radiology department and works closely with radiology personnel to maintain system integrity.

The duties of a PACS administrator are tailored to the needs of individual departments depending on the variety of digital image acquisition systems and PACS. The tasks or duties, as Oosterwijk (2004) points out, fall into three major categories: project management, system maintenance, and image and information management. A few examples of specific tasks would be to:

1. Ensure that the PACS is working according to the needs of the department and the system specifications.

2. Check that workstations are functioning properly with optimum display of image brightness and contrast.

3. Assign and update passwords for staff.

4. Set up standards for using the system.

5. Maintain effective communications with other departments using the PACS.

6. Communicate with the facility's information systems (IS) or IT department.

7. Provide ongoing education and training for system users.

8. Liaise with PACS vendors and relate new developments to the facility's administrators and managers.

9. Map workflow.

10. Perform quality control of system components.

PACS Administrator Professional Certification

The PACS administrator role has become so commonplace in digital radiology departments that already efforts are being made to provide certification for individuals interested in assuming this position. One such major effort is that of the PACS Administrators Registry and Certification Association (PARCA). This independent organization plays an active role in not only developing the skill set for PACS Administrators but also providing access to certification examinations.

Skill sets are established by an advisory group with members who have extensive experience and knowledge in PACS and imaging informatics. PARCA offers certificates along two distinct paths. While one path is intended for individuals with a clinical background (radiological technologist, for example), the other path is for individuals with an IT knowledge base. Three types of certification are offered: the Certified PACS Interface Analyst (CPIA), the Certified PACS System Analyst (CPSA), and the Certified PACS System Manager (CPSM). For further details, the interested reader should refer to the PARCA Web site at http://www.pacsadmin.org.

Radiology Informatics Curriculum

In the total digital imaging and digital health care environments, it will become increasingly important that the education and training of radiologic technologists focus on curriculum that includes medical informatics and radiology informatics. Specifically, there should be courses dealing with digital image acquisition technologies, digital image processing, computer hardware and software, networking and connectivity, storage and display technologies, teleradiology, and telemedicine. In other words, programs will have to prepare students to assume the role of technologist as informaticist. This means that educators will also have to assume increasing roles in teaching radiology informatics, or medical imaging informatics, which will be described further in Chapter 9.

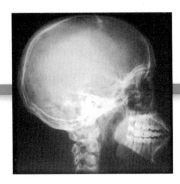
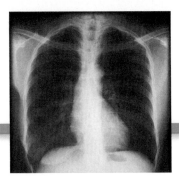
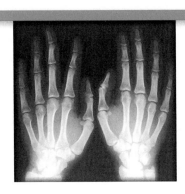

REVIEW QUESTIONS

1. Write out a definition of the term "picture archiving and communication systems" (PACS).

2. Briefly trace the historical development of PACS.

3. Draw and label the major system components of PACS.

4. What are two communication standards used in PACS?

5. Explain what happens when an image is sent to PACS from the image acquisition modality.

6. What is a computer network? List several examples of computer networks.

7. Describe how images are stored in a PACS.

8. What is image compression, and what is its main purpose?

9. Define the term "compression ratio."

10. What are the differences between lossless and lossy image compression?

11. What are the differences among the different types of image display workstations used in a PACS environment?

12. What is the purpose of each of the following:

    a. RIS/PACS Broker

    b. Web server

13. Explain the elements of the term "workflow" in a PACS environment.

14. List five types of information systems used in a digital radiology department/digital hospital.

15. What are the primary characteristics of a radiology information system (RIS)?

16. What is DICOM and what is its purpose in digital imaging?

17. What is IHE and what is its purpose?
18. What is meant by the term "enterprise-wide image distribution"?
19. List four remote access technologies used for enterprise-wide image distribution.
20. What is a PACS administrator? List several tasks of the PACS administrator.

REFERENCES

Arenson, R.L., Andriole, K., et al. (2000). Computers in imaging and healthcare: Now and in the future. *Journal of Digital Imaging, 13*(4), 145–156.

Andriole, K. (2002). Image Acquisition. In K.J. Dreyer, A. Mehta, & J.H. Thrall (Eds.), *PACS: A Guide to the Digital Revolution.* New York: Springer-Verlag New York Inc.

Bidgood, D., Bray, B., et al. (1999). Image Acquisition context. *Journal of the American Medical Informatics Association, 6*(1), 61–75.

Bushberg, JT., Siebert, A., et al. (2002). *The Essential Physics of Medical Imaging.* Williams & Wilkins. Philadelphia, PA.

Chang, P. (1999). Enterprise-wide image distribution. *Decisions in imaging economics,* Vol 1, 15–18.

Clunie, D.A., & Carrino, J.A. (2002). DICOM. In K.J. Dreyer, A. Mehta, & J.H. Thrall (Eds.), *PACS: A Guide to the Digital Revolution.* New York: Springer-Verlag New York Inc.

Dandu, R. V. (2008). Storage media for computers in radiology. *Indian Journal of Radiology and Imaging, 18*(4), 287–289.

Dreyer, K.J. (2002). Enterprise Imaging. In K.J. Dreyer, A. Mehta, & J.H. Thrall (Eds.), *PACS: A Guide to the Digital Revolution.* New York: Springer-Verlag New York Inc.

Emig, D. and Kijewski, J. (2001). The application service providers in health care. *Electomedica, 69*(1), 2–4.

Eng, J. (2001). Computer network security for the radiology enterprise. *Radiology, 220,* 303–309.

Honeyman, J.C. (1999). Information systems integration in radiology. *Journal of Digital Imaging, 12*(2), 218–222.

Hori, S.C. (2004). In K.J. Dreyer, A. Mehta, & J.H. Thrall (Eds.). *PACS: A Guide to the Digital Revolution.* New York: Springer-Verlag New York Inc.

Huang, H.K. (1999). *PACS-Basic Principles and Applications.* New York: Wiley-Liss.

IHE Changing the Way Healthcare Connects (2009) http://www.ihe.net/

Indrajit, I. K. (2007). Digital imaging and communications in medicine: A basic review. *Indian Journal of Radiology and Imaging, 17*(1), 5–7.

Indrajit, I.K., & Verma, B. S. (2007). DICOM, HL-7 and IHE: A basic primer on healthcare standards for radiologists. *Journal of Radiology and Imaging, 17*(2), 66–68.

Kalyenpur, A., Neklesa, V.P., et al. (2000). Evaluation of JPEG and Wavelet compression of body CT images for direct digital teleradiologic transmission. *Radiology, 217,* 772–779.

Mann, S. (2002). Image Compression. In K.J. Dreyer, A. Mehta, & J.H. Thrall (Eds.). *PACS A Guide to the Digital Revolution.* New York: Springer-Verlag New York Inc.

Margolin, K. (2001). Web technology and its relevance to PACS and teleradiology-Take II. *Applied Radiology,* Vol 2, 28–32.

McGeary, D. (2009). PACS-An Overview. *Biomedical Instrumentation & Technology, 343*(2), 127–130.

Mosby's Medical Dictionary (8th ed.). (2009). Elsevier. St Louis, MO.

Nagy, P. (2007). The future of PACS. *Medical Physics, 34*(7), 2676–2682.

Roszkowski, S., Slaughter, R., & Sterling, D. (2000). Acceptable levels of digital image compression in chest radiology. *Australasian Radiology, 44,* 32–35.

Seeram, E. (2009). *Computed Tomography-Physical Principles, Clinical Applications, and Quality Control.* Philadelphia: WB Saunders–Elsevier.

Seeram, E., & Seeram, D. (2008). Image postprocessing in digital radiology: A primer for technologists. *Journal of Medical Imaging and Radiation Sciences, 29*(1), 23–43.

Seeram, E. (2006) Irreversible Compression in Digital Radiology: A Literature Review. *Radiography, 12,* 45–59.

Seeram, E. (2007) Using Irreversible Compression in Digital Radiology: A preliminary study of the opinions of radiologists. *Progress in Biomedical Optics and Imaging-Proceedings of SPIE.* San Diego, CA. 245–249

Siegel, E., & Kolodner, R.M. (Eds.). (1999). *Filmless Radiology.* New York: Springer-Verlag New York Inc

Siegel, E., & Reiner, B. (2002). Image Workflow. In K.J. Dreyer, A. Mehta & J. H.,Thrall (Eds.). *PACS: A Guide to the Digital Revolution.* New York: Springer-Verlag New York Inc.

Siegel, E., & Reiner, B. (2002) Radiology reading room design: The next generation. *Applied Radiology,* April, 11–16.

Reiner, B., & Siegel, E. Psychological factors affecting the adoption of PACS. *Applied Radiology,* April, 17–20.

Tucker, D. and Mehta, A. (2002). Storage and Achieves. In K.J., Dreyer, A., Mehta & J. H., Thrall (Eds.). *PACS: A Guide to the Digital Revolution.* New York: Springer-Verlag New York Inc.

Van Bemmel, J.H., & Musen, M.A. (Eds.). (1997). *Handbook of Medical Informatics.* Heidelberg: Springer-Verlag.

Wiggins, R.H., Davidson, H.C., et al. (2001). Image file formats: Past, present and future. *Radiographics, 21*, 789–789.

Wirsz, N. (2000). Overview of IT-Standards in Healthcare. *Electromedica, 68*(1), 21–24.

Whitby, J. (2007). The DICOM standard. BARCO NV, 4-13. Kertnij. Belgium.

Yoshihiro, A., Nakata, N., et al. (2002). Wireless local area networking for linking a PC reporting system and PACS clinical feasibility in emergency reporting. *Radiographics, 22*, 721–728.

What is HIPAA? (2009). Available at http://www.hipaaplus.com/abouthippa.htm.

CHAPTER 9

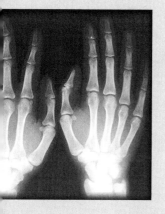

Medical Imaging Informatics: An Overview

OBJECTIVES

Upon completion of this chapter, the student should be able to:

1. Define the term information technology (IT)

2. Identify and describe briefly the main characteristic features of computer hardware and software

3. Identify and describe briefly the main characteristic features of communications technology

4. State the meaning of the term informatics and list several informatics subspecialties

5. Identify the basic elements and scope of health care/medical informatics

6. Define the term medical imaging informatics

7. Identify the major components of a medical imaging informatics framework

8. Explain how PACS fall within the scope of medical imaging informatics

9. Identify the basic elements of health information systems, such as a hospital information system (HIS) and a radiology information system (RIS)

10. Define the term electronic health record (EHR) and identify its major components

11. Discuss the importance of systems integration in a medical informatics environment

12. Explain the basics of IT security in terms of security threats and security methods

13. Discuss the skills and certification requirements of the PACS technologist

14. State the benefits of imaging informatics

KEY TERMS

American Board of Imaging Informatics (ABII)

Algorithms

Certified Imaging Informatics Professional (CIIP)

Communications technology

Computer technology

Electronic health record (EHR)

Framework for MII

Hardware

Health care information systems

Imaging informatics

Information security

Information system

Input

Modem

Output

PACS certification

Processing

Security threats

Software

Storage

Introduction

The term "informatics" is a relatively new term and was derived from the term "information." For computer applications in general, information refers to useful, meaningful, and organized data. In other words, computers convert data into information to be used by humans for solving problems in the real world.

The computer applications in medical imaging described in this book include modalities such as computed radiography (CR), digital radiography (DR) using flat-panel digital detectors, digital mammography (DM), and digital fluoroscopy (DF). These digital imaging methods acquire raw data from the patient that are processed by computers to produce useful information. This information is, of course, the images that radiologists use to make a diagnosis of the patients' medical conditions. In addition, the computer is used to produce textual information that goes hand-in hand with the image information. Subsequently, both types of information are sent to the picture archiving and communication system (PACS) for display, viewing and image processing, storage, and communication to remote sites to other physicians who play an integral role in the medical management of the patient.

The purpose of this chapter is to outline the major elements of imaging informatics, the application of information technology (IT) to imaging. In particular, this chapter will illustrate the contributions of various technologies that enable PACS and digital imaging to participate in the evolution and growth of a new medical subspecialty for the 21st century known as imaging informatics.

Information Technology

The production of vast amounts of information in all walks of life, from the National Aeronautics and Space Administration (NASA) space program to Internet vocations to health care and medical imaging, has created a need for effective and efficient use and management of this information. This task is accomplished through the use of information technology, or, IT as it is popularly referred to.

Definition

IT is currently commonplace in medicine and is routinely used in hospitals, in almost all departments. IT now plays an important and significant role in the digital imaging department. Digital devices must be able to communicate with each other regarding images and textual information, and this function requires the use of IT.

There are several definitions of IT, but one that is perhaps best suited to this chapter is one offered by Williams (2007). He defines IT as "a general term that describes any technology that helps to produce, manipulate, store, communicate, and/or disseminate information." IT, therefore, involves the use of two major technologies, computer technology and communications technology, to solve problems in society.

Computer technology deals with the structure and function of a computer, and how it can be used to solve problems. Communications technology deals with the use of electromagnetic devices and systems for communicating over long distances. (Williams, 2007).

It is not within the scope of this book to describe the details of computer and communication technologies; however, a brief outline of the essential elements of each technology will be provided.

Computer Technology Basics

A computer is an electronic machine for solving problems through the use of a number of characteristic elements. The following points are noteworthy:

- Computers consist of various electronic devices for converting raw data into information in a form that can be used to solve problems.

- A computer is made up of hardware and software. Hardware is the physical components used to process data and software is the computer programs (algorithms) that direct all hardware components to solve problems and thus derive useful practical solutions. Hardware devices include the keyboard and mouse; the central processing unit (CPU); memory chips such as random access memory (RAM); storage devices, such as magnetic disks and tapes and optical disks; and monitors and printers. Software includes system software and applications software. System software refers to operating systems such as Windows NT and XP, MacOS, UNIX, and LINUX; applications software refers to algorithms that perform specific tasks. These include, for example, Microsoft Word® for word processing and Adobe Photoshop® for image processing and manipulation.

- Computers use at least five fundamental operations to process data and disseminate information. These include, in a linear order:

  1. Input. This refers to data entry using hardware devices such as a keyboard or a mouse, etc.

  2. Processing. This involves the use of hardware devices such as the CPU to process data entered into the computer. Processing converts data to information that can be used by human observers to solve problems, such as diagnosing a patient's medical condition.

  3. Storage. Once information is obtained, it can be stored temporarily inside the computer (internal storage or memory) or it can be stored permanently outside the computer (external storage). External storage can hold a larger amount of information than internal storage.

  4. Output. The results of computer processing can be displayed on monitors for viewing by a human observer. For example, computed radiography data from the imaging plate is processed and displayed on a monitor as an image for viewing and interpretation by a radiologist. Output images can be post-processed to enhance the interpretation skills of the radiologist.

  5. **Communications.** Computer data and output information (images for example) can be transmitted to other individuals anywhere in the world, using the Internet, for example, as the communications vehicle.

Communications Technology Basics

Communications technology dates back to 1592 with the invention of the first newspaper in Italy. Popular devices that make use of communications technology include telephones, radios, movie cameras, televisions, cell phones, WebTV, Internet telephones, and wireless services such as Wi-Fi and Bluetooth.

- Computer communications technology consists of the following key elements:

- Modem. This is a contraction for modulate/demodulate. The modem is used to send and receive signals from computers by converting a digital signal from the computer (modulate) into an analog signal. This analog signal is transmitted over a communications link (phone line for example) to a receiving computer. The analog signal must be converted back to a digital signal (demodulate) for processing by a digital computer. Modems can be external or internal to the computer and transmit data in bits per second (bps). The bps will vary depending on the type of technology used.

- **Communications media.** Data transmission requires some sort of medium to do the task. The phone line is one such medium. Other communications media include wire pairs (twisted pairs), coaxial cables, fiber optics, microwave, and satellite transmission. Wireless transmission is also used to send data using radio frequencies to connect various physical devices. Protocols are essential tools for devices to communicate with each other. A protocol "is a set of rules for the exchange of data between a terminal and a computer or between two computers. Think of protocol as a sort of precommunication agreement about the form in which a message or data is to be sent and receipt is to be acknowledged. Protocols are handled by hardware and software to the network so users need worry only about their own data" (Capron & Johnson, 2006). The protocol used with Internet communications is the transmission control protocol/Internet protocol (TCP/IP). Standards also help to facilitate communication among different systems. DICOM is an example of one standard used in medical imaging to address, in particular, communication of images.

- **Communication Networks.** A network allows several devices (computers for example) to be connected together to utilize data and information. The layout or configuration of the network is called a topology. Three typical networks—the bus, star, and ring networks—were described in Chapter 8 on PACS. A network consists of several components including a host computer and nodes (any device coupled to the network); packets (block of data to be transmitted); protocols; and other devices such as hubs, switches, bridges, routers, and gateways. There are several types of networks, based on the size of the network, ranging from the smallest, the local area network (LAN) to the largest, the wide area network (WAN). The metropolitan area network (MAN) falls in between the LAN and the WAN. As well as the wired communications media described above, wireless communications media have become commonplace. These media include infrared transmission broadcast radio, microwave radio, and communications satellites. These media utilize different frequencies from the radio frequency of the electromagnetic spectrum. For example, all cell phones utilize a frequency range of 824–900 MHz (William & Sawyer, 2007).

- Computer communications technology also involves topics such as cyber-threats, security, and safeguarding issues; however, these topics are not within the scope of this book.

Digital medical imaging (or digital imaging for short) utilizes several aspects of IT, and therefore it is important for the technologist to have a firm understanding of the general concepts of IT. IT now has a great impact on the practice of medicine and, more importantly, on digital imaging. For example, IT is applied to information systems, standards for communicating both textual data and image data sets, communication networks, Web technology, privacy, confidentiality, and security of medical information, to mention only a few.

What Is Informatics?

As noted in the discussion above, the term "informatics" is closely linked with IT. The term dates back several decades and its origin can be traced back to Russian writings (VanBemmel & Musen, 1977). Informatics refers to the process of changing data to information, and therefore computers and communications technologies are central elements to the process.

Informatics Subspecialties

Informatics is now applied to several disciplines and has led to new subspecialties such as medical informatics, health care informatics, biomedical informatics, nursing informatics, imaging informatics (radiology informatics), cardiology informatics, clinical informatics, and so on. Health care and medical informatics will be described here.

Health Care Informatics/ Medical Informatics

The application of IT to health care or medicine is referred to as health care informatics and medical informatics, respectively. There are several definitions in the literature and on various medical informatics Web sites. The British Medical Informatics Society provides the following overview of the terms:

"The terms 'medical informatics' and 'health informatics' have been variously defined, but can be best understood as the understanding, skills and tools that enable the sharing and use of information to deliver healthcare and promote health. 'Health informatics' is now tending to replace the previously commoner term 'medical informatics' reflecting a widespread concern to define an information agenda for health services which recognizes the role of citizens as agents in their own care, as well as the major information handling roles of the non-medical healthcare professions.

Health informatics is thus an essential and pervasive element in all healthcare activity. It is also the name of an academic discipline developed and pursued over the past decade by a world-wide scientific community engaged in advancing and teaching knowledge about the application of information and communication technologies to healthcare—that place where health, information and computer sciences, psychology, epidemiology and engineering intersect." (www.bmis.org, 2008)

Scope of Health Informatics

The scope of health informatics covers a wide and varied range of topics. Several textbooks on health informatics for example, provide some direction in this regard (Coirea, 1977; Englebardt & Nelson, 2002; Hebda et al., 2005; Norris et al., 2002; Shortliffe & Perreault et al., 2001; Van Bemmel & Musen, 1997). In general, the common themes that emerge are centered on four major components: core introductory concepts, IT, health care information systems, and specialized applications.

Health informatics core concepts include the basic concepts of informatics relating to models, data, information, and systems theory, which are essential in order to understand information and communication systems (Coiera, 1997). The IT component should address computer technology such as hardware and software, data integrity and management, electronic communication (computer networks and protocols, for example), and Internet technologies (Hebda et al., 2005).

Health care information systems is an important topic, and includes a study of clinical information systems, such as nursing, laboratory, cardiology, and radiology information systems, and administrative systems, which deal with such functions as patient registration and scheduling. Additionally, topics relating to information systems include training, security and confidentiality issues, system integration, the electronic health record, regulatory issues, and disaster recovery, to mention only a few (Hebda et al., 2005).

Finally, the topic of specialized applications in a health care informatics curriculum will deal with the use of computers in education and research. In addition, telehealth concepts and issues, as well as decision support systems, are mandatory topics in health care informatics. (Hebda et al., 2005).

Medical Imaging Informatics

Medical imaging includes several modalities such as diagnostic radiography, fluoroscopy, computed tomography, magnetic resonance imaging, medical sonography, and nuclear medicine. More recently, radiation therapy incorporates some degree of imaging (using a CT scanner for example) into its practice. It is clearly apparent that medical imaging plays a significant sole in health care since it is used for diagnosis, assessment and planning, guidance of procedures communication, education, training, and research (Greens & Brinkly, 2001).

Definition

The application of IT to medical imaging is referred to as medical imaging informatics (MII) or, simply, imaging informatics. MII is a new subdiscipline in radiology proposed several years ago by Kulikowski (1997), who felt that the tasks performed by computers in a digital imaging department form the basis of this subspecialty. In particular, these tasks include digital image acquisition, digital image processing and image display, image storage and archiving, computer networking, and image transmission.

More recently, the use of picture archiving and communication systems (PACS) (Chapter 8) has become commonplace in digital imaging all over the world. As mentioned earlier, the use of PACS is now a routine part of the duties of the technologist (Fridel et al., 2009). PACS has been labeled by Huang (2004) as an "image information technology (IT) system for transmission and storage of medical images . . ." and as "an IT system of components." In this regard, he views imaging informatics as "the use of informatics methods to extract and synthesize the information-rich PACS and other patient-related data based to further advance medical research, education, and clinical services" (Huang, 2004).

Imaging informatics has been evolving through the years, as digital imaging departments become more and more efficient and commonplace. For example, several authors have described evolving

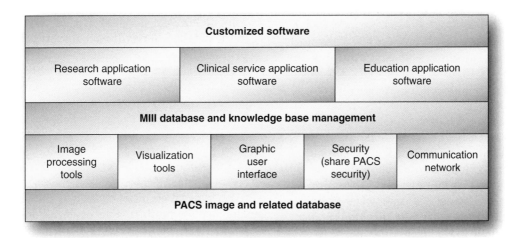

Customized software		
Research application software	Clinical service application software	Education application software

MIII database and knowledge base management

Image processing tools	Visualization tools	Graphic user interface	Security (share PACS security)	Communication network

PACS image and related database

FIGURE 9-1. The major components of a medical imaging informatics infrastructure (MIII) and their logical organization.
Source: *Huang, H. K. (2004).* PACS and Imaging Informatics. *John Wiley and Sons. New York, NY. Reproduced by permission*

nature of imaging informatics and its role in the 21st century (Bartholmai et al., 2002; Branstetter et al., 2004; Huang, 2004; Seeram, 2004; Wiggins, 2003). More recently, imaging informatics has been identified as one of the biomedical imaging research opportunities that "has the potential to enhance the roadmap themes of the National Institutes of Health" in the United States (Hendee, 2006). Of the several recommendations of the third Biomedical Imaging Research Opportunities Work Shop (BIROW III) held in Bethesda, MD, the following two are important to the continuing education of imaging technologists:

1. "Create educational programs in imaging informatics" (Hendee, 2006)

2. "Establish training programs in the routine use of imaging informatics by healthcare professionals . . ." (Hendee, 2006)

This chapter offers a small step in that direction.

Framework for MII

A framework for MII has been conceptualized and described by Huang (2004), a notable expert in the area of PACS and imaging informatics. The major components and their organization are illustrated in Figure 9-1. As can be seen, there are three major sections: customized software, the imaging informatics database and knowledge base management, and the PACS image and related database.

The customized software is application-oriented software intended to deal with issues related to research, education, and clinical services. The MII database and knowledge-base management section address the use of software tools to manage image processing and visualization, communications, graphical user interface, and data and knowledge (Huang, 2004). The third major section of Huang's informatics infrastructure addresses the management of images and associated text information in the PACS database, using standards such as DICOM (Chapter 8) for the communication of images. In addition, data such as patient demographics, diagnostic reports, etc., commonly associated with information systems (RIS, for example) are addressed using the HL-7 (Chapter 8) standard to communicate text data.

This framework provides the basis for topics that are essential to an imaging informatics curriculum for radiologists and technologists. Such curriculum elements and associated credentialing will be highlighted later in the chapter.

PACS Technology

As mentioned earlier, IT involves two technologies computer technology and communications technology. PACS is an example of an electronic system that is based on the use of computer and communications technologies. PACS, therefore, is an informatics-rich environment (Huang, 2004). The essential elements of PACS were described in Chapter 8; however, PACS will be briefly summarized here to emphasize the technical components relating to imaging informatics.

PACS is a computer-based system for storing and transmitting images to remote locations for use by others involved in the medical management of the patient. PACS is also coupled to various information systems and, more importantly, to image acquisition modalities.

The major components of PACS include digital image acquisition modalities, a computer network database server, an archival system, and a soft-copy display workstation. In addition, a PACS is often connected to health information systems such as a radiology information system (RIS) and a hospital information system (HIS).

The images produced by the image acquisition modalities (CR, DR, CT, MRI, and so on) are sent to the PACS for storage and archiving and subsequent transmission to remote locations. In this regard, a computer network is used for image transfer using the DICOM standard. The images are stored in the database server (image server) "the 'brain' of a centralized PACS" (Samei et al., 2004). Images are stored in an archival system consisting of short-term, long-term, or duplicate storage. Storage devices range from magnetic disks, optical disks, magneto-optical disks, and digital videodisks (Samei et al., 2004).

Display systems in a PACS environment fall into two categories: cathode-ray tubes (CRTs) and liquid crystal displays (LCDs). The goal of image display is to facilitate image interpretation by the radiologist. The display monitor is an essential component of the PACS workstation. A display workstation used by radiologists features various tools used to enhance productivity. These tools, described in Table 9-1, are all informatics-related tools, such as prefetch algorithms, hanging protocols, image processing algorithms, and decision support tools (Samei et al., 2004).

The final component of a PACS involves access and distribution of images in the PACS to interested parties, not only in the radiology department but also to others throughout the health care enterprise. While the former is referred to as a traditional radiology-centric PACS model, the latter is called the enterprise-wide image distribution model (Samei et al., 2004).

TABLE 9-1. Several functionalities of display workstations for use in a PACS environment.

Option of Function	Purpose
Prefetch algorithms	Software programs that automatically retrieve historical examination results and reports for correlation with the current study
Hanging protocols	Intelligent image display guidelines based on the anatomic region, examination type, technique, and pathologic condition; customized based on the preferences of individual radiologists and linked to the user's sign-on
Image processing	Specialized processing algorithms used to enhance specific anatomic features or types of pathologic condition (i.e., disease-specific processing); incorporated into the workstation via keyboard presets to enhance radiologists' productivity
Decision-support tools	Diagnostic aids to assist in soft-copy interpretation, such as software for computer-aided detection, segmentation, and textural analysis and additional artificial intelligence techniques to reduce the "human weaknesses" of bias, fatigue, and inconsistency

Source: *Samei E. et al. (2004). General guidelines for purchasing and acceptance testing of PACS equipment.* Radiographics, 24, 313-334. Reproduced by permission of RSNA and the authors

Within a PACS environment, it is mandatory that the PACS be integrated with information systems, since these systems contain data and information related to the patient whose images are stored in the PACS. The health information system in Huang's (2004) MIII framework is an essential technical component, and therefore it will be reviewed briefly below.

Health Information Systems

An information system is a computer-based system used to collect and process data to provide its users with information needed for problem solving and decision-making. As noted by Hebda et al. (2005) "the terms health care information system and hospital information system (HIS) both refer to a group of systems used within a hospital or enterprise that support and enhance healthcare."

There are two major component systems of the HIS; Clinical information systems (CISs), and administrative information systems (AISs). CISs include a number of information systems such as for example; order entry system, monitoring system, nursing information system, laboratory information system, and a radiology information system (RIS). AISs include information systems dealing with registration, scheduling, financial payroll and human resources, quality assurance, and contract management (Hebda et al., 2005). It is not within the scope of this book to describe these information systems: however, brief elements of the RIS will be highlighted to illustrate that the RIS is an essential component of imaging informatics.

The characteristic features of an RIS are as follows:

- Order entry: requested radiology examinations ordered by physicians are entered into the system. This is also known as registration of patients.
- Scheduling of various imaging procedures.
- Report generation: radiologists enter image interpretation reports. These reports are linked to the appropriate patient and examination.

- Billing preparation: costs associated with various procedures performed on patients are generated and sent to a billing system.
- Other related functions: these include quality assurance, inventory monitoring, and statistical analysis, as well as communications that are important to the daily operations of the imaging department.

Since the information contained in the RIS can be shared with the HIS, physicians in the hospital, for example, can access related information on their patients from their offices, if required.

The Electronic Health Record

With the widespread use of HIS, RIS, and PACS, the paper-based medical record is being replaced by the electronic health record (EHR) to overcome the limitations of paper-based records. One such major limitation is that the paper-based record cannot include images (such as those stored in the PACS) "nor do they make use of decision support systems" (Hebda et al., 2005).

Definition and Components

The Healthcare Information and Management Systems Society (HIMSS) defines the EHR as a "secure, real-time, point-of-care, patient-centric information resource for physicians." The EHR contains a vast amount of medical information, data about the patient (demographic information, for example), and, of course, other related health information such as images from medical imaging procedures. The EHR contains data and information that can fall basically in one of its six components (Hebda et al., 2005):

1. Order entry
2. Clinical documentation
3. Data repository
4. Decision support
5. Results reporting
6. Clinical messaging and e-mail

The EHR provides a wide range of benefits to health care professionals, including physicians, but it also has benefits that are available to the health care enterprise in general, such as improved data integrity and quality of care, as well as increased productivity from satisfied health care providers (Hebda et al., 2005).

The EHR will not be described further in this book; however, the interested student may refer to the textbook by Hebda et al. (2005).

Systems Integration Overview

Systems integration is an important concept in imaging informatics, for it deals with the notion that to be effective and efficient, imaging modalities (data acquisition devices), PACS, and information systems must be able to communicate (exchange data) with each other in a seamless manner.

Requirements for Systems Integration

There are several requirements for effective and efficient systems integration. These include an interface, data dictionary, uniform language, master patient index (MIP), and communication (data exchange) standards (Englebardt & Nelson, 2002; Hebda et al., 2005; Shortliffe et al., 2001).

An interface serves to connect systems so that they can exchange data. The early interfaces were known as point-to-point interfaces because they allowed two systems to communicate with each other. Today, more sophisticated computer software interfaces called interface engines facilitate the exchange of data among several systems. Such communication is made possible through the use of a clinical data repository and a technique referred to as mapping. "Mapping is the process in which terms defined in one system are associated with comparable terms in another system" (Hebda et al., 2005).

While a data dictionary provides the definition of terms used in the particular enterprise (a health care enterprise, for example), the MIP is a database that contains all information (demographics, for example) about the patient and plays an

important role in identifying and locating the records belonging to the patient under study.

The use of standards for data exchange in imaging informatics is a mandatory concept for radiologists and technologists, as well as related personnel working in the imaging department (physicists and biomedical engineers and IT personnel, for example) to understand. As noted earlier in the chapter, the two standards that are used in the imaging department to communicate images and textual data are DICOM (Digital Imaging and Communications in Medicine) and HL-7 (Health Level-7), respectively. DICOM has been developed specifically for communication of images from the image acquisition devices to the PACS and from the PACS to others within the enterprise; HL-7 has been developed to handle text data exchange among various information systems, such as the RIS and HIS (Whitby, 2007).

Finally, it is important to note that the Integrating the Healthcare Enterprise (IHE) initiative (Chapter 8) is also an important imaging informatics topic. This initiative dates back to 1998 through a joint venture between the Radiological Society of North America (RSNA) and the HIMSS. The overall objective of the IHE initiative is to ensure that image acquisition devices, PACS, and information systems from different vendors, communicate (exchange data) with each other in a seamless fashion (Indrajit, 2007; Indrajit and Verma, 2007). A comparative overview of these standards and initiatives is provided in Table 9-2.

IT Security Fundamentals

As health care informatics continues to develop and become more and more commonplace, the topic of security becomes increasingly important. In this regard, the Health Insurance Portability and Accountability Act (HIPPA) has drawn serious attention to the need for system security. In addition, HIPPA security rule requires that health care institutions determine threats and take action to protect information (Gillespie, 2003; Joachim, 2003).

What Is Security?

In terms of IT, the U.S. National Information Systems Security defines **information security** as: "the

TABLE 9-2. A comparative overview of healthcare standards and initiatives relevant to radiology.

Parameter	DICOM	HL-7	IHE
Nomenclature	Digital Imaging and Communications in Medicine	Health Level Seven, INC	Integrating the Health Enterprise
Origin	Developed by American College of Radiologists (ACR) and National Electrical Manufacturers Association (NEMA)	Not for profit volunteer organisation headquartered in Ann Arbor MI	Developed by Radiological Society of North America (RSNA) and Healthcare Information Management Systems Society (HIMSS)
Founding Year	1985	1990	1998
Latest Version	DICOM Version 3 (2007)	HL-7 Version 3	Each year new profiles are selected
Role	Provides protocols for integration of image data between imaging, nonimaging modalities, devices and systems	Provides protocols for exchange, management, and integration of varied data in electronic health records	Provides implementation profiles based on existing standards like HL-7 and DICOM
Data	Image information objects and nonimage information objects	Clinical and administrative electronic healthcare data	Functional integration workflow elements
Functional Elements	Protocols, Objects, Services, Service Class, Conformance	Act, Participation, Roles	Actors, Transactions, Integration profiles
Key Area	Image and few nonimage data interoperability	Health record and Clinical interoperability	Integration of systems and standards

Source: *Indrajit, I. K., & Verma B. S. (2007). DICOM, HL-7 and IHE: A basic primer on Healthcare Standards for Radiologists.* Indian Journal of Radiology and Imaging, 17, 66-68. *Reproduced by permission*

protection of information systems against unauthorized access to or modification of information, whether in storage, processing or transit, and against the denial of service to authorized users, including those measures necessary to detect, document, and counter such threats." This definition simply means that security is intended to protect system data and information and to maintain information integrity. Security allows authorized users to have access to the information and prevents unauthorized users from accessing it (Capron & Johnson, 2007; Hebda et al., 2005; Rizzo, 2005).

The topic of IT security is wide and varied and cannot be described here in any detail. This section will introduce the student to the nature of computer security and to demonstrate that it is an important component of imaging informatics.

Security Threats

According to Rizzo (2005), security threats fall into three categories: social engineering attacks, hardware attacks, and software attacks. Social engineering attacks seek to obtain data and information "from authorized users through deception"; hardware attacks refer to attacks on hardware components, such as the theft of a computer; software attacks deal with attacks on operating systems and application software, for example. The means of attack include viruses, worms, Trojan horses, malicious programs, and denial of service. The more ambitious student should refer to the works of Rizzo (2005), Halberg (2001), Hebda et al. (2005), Englebardt and Nelson (2002), Aron and Sampler (2003), and Williams and Sawyer (2007) for more information.

Security Methods

The vast array of security risks provides a significant rationale for security methods. Home computer users, for example, ensure that their computer system is protected to a certain degree through the use of antivirus and spyware detection programs. Similarly, organizations ensure that their IT systems are secured.

Security methods range from physical security, authentication, passwords, firewalls, and antivirus software, to spyware detection software, encryption and keys, and wireless security measures. These topics are not within the scope of this book. For those who are interested in reading about the classical basis for network security for the imaging enterprise, refer to the paper by Eng (2001). This paper also provides a summary of HIPPA security rules.

The Technologist as Informaticist

The notion of the radiologist as informaticist was identified as early as 2000 with the evolution and rapid growth of digital imaging technologies (Arenson et al., 2000). Likewise, this notion should be extended to the radiologic technologist, as was identified by Seeram (2004), for several reasons:

1. The imaging technologist works routinely on a daily basis with digital image acquisition modalities, by producing images in the imaging room. In digital fluoroscopy, the technologist provides technical assistance to the radiologist and should be well versed in related technical matters.

2. The technologist works routinely with PACS, by first assessing all images acquired and analyzed at the acquisition workstation and subsequently sending them to the PACS.

3. The technologist performs quality control on image acquisition devices, display devices, and on the PACS itself.

4. The technologist educates others in the role of the digital imaging department, the hospital in general, and the health care enterprise, and therefore must keep up with advances through ongoing continuing education.

5. Advanced imaging technologists are beginning to play an important role in image post-processing, imaging research, and publishing ventures.

The above role function provides a rationale for a new subspecialty in the digital imaging department in which the imaging technologist can evolve into an informaticist.

The PACS Technologist

The developments and rapid growth of digital imaging is coupled with the emergence of new roles for the technologist. One such role was identified as the PACS technologist (Cabrera, 2002). Bartholmai et al. (2002) identified a new radiology subspecialty for the 21st century, the electronic imaging technology (EIT) specialist. Specifically, they developed an EIT Fellowship curriculum for radiologists that includes image analysis and processing; image display technologies; PACS, including storage, networks, and PACS administration; IT and systems integration issues; information systems; data security; economics; legal issues, and research. (Bartholmai et al., 2002).

In 2004, Branstetter et al. (2004) published a paper entitled "Reviews in Radiology Informatics: Establishing a core curriculum" in which they described the need for radiologists to have IT skills in order to provide leadership in applying IT to radiology. They called this new subspecialty "radiology informatics." Once again, this notion can be extended to technologists, that is, technologists should have IT skills in order to provide technical leadership in perhaps a similar manner to the radiologist.

The lack of a curriculum in radiology informatics prompted the Society of Imaging Informatics in Medicine (SIIM) to develop one. The SIIM curriculum essentially identified four major subject areas: IT, clinical informatics, PACS administration, and academics. Examples of subtopics identified include networks, storage and archiving, security, information systems, image display, system integration, quality control, and research and education, to mention only a few.

Skills for PACS Administrators

As digital imaging technologies and PACS continued to grow and replace film-based imaging, it became clearly apparent that another technically specialized individual was needed in the digital imaging department (Nagy et al., 2005). This individual was labeled the PACS administrator. In an effort to define the skills and tasks related to PACS administration, Nagy et al. (2005) developed a model to address this need. Their model consists of three areas that include behavioral, business, and technical competencies. As stated by Nagy et al. (2005), "The model seemed especially appropriate because each area of competency corresponds with an educational profile of RTs, radiology administrators or IT specialists who currently work as PACS administrators."

While the behavioral area addresses competencies focused on training, workflow analysis, reading environment and customer relations management, the business area examines competencies in PACS readiness, economics, strategic vision, vender selection, and sustaining PACS. Finally, the technical area addressed competencies in the technology, troubleshooting, systems management, modalities, and security competencies (Nagy et al., 2005).

Certification in PACS

The increasing growth and utilization of PACS in imaging have provided the need for individuals actively working in a PACS environment to become certified. In this regard, the PACS Administrators in Radiology Certification Association (PARCA) provides PACS certification at four different levels to address the extent of an individual's involvement in PACS. These different levels include:

1. Certified PACS Associate (CPAS)
2. Certified PACS Interface Analyst (CPIA)
3. Certified PACS Systems Analyst (CPSA)
4. Certified PACS System Manager (CPSM)

The CPAS certification requires that an individual pass two examinations; one, a clinical examination and the other, a technical examination. Once CPAS certified, an individual can ladder into either the CPIA or the CPSA certification. Finally, individuals who complete both CPIA and CPSA can apply to write the CPSM examination.

Details of the PARCA certification process are available at their Web site www.pacsadim.org (at the time of writing this chapter).

 ## Certification in Imaging Informatics

The idea of going beyond the PACS administrator certification has led to the creation of the Certified Imaging Informatics Professional (CIIP). The CIIP certification is a venture between SIIM (formerly called SCAR) and the American Registry of Radiologic Technologists (ARRT) (Honeyman-Buck, 2006; Socia, 2006). Details such as the mission, goals, eligibility criteria, examination development process, and content are available on the SIIM Web site. Additionally, Honeyman-Buck (2006) provides a set of references and reading lists for imaging informatics professionals that can be used to prepare them for certification.

In 2007, the American Board of Imaging Informatics (ABII) was founded by the SIIM and the ASRT. The mission of ABII is "to enhance patient care, professionalism, and competence in imaging informatics. ABII has created and manages the Imaging Informatics Professional (IIP) certification program and awards the Certified Imaging Informatics Professional (CIIP) designation to qualified candidates" (www.abii.org). The current outline of the topics covered on the examination on the Web site. The questions are based on the following major content areas: procurement (5%); project management (5%); operations (10%); communications (10%); training and education (5%); image management (20%); IT (15%); systems management (10%); clinical engineering (10%); and medical informatics (10%).

The Benefits of Imaging Informatics

Imaging informatics evolved as the technologies of digital image acquisition, image processing, image display, storage, and communications became widespread and commonplace. The evolution of the electronic medical record (EMR) coupled with the information that accompanies a patient in radiology (imaging), known as the "entire patient entity" (EPE) (Geis, 2007), have led to the reality that imaging informatics provides benefits that are significant not only to the imaging department but to the health care enterprise.

For example, in radiology, Nagy (2008) describes three informatics tools that can enhance the efficiency and quality of radiology services: quality control reporting, technologist peer review, and communication between radiologists and referring physicians.

The more educated individuals who work with patients for the purpose of restoring their health become, the more they are able to contribute efficiently, effectively, and reliably to patient care. Individuals trained in imaging informatics as a subspecialty of radiology provide such contribution (Brastetter, 2007; Geis, 2007), and in the end the patient will benefit from their wisdom.

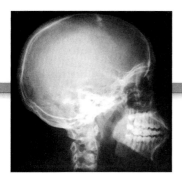

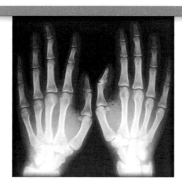

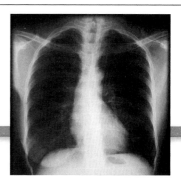

REVIEW QUESTIONS

1. What is meant by the term "information technology"?
2. Explain the fundamental differences between computer hardware and computer software.
3. What are the five basic operations that computers use to process and disseminate information?
4. What are four key elements of computer communications technology?
5. What is the meaning of the term "informatics"? List several informatics subspecialties.
6. Distinguish between health care informatics and imaging informatics.
7. Review the major elements of a medical imaging informatics framework.
8. Identify the key features of PACS and relate how it fits into a medical imaging informatics framework.
9. Explain how information systems such as a radiology information system fits into the framework of medical imaging informatics.
10. What are the main characteristics of the electronic health record?
11. Explain the need for systems integration in imaging informatics.
12. Briefly identify what is meant by IT security, security threats and methods of attacks on security.
13. Explain the concept of the technologist as an informaticist.
14. Outline the certification process for imaging informatics personnel.

REFERENCES

Arenson, R. L. et al. (2000). Computers in imaging and healthcare: Now and in the future. *Journal of Digital Imaging, 13*(4), 145–156.

Aron, D., & Sampler, J. L. (2003). *Understanding IT: A Manager's Guide.* London: Pearson Education Ltd.

Brandstetter, B. (2007). Basics of imaging informatics. *Radiology, 243*(3), 656–667.

British Medical Informatics Society (2008). *www.bmis.org.*

Capron, H. L., & Johnston, J. A. (2007). *Computers: Tools for an Information Age* (9th ed.). New Jersey: Prentice Hall.

Englebardt, S. P., & Nelson, A. (2002). *Healthcare Informatics: An Interdisciplinary Approach.* St Louis: Mosby.

Eng, J. (2001). Computer network security for the radiology enterprise. *Radiology, 220,* 303–309.

Fridell, K., Aspelin, P., & Edgren, L. et al. (2009). PACS influence the radiographer's work. *Radiography, 15*(2), 121–133.

Geis, J. R. (2007). Medical imaging informatics: How it improves radiology practice today. *Journal of Digital Imaging, 20*(2), 99–104.

Gillespie, G. (2003). CIOs coming in for a pit stop in the HIPPA compliance race. *Health Data Management, 11*(8), 34.

Greens, R. A., & Brinkley, J. F. (2001). Radiology Systems. In E. Shortcliff & L. E. Perreault (Eds.), *Medical Informatics* (2nd ed.). New York: Springer-Verlag.

Halberg, B. (2001). *Networking: A Beginner's Guide.* (2nd ed.). Osborne/McGraw-Hill, New York, NY.

Hendee, W. R. (2006). Biomedical imaging research opportunities workshop III: Summary of findings and recommendations. *Radiology, 238*(2), 402–404.

Honeyman-Beck, J. (2006). References and reading lists for imaging informatics professionals: Preparing for certification. *Journal of Digital Imaging 19,* Suppl 1, 1–5.

http://www.abii.org

http://www.cpupedia.com/definition/information and technology.aspx

Huang, H. K. (2004). *PACS and Imaging Informatics.* New Jersey: John Wiley & Sons.

Indrajit, I. K., & Verma, B. S. (2007). DICOM, HL-7, and IHE: A Primer on Healthcare Standards for radiologists. *Indian Journal of Radiology and Imaging, 17,* 66–68.

Indrajit, I. K. (2007). Digital Imaging and Communications in Medicine: A Basic Review. *Indian Journal of Radiology and Imaging, 17,* 5–7.

Joachim, D. (2003). Hospitals get HIPPA. *Network Computing, 14*(13), 54–60.

Kulikowski, C. A., & Jaffe, C. C. (Eds.). (1997). Focus on imaging informatics. *Journal of the American Medical Informatics Association, 4*(3), 165–256.

Nag, P. G. (2008). Using Informatics to Improve the Quality of Radiology. *Applied Radiology Supplement*, Dec, 9–14.

Rizzo, J. V. (2005). IT security basics: What you need to know. *Biomedical Instrumentation Technology*, Nov/Dec, 454–458.

Samei, E. et al. (2004). General guidelines for purchasing and acceptance testing of PACS equipment. *Radiographics, 24*, 313–334.

Seeram, E. (2004). Digital image processing. *Radiologic Technology, 75*(6), 435–455.

Shortliffe, E. H., & Perreault, L. E. et al. (2001). *Medical Informatics: Computer Applications in Health Care and Biomedicine.* New York: Springer-Verlag New York, Inc.

Socia, C. W. (2006). Credentialing imaging informatics professionals: Creation of items for the CIIP examination. *Journal of Digital Imaging, 19*, Suppl 1, 6–9.

Van Bemmel, J. H., & Musen, M.A. (1997). *Handbook of Medical Informatics.* New York: Springer-Verlag.

Whitby, J. (2007). The DICOM Standard. Barco N.V. Kortrijk, Belgium, pp 4–13.

Williams, B. K., & Sawyer, S. C. (2007). *Using IT: A Practical Introduction to Computers and Communications.* New York: McGraw-Hill.

CHAPTER 10

Quality Control for Digital Radiography

Charles Willis, PHD

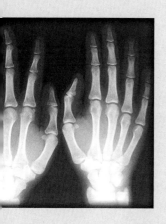

OBJECTIVES

Upon completion of this chapter, the student should be able to:

1. Outline the differences between quality control in conventional and digital radiography.

2. Explain how errors arise in digital radiography.

3. Recognize quality control methods for detecting and avoiding errors.

4. Integrate specific quality control methods into a quality assurance program for digital radiography.

KEY TERMS

Control limits
Diagnostic quality
Exposure factor creep
Flat field
Ghost image
Gray scale display function (GSDF)
Indicators
Latitude

Metadata
Modality worklist (MWL)
Process map
Range-of-adjustment
Reusable image media (RIM)
Shading correction
Task allocation matrix

Introduction

Quality control (QC) includes all those activities undertaken to get an indication of how well the imaging operation is working. Considering the amazing capability of digital radiography to produce consistent, diagnostic quality images under the most challenging conditions, some may wonder why QC is still necessary. Although most of the chain of events that results in a digital radiographic image has been automated, errors still occur. If the goal is to provide the highest quality medical care, QC processes must be in place in order to detect and correct these errors.

Why is Quality Control still needed in Digital Radiography?

Perhaps the best answer to this question is that the world is not perfect. So long as human beings are involved with the process of creating a digital radiographic image, mistakes will be made. This is not to suggest that automated processes are perfect. Human errors tend to be spontaneous and random. Machine errors tend to be systematic. Even when machines are initially set up to perform properly, performance can degrade over time. The combination of humans and machines can improve performance, since machines are fast and humans can recognize errors though inductive reasoning. Conversely, the combination of humans and machines can magnify errors. For example, if the operator interface to the machine is extremely complex, human errors will increase exponentially. A popular proverb known as Murphy's Law states that "Anything that can go wrong, will go wrong."

National professional organizations recognize the need for QC in radiology and have included requirements for QC in their standards of practice. Some state and federal regulations, such as the Mammography Quality Standards Act of 1992, contain specific requirements for QC. How is it possible to know whether the imaging operation is going badly or efficiently without active and objective measurements of performance?

Distinctions between Quality Control and Quality Assurance

In radiology, QC is the visible, ongoing effort to collect information about an imaging operation. QC is part of an overall quality assurance (QA) program, which seeks to get the most efficient performance from both the imaging facility and the physician. Wise radiology administrators understand that an investment in QC is more than compensated for by improvements in efficiency and quality. The cost of QC is trivial compared to the potential cost of a single malpractice claim.

Components of Quality Control

QC is accomplished through four steps, namely, acceptance testing (AT), establishment of baseline performance, diagnosis of changes in performance, and verification of correction of deterioration. AT is the first opportunity to determine whether the imaging equipment meets the requirements of state and federal regulatory agencies, as well as special requirements that may have been written into the purchase contract. AT should be conducted *before* the imaging device is used for patients. It is smart to conduct AT with the vendor service engineer present, so that deficiencies can be corrected immediately if possible. AT is generally the responsibility of a medical physicist. Because of the novelty of digital radiographic technology, some traditional tests had to be modified for DR and new tests were needed. The American Association of Physicists in Medicine (AAPM) has defined specific tests for computed radiography (CR) and for displays intended for diagnostic interpretation.

AT is often used as an opportunity to establish baseline performance. Certainly, we should expect the new device to perform well upon installation. Usually, some observation of performance is required while the device is in routine use in order to establish nominal performance and normal fluctuations in performance. This period of observation is important in deciding upon which indicators of changes in performance we are going to monitor routinely. The fluctuations in performance are translated into control limits, the maximum deviation from normal that we are going to allow before initiating corrective action. Technologists are most familiar with this methodology as it applies to film processor QC. The indicator is optical density (OD) of a test film, and the control limits are plus or minus OD from the average OD that is tolerated before a service call is initiated.

When deterioration in performance is observed, and corrective action is taken, it is important to verify that performance has returned to normal levels. This may include more comprehensive tests than the usual performance indicators, perhaps even a repeat of the complete AT procedures.

A Definition of "Quality"

In its broadest sense, a "quality" image is one that makes accurate diagnosis possible. This is known as "diagnostic quality." The quality of any image can be described in terms of contrast, resolution, and noise. For imaging that makes use of ionizing radiation, the dose to the patient must be considered. Artifacts that can mask or mimic clinical features are another aspect of diagnostic image quality. An image of exquisite quality that does not make its way to the physician for interpretation is of no value in the diagnostic process. QC must therefore address errors that affect both image quality and availability.

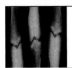

Understanding Processes and Errors in Digital Radiography

The ultimate product of the radiology operation is not the images, but rather the physician's interpretation of the images. The quality of the report is beyond the scope of this chapter; however, it is important to recognize that QC activities in hospitals routinely monitor the quality of reporting, and national standards address the content and timeliness of communications between radiologists and clinicians. In order to determine where errors can occur and where QC measures should be instituted, it is helpful to consider each step in the process of performing a digital radiographic examination and producing the report.

Process Map for a DR Examination

A flowchart of the steps involved in performing a DR exam can be created, such as the one shown in Figure 10-1. This flowchart is also known as a process map. Constructing a process map is a way to understand the interrelationships between activities within the imaging operation. The individual steps can be very general or very detailed, depending on the purpose of the map. Maps for the same process differ depending on the specifics of the local imaging operation. For example, an imaging facility that has an automated radiology information system (RIS) will have a different process map than a facility that uses manual methods for scheduling examinations. An imaging facility with a cassette-based DR system will have a different process map than a facility that uses an integrated DR system. For example, consider the process from arrival of the patient in the imaging department to release of the patient.

The process begins with the arrival of the patient in the imaging department. Steps 3 and 4 ensure that for a "walk-in" patient, the appropriate examination is scheduled in the RIS. This is an example of a QA activity, although no data was collected for QC purposes. Other QA activities are accomplished through interactions between the technologist and the patient, such as Step 7, where the exam is explained to the patient. At this time the technologist may verify that the patient is in fact the person identified in the exam request, that the anatomy to be examined matches the exam request, and other information about the patient such as pregnancy status, restricted motion, allergies if contrast is to be used, and appliances that may interfere with the radiographic projection or its development. A simple QC method is to include a checklist on the exam request that the technologist annotates to indicate that all these actions were taken. Step 12 is an inspection of the image for gross positioning errors that might require repeating a view. Step 14 is a more comprehensive review of the image at a workstation that is more capable of displaying subtle problems that might not be apparent at a preview station. The QC workstation in Step 14 might also have more sophisticated capabilities for modifying a

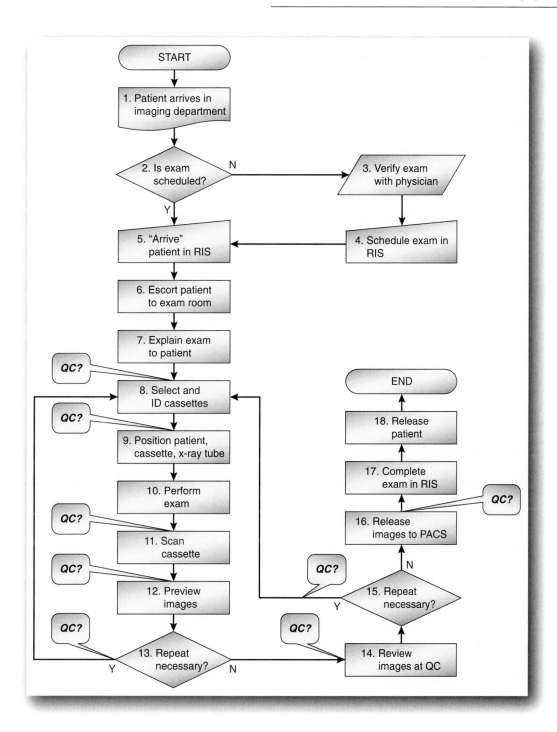

FIGURE 10-1. Process Map for DR Examination. Each step of the process of performing a DR exam is depicted in the flowchart, with arrows indicating the sequence of steps. Places in the process where QC questions arise are annotated.

Source: *Delmar, Cengage Learning*

substandard image without requiring a repeated exposure. The process map is designed so that images are released to the picture archiving and communications system (PACS) in Step 16, only after all have been reviewed and approved at the QC workstation.

Superimposed on the process map, eight boxes indicate places in the process where questions about QC arise. For example, before the cassettes are selected for the exam in Step 8, is each image receptor properly erased and ready to record another exposure? Is the correct patient identification associated with each cassette? Before positioning the patient in Step 9 for the examination, is the imaging system ready to make an appropriate exposure? Before the cassette is scanned in Step 11, is the scanner properly calibrated to develop the latent image in the receptor? When the images are viewed in Steps 12 and 14, how good is the fidelity of the image display? Since the decision to repeat images in Steps 13 and 15 involves additional radiation exposure to the patient, how often does this occurs and for what reasons? Once the images are released to the PACS in Step 16, did any or all of the images actually arrive at their intended destination? These questions can be answered by QC activities that are performed either as an integral part of the process map for each exam, or periodically to avert or detect errors.

Errors in the Association of Demographic and Exam Information

In Step 8 of our process map, the technologist identifies both the patient and the exam to the imaging system. This usually occurs before the exam as shown in Figure 10-1, but sometimes can be done after the examination is performed.

Every radiographic image has associated patient demographic and examination information, including patient name, patient date of birth or age, patient sex, a unique patient identification number, an exam accession number, the type of exam performed, the date and time of exam, and other information. In conventional screen-film radiography, the patient and exam information appears directly on the developed film. A window in the cassette allows the shadow of a printed version of the data to be flashed directly on the film. After the exam, when the film is developed, the data is visible. If the data is illegible, or incorrect, or no flash device is available, the data can be written onto the film with an indelible marker.

In DR, demographic and exam data accompany the DR image in an electronic file header. This is called "metadata," and it contains much more specific information about the image, including how it was acquired and processed. The Digital Imaging and Communications in Medicine (DICOM) standard specifies the format and content of the header file. These fields, or tags, are named by group and element. For example, (0010,0020) is "Patient ID." A portion of metadata from a DR exam is shown in Figure 10-2.

Where does all this demographic and exam information come from? Demographic information may originate in the hospital information system (HIS) when the patient is registered. Demographic and some exam information may be present in the radiology information system (RIS) when the exam is scheduled, or when the patient arrives. Some information may be provided in the exam request form. Some or all information may be recorded by the technologist at the time of the exam.

The simplest system is for the technologist to input all demographic and exam information into DR at the time of exam. Each DR system has some sort of registration device that allows direct manual input of demographic and exam information. Three basic drawbacks to this approach are the potential for human typographical errors, the fact that this is time-consuming, and that the data may already have been input by another person in the HIS or RIS, introducing an inefficiency of "duplicate entry" and the possibility of discrepant information in the two automated systems.

Some vendors of cassette-based DR systems provide manual demographic association aids, as shown in Figure 10-3. Special labels are affixed to the outside of the cassettes. The labels can be marked with a china marker or dry-erase marker to avoid confusion between patients and views.

Where demographic and exam information exists in the RIS, an automated query to the RIS using the accession number as a key field can return all associated data to the DR acquisition station. The technologist still has to manually enter the accession number, which may be many digits, and verify that appropriate data is retrieved. The technologist may still have to manually enter some exam data. It is clear that RIS queries improve the accuracy of demographic and exam information, as well as reducing the technologist's time.

In imaging departments where the exam request is printed, a bar code of the accession number can also be printed. A bar-code scanner can be added to the DR acquisition station as a substitute for the keyboard to reduce typographical errors. Some systems default to the previous patient's demographic information in the event of an unsuccessful query, so the technologist still must verify that the appropriate data was retrieved. The technologist may still have to manually enter some exam data.

DICOM modality worklist (MWL) is a feature designed specifically to take advantage of information that already exists in the RIS. When an exam is scheduled for a particular imaging resource, the RIS makes a list of patients available to the DR acquisition station. The technologist only has to select the proper patient from the worklist in order to load all the demographic and exam information. When properly implemented, MWL makes a

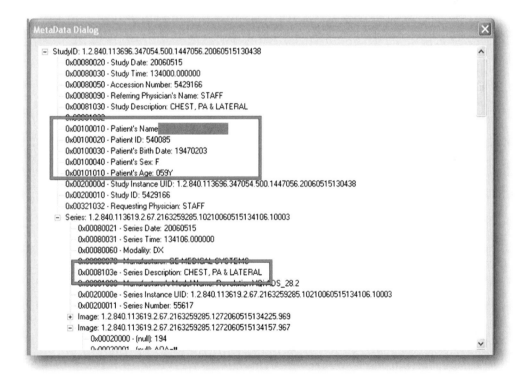

FIGURE 10-2. Metadata from a DICOM image file. Each data element, or "tag," is identified by an eight-digit "group" and "element." Red outlines data concerning patient information and type of exam, orientation and time of exam, and details about how the image was acquired and how it should be displayed. This metadata is from a DICOM "DX" modality type. Some DR images are identified according to an older format for "CR" modality type.
Source: Delmar, Cengage Learning (continues)

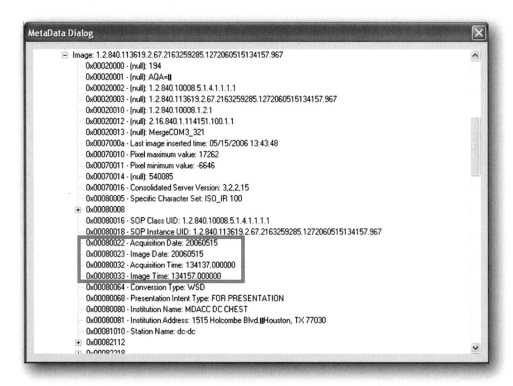

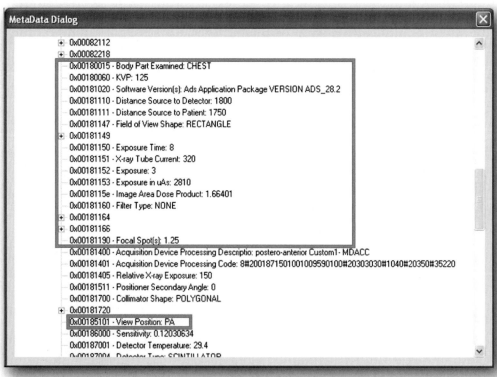

FIGURE 10-2. *(continues)*

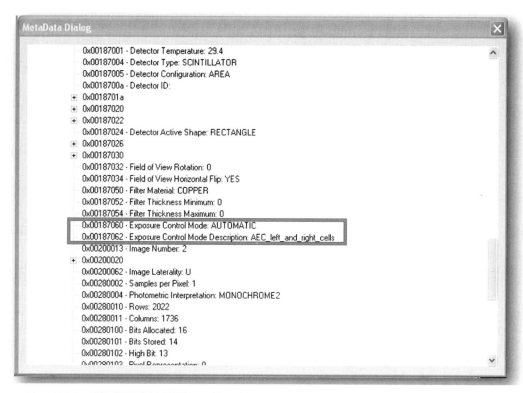

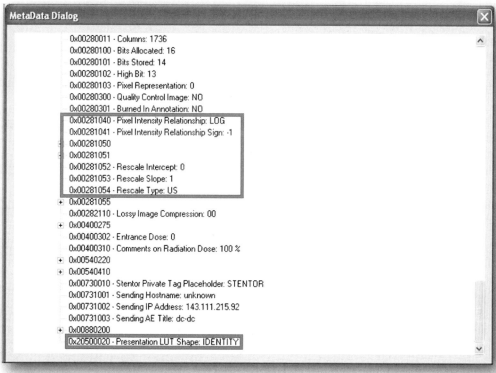

FIGURE 10-2. *(continued)*

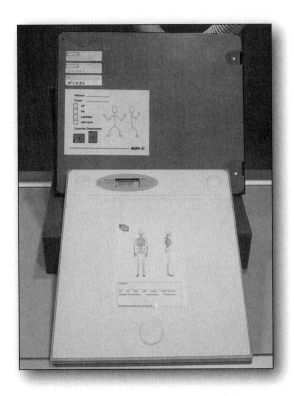

FIGURE 10-3. Demographic association aids for cassette-based DR systems.
Source: *Delmar, Cengage Learning*

dramatic improvement in the accuracy of associations. Although MWL is a tremendous time-saver, it does not relieve technologists fully from the need for vigilance over demographic and exam information. MWL has limitations; for example, in the case of an unscheduled exam, there may be a delay between scheduling the exam in the RIS and making it available to the acquisition station. Another limitation of MWL is resource reallocation, where although an exam was scheduled for one imaging resource, for some reason the exam must be conducted at another resource. A frequent practical example is when there is a delay in obtaining a post-void image, so that the next patient must be examined in another room. For this reason, similar resources are often pooled so that they share the same MWL; however, where all resources have been pooled a search of the worklist is lengthy. Some patients have multiple exams scheduled for the same day, so the technologist must exercise care to select the proper exam from the MWL. MWL introduces a new type of error, that is, proper demographic and exam information that are associated with the wrong patient images. A simple technologist error in selecting the wrong patient or wrong examination from the worklist creates a condition that may be more difficult to detect than a typographical error. During an interruption in RIS services, MWL is not available, but the imaging operation may still need to continue. Therefore, a manual means to input and correct demographic and exam information must still be provided. MWL must be supported by both the DR acquisition station and the RIS, and must be properly configured.

What are the consequences of misassociation of demographic and exam information and DR images? Incorrect information can cause the image to be unavailable for viewing. In a PACS, a mismatch between the image header and image database information from RIS generates what are known as "exceptions," "broken studies," or "orphans." These studies are usually sequestered and cannot be viewed by normal methods until the discrepancies are corrected. The clinical result is a "delay of diagnosis," which can have dramatic consequences for the outcome of the patient. Incorrect exam information can also affect image development. A chest image processed as a "skull" exam usually looks bad. A single exposure processed as a multiple exposure field exam is likely to be inappropriately developed. As mentioned previously in the discussion of MWL, misassociation also complicates error detection. Images assigned to a valid, but wrong, patient identifier are "lost." Images assigned to valid, but wrong, patient introduces the possibility of misdiagnosis. Proliferation of digital images within a PACS complicates correction. When a misassociation is discovered, how many other copies are floating around? Image caches on servers, workstations, web servers, gateways, remote sites, archives, all must be corrected.

Errors that can be Avoided by Periodic Testing

Returning to Figure 10-1, only one of the QC questions that arose during analysis of the process map has been addressed. Most of the remaining questions concern the readiness of the DR system to acquire and display images. Because verifying every performance parameter before each exam would interfere with clinical operations, periodic measurements assure that the system is properly configured and calibrated and that performance has not degraded. This is precisely how the quality of other x-ray imaging equipment is managed. For example, the medical physicist performs annual tests of the x-ray generator to verify performance. These tests may be repeated following a service event. The technologist performs periodic tests, such as film processor sensitometry, to verify performance.

When performing the exam in Step 10, a number of potential errors can arise from improper configuration and calibration or degraded performance. These include inadequate erasure, improper compensation for nonuniform gain, incorrect gain adjustment, incorrect exposure factor selection, and artifacts. Artifacts arise from interference with the projected x-ray beam, image receptor defects, and interference with conversion of the captured projection into a digital image. These errors may be detected by inspecting the image at the acquisition station or at a QC workstation. Correction may be possible by digital image processing or it may require a repeated exam. Most of these errors can be avoided by active QC measures, such as periodic testing. Some errors are the result of improper practice by the technologist, such as incorrect technique factor selection and artifacts from patient clothing or jewelry that interfere with the projected beam.

Unlike conventional screen-film image receptors, DR detectors are all inherently nonuniform. An example of an uncorrected image using an integrated DR receptor is shown in Figure 10-4. Cassette-based systems have uniform surfaces to capture the radiographic projection, but the efficiency of collection of stimulated emissions is highly nonuniform across the field of view. Both integrated and cassette-based DR systems require that a uniformity correction is applied to compensate for differences in gain across the receptor. This calibration for nonuniformity, also known as a shading correction, must be repeated on a periodic basis. The frequency of calibration depends on the specific DR device, and ranges from daily

A

B

FIGURE 10-4. Integrated DR receptor. (A) DR receptors are inherently nonuniform. (B) A uniformity correction must be calibrated on a periodic basis to compensate for differences in gain and artifacts, such as dead pixels. Source: *Delmar, Cengage Learning*

to semi-annually. A QC test for nonuniformity is easy to perform. All that is required is to expose the receptor to a uniform field of radiation, or flat field, which can be accomplished by using a large SID, such as 180 cm, opening the collimator to cover the receptor, and then developing the image. Viewing the image reveals defects and improper uniformity calibration. During viewing, care should be taken in adjusting the contrast. At extremely high contrast, any DR image will appear nonuniform. This is illustrated in Figure 10-5. Correction of nonuniformity improves both the contrast and sharpness of the DR image, as shown in Figure 10-6.

Another simple QC test helps answer the question raised in Step 8, concerning the readiness for the receptor to acquire another image. DR receptors are reusable image media (RIM), that is, they are not consumed in the process of acquiring an image. Instead, after the digital image is transferred, any signal remaining in the receptor is erased, so that the receptor can be used to acquire another image.

If erasure is inadequate, the previous exposure is superimposed as a ghost image on the current image, as seen in Figure 10-7. Developing an unexposed receptor, sometimes using a higher than normal gain setting, can reveal residual signal that has not been removed during erasure.

Inadequate erasure can arise from a variety of sources. For cassette-based systems, the duration of erasure could be too short or the intensity of the erasure could be too low, perhaps from burned out erasure lamps. Scattered radiation from other examinations can fog a DR receptor in the same way that screen-film can be fogged. Fog can build up over time on DR receptors from environmental sources of radiation. Even with a proper erasure cycle, gross overexposure on the previous exam can leave residual signal. Ghost images can occur in both direct and indirect DR systems, although the

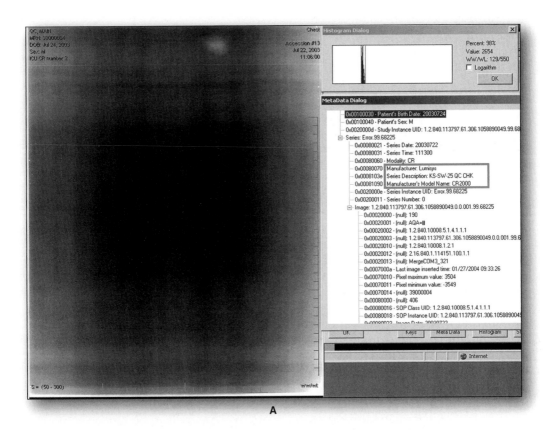

A

FIGURE 10-5. Flat-field images on several DR systems. (A) Lumisys cassette-based DR. (B) and (C) SwissRay integrated DR. (D) Canon integrated DR. Acceptable uniformity on (A) and (B) Unacceptable uniformity on (C) and (D).
Source: *Delmar, Cengage Learning (continues)*

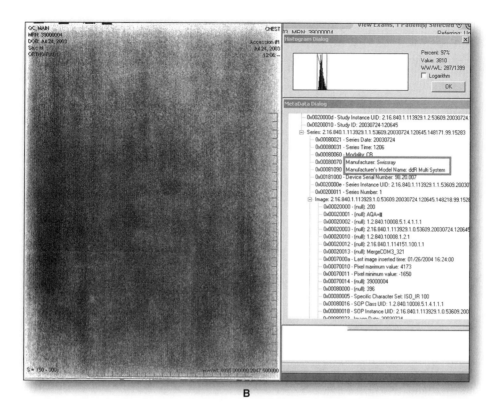

B

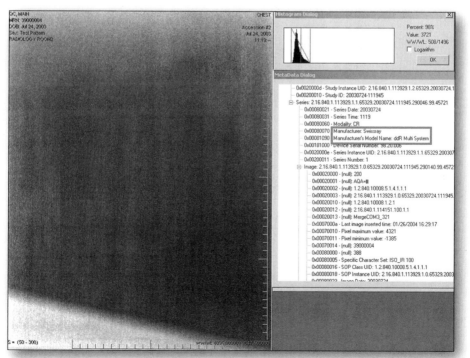

C

FIGURE 10-5. *(continues)*

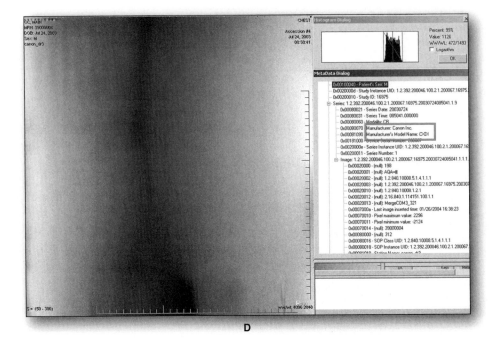

D

FIGURE 10-5. *(continued)*

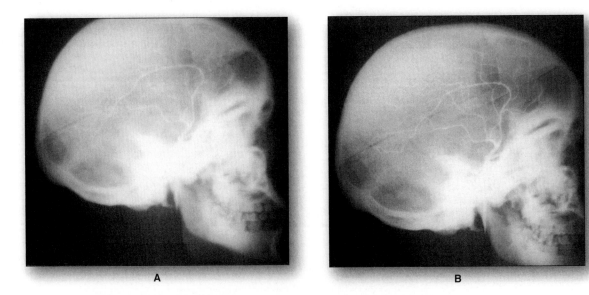

A

B

FIGURE 10-6. Correction of nonuniformity on a cassette-based DR system. (A) The lateral view of a skull angiography phantom before nonuniformity correction. (B) After nonuniformity correction, contrast and sharpness are improved. Source: *Delmar, Cengage Learning*

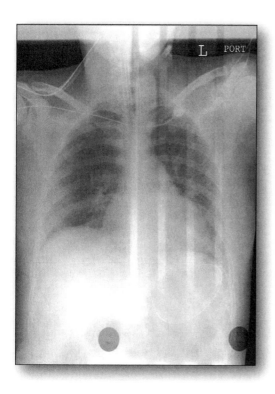

FIGURE 10-7. Ghost image on cassette-based DR receptor.
Source: *Delmar, Cengage Learning*

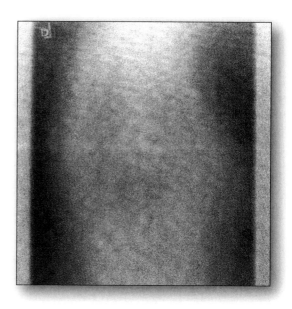

FIGURE 10-8. Ghost image on indirect DR system.
Source: *Delmar, Cengage Learning*

specific mechanisms differ. Ghost images are usually associated with high exposures levels with thick body parts and short times between exposures. Nonuniformity calibration when residual images are present can also cause ghost images that are reproduced many times, as seen in Figure 10-8.

Because DR receptors are reused, artifacts arising from receptor defects, dust and debris that interfere with the collection of light for CR and indirect DR systems, and contaminants such as barium contrast will show up on all subsequent images from that receptor until the problem is corrected, as shown in Figure 10-9. Often the appearance of debris on the imaging receptor in a clinical image is difficult to distinguish from foreign bodies. With cassette-based systems, a visual inspection inside the cassette usually identifies the interfering material. With integrated systems, the receptor needs to be re-exposed to a uniform field to detect the presence of debris.

Every DR system has a gain adjustment, which determines how much signal will be produced

when the receptor is exposed to a specific amount of radiation. A flat-field produced by specific exposure conditions of kVp, additional filtration, and measured radiation exposure to the receptor is needed to measure and to adjust gain. Each DR manufacturer has different conditions for the gain adjustment. The gain must be checked periodically and adjusted as required. Because the exposure conditions are critical for the gain adjustment, someone skilled in radiation dosimetry, such as a medical physicist, should be involved in the procedure.

In addition to checking gain, the same flat-field exposure serves to check the value of the DR exposure indicator. With screen-film radiography, the optical density (OD) of the developed film indicates how much radiation had been used in the examination. Because DR systems adjust their output signal to compensate for variations in exposure level, there is no convenient method for determining the amount of radiation that was used to produce the image. Almost every commercial DR system calculates some sort of exposure indicator. At this writing, there is no standardization in the mathematical form or units of commercial exposure indicators.

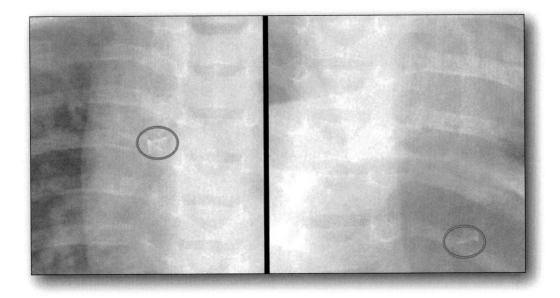

FIGURE 10-9. Defect on image receptor. Artifact, circled in red, is visible in two clinical images of different orientation.
Source: *Delmar, Cengage Learning*

Table 10-1 lists exposure indicators, units, and calibration conditions for some commercial DR systems. The AAPM Task Group 116 is working with DR manufacturers and the International Electrotechnical Commission (IEC) to standardize exposure indicators and their calibration conditions. Appendix A provides a brief description of the AAPM on standardization. It is important for technologists to understand the exposure indicator particular to the DR systems in their imaging facility, because this is the only feedback provided to indicate overexposure or underexposure.

By acquiring the flat-field image according to the specific conditions of the manufacturer, it is possible to verify uniformity, absence of receptor defects, gain, and the value of the DR exposure indicator. In addition to periodic flat-field exposures, a list of proactive QC countermeasures can be compiled that emphasizes avoiding rather than correcting errors. When possible, all receptors could be erased at the start of each shift. The equipment and its environment could be cleaned periodically. A properly calibrated exposure indicator could be used to conduct periodic checks of the automatic exposure control (AEC). Likewise, the exposure indicator is crucial for validating a technique guide for manual exposure factor selection. Thorough AT could be conducted for all new receptors. Checks of DR system performance could be repeated immediately following service events and software upgrades.

The AAPM Task Group 10 worked with CR vendors to specify AT and periodic QC tests for CR. Although AT and QC for other DR systems has not been defined at this writing, the CR tests constitute a reasonable starting point. DR manufacturers have developed a variety of phantoms and automated tests to assist us in assessing performance on a periodic basis. Some of these are shown in Figure 10-10. Figure 10-11 demonstrates the gradual degradation of sharpness in a DR detector indicated by automated QC tests. It is interesting to note the large amount of variation in the data.

Errors in Performing the Examination

The one test that can and should be done for every DR image is a visual assessment of image quality before release. In Steps 12 and 14 of the process map, each image is reviewed to determine whether image quality is satisfactory or whether the projection should be repeated. Inspection of the images

TABLE 10-1. DR Exposure Indicators, Units, and Calibration Conditions.

Manufacturer	Indicator Name	Symbol	Units	Function	Calibration Conditions
Fujifilm	Sensitivity, S Value	S	unitless	200/S α X (mR)	1 mR at 80 kVp (3mm Al) => 200
Kodak	Exposure Index	EI	mbels	EI + 300 = 2X	1 mR at 80 kVp + 1.0 mm Al and 0.5 mm Cu => 2000
Agfa	log of Median of Histogram	lgM	bels	lgM + 0.3 = 2X	2.5 µGy at 75 kVp + 1.5 mm Cu => 1.96 (at 400 Speed Class)
Konica	Sensitivity Number	S value	unitless	for QR = k, 200/S α X (mR)	for QR = 200, 1 mR at 80 kVp => 200
Canon	Reached Exposure Value	REX	unitless	for Brightness = c1, Contrast = c2, REX α X (mR)	for Brightness = 16, Contrast = 10, 1 mR => 106 (≈)
Philips	Exposure Index	EI	unitless	100/S α X (mR)	70 kVp + 21 mm Al
GE	Uncompensated Detector Exposure	UDExp	µGy Air KERMA	UDExp α X (µGy)	80 kVp
GE	Compensated Detector Exposure	DExp	µGy Air KERMA	UDExp X (µGy)	
GE	Detector Exposure Index	DEI	unitless	DEI ≈ 2.4X (µGy)	
SwissRay	Dose Indicator	DI	unitless		
Imaging Dynamics Corporation	Accutech	f#		$2^{f\#} = X_{relative}$	80 kVp + 1 mm Cu
Seimens Medical Systems	Exposure Index	EXI	µGy Air KERMA	X(µGy) = EI/100	70 kVp + 0.6 mm Cu
Alara CR	Exposure Indicator Value	EIV	mbels	EIV + 300 = 2X	1mR at 70kVp + 21 mm Al =>2000
iCRco	Exposure Index	none	unitless	= log[X(mR)]	1mR at 80kVp + 1.5 mm Cu => Index = 0

reveals errors that might be made by the technologist positioning the patient in the radiation field and performing the examination in Step 9, such as mispositioning, patient motion, incorrect radiographic technique selection, poor inspiration, improper collimation, incorrect alignment of x-ray beam and grid, wrong exam performed, and double exposure. There is little that digital image processing can do to improve these substandard images. Correction of these errors is likely to require repeated views.

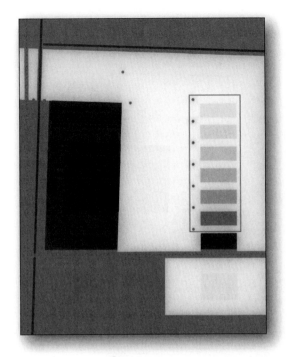

Agfa System Linearity

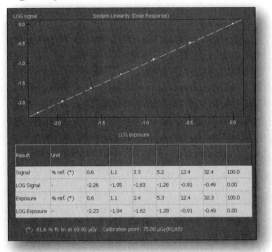

Result	Unit							
Signal	% ref. (*)	0.6	1.1	2.3	5.2	12.4	32.4	100.0
LOG Signal	-	-2.26	-1.95	-1.63	-1.28	-0.91	-0.49	0.00
Exposure	% ref. (*)	0.6	1.1	2.4	5.3	12.4	32.3	100.0
LOG Exposure	-	-2.23	-1.94	-1.62	-1.28	-0.91	-0.49	0.00

(*) 61.6 % fs lin at 69.90 μGy Calibration point: 75.00 μGy(RQA5)

Agfa Step Wedge

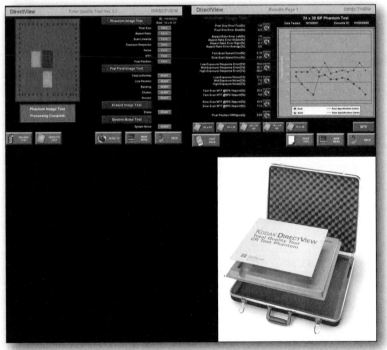

Kodak Direct View

FIGURE 10-10. DR vendor automated QC test kits.

Source: *Reprinted with permission from Agfa HealthCare, Carestream Health, Inc., Rochester, N.Y., and Fujifilm Medical Systems USA, Inc. (continues)*

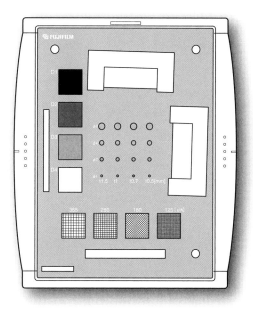

Fuji One Shot
Phantom Plus

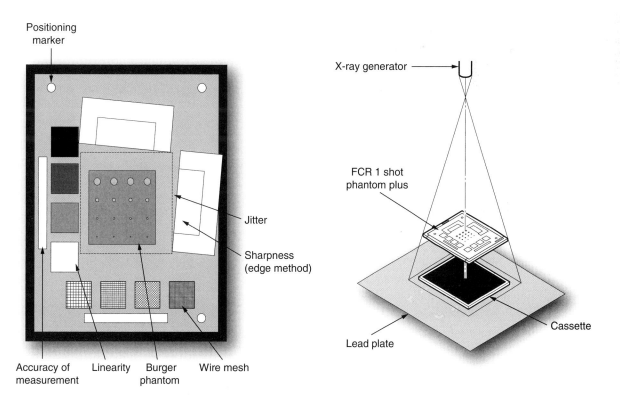

FIGURE 10–10. *(continued)*

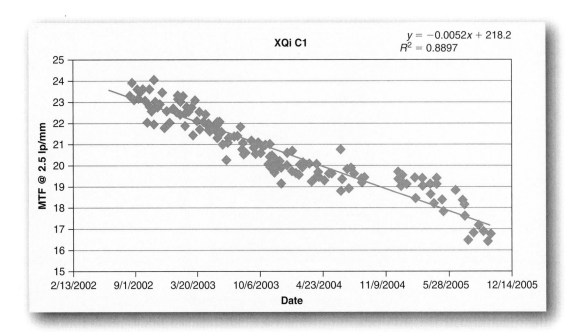

FIGURE 10-11. Results of automated QC testing of a DR system. The graph shows a general decrease in the value of modulation transfer function (MTF) at 2.5 line pairs per mm calculated automatically in tests over several years. The minimum acceptable value established by the manufacturer is 17%. The detector required replacement. Source: *Delmar, Cengage Learning*

Other errors can arise when the image receptor renders the captured projection for viewing, which would be during Step 11 in the process map. Potential errors include incorrect recognition of the exposure field resulting in incorrect determination of the values of interest (VOI) in the image, incorrect histogram rescaling, incorrect grayscale rendition, incorrect edge restoration, inappropriate noise reduction, and incorrect reorientation for the projected anatomy. Correction of these errors is usually possible at the QC workstation without a repeated exam.

Sometimes improper operation of the DR system is the underlying cause of a failure to detect the radiation field. When the technologist employs nonparallel collimation, multiple exposure fields on a single cassette-based receptor, poor centering of the anatomy on the receptor, or violates collimation rules, and in some instances where an implant or auxiliary shielding overlies one or more collimation boundaries, the algorithm that detects the edges of the radiation field is confounded. The result is inappropriate histogram analysis and incorrect rescaling of the image for display.

Since a key aspect of QC is a visual inspection of the DR image, it is important to consider the capabilities of the QC workstation where we are making decisions in Step 14 about repeating or correcting images. In some DR systems these functions are incorporated into the acquisition station or identification station that is used for performing the exam or developing the DR image. Traditionally, QC workstations allow the technologist to modify image processing, modify demographic and exam information, imprint demographic overlays, add annotations, apply borders or shadow masks, flip and rotate images, increase magnification, conjoin images to make composite images for scoliosis and full leg exams, modify the sequence of views, verify the exposure indicator, and select images for archive or transmission to PACS. The QC workstation usually includes the capability of deleting images.

Bad electronic images can disappear without a trace; bad films can also disappear, but leave a signature. Technologist supervisors learn quickly to count how many films are in the box at the start-of-shift, count again at the end-of-shift, and compare against the number of views produced by all exams during the shift. Some manufacturers have begun to incorporate in their QC workstations the capability to collect data on repeated and rejected images for reject analysis. If this feature is not available on the QC workstation, an alternative method will need to be developed for documenting the number and causes of rejected or repeated images.

Reject analysis is a time-honored method for assessing and improving quality of imaging operations. It is not enough to simply collect the data: the data must be analyzed to reveal recurring causes, the results need to be reported to management and staff, and action needs to be taken based on the results in order to effect any improvement. Management should implement remedial training as indicated. It is worthwhile to share the results with the DR vendor, because they may be able to provide advice or modify image processing settings for problematic exams.

Early adopters of DR technology claimed few or even no rejected images. Considering the number of technical errors that can be made in projection radiography that are independent of the acquisition technology, an unrealistically low repeat rate implies that the standards for acceptable quality were also low. The results of DR reject analysis from one hospital are shown in Table 10-2. These are fairly typical in cause and frequency to the results of reject analysis in conventional screen-film operations. Positioning errors are by far the most frequent cause of repeated exams.

One of the tasks of the technologist after the DR image is acquired is to determine whether the image is underexposed or overexposed. You can see from Table 10-2 that only a small proportion of repeated images were caused by improper exposure. This is normal for an imaging operation that has appropriate targets for DR exposure. As mentioned previously, because of automatic rescaling of the digital image, the "darkness" or "lightness" of the DR image is not a reliable way to assess exposure factor selection. When few x-rays are used to produce a DR image, the image appears noisy. As more x-rays are used to produce the DR image, the image appears less and less noisy. Technologists are quick to learn that physicians are less likely to reject overexposed DR images than underexposed DR images. Since repeating exams is an unpleasant experience,

TABLE 10-2. Reject Analysis For One Month From a Hospital Using DR (Willis, 1999).

Reason	Number	%
Positioning	489	46.9%
Overexposed	122	11.7%
Underexposed	105	10.1%
Reprinted	89	8.5%
Motion	57	5.5%
Over-collimated	40	3.8%
Artifact	23	2.2%
No exposure	21	2.0%
Double exposed	17	1.6%
No marker	10	1.0%
Marker over part	8	0.8%
Other	8	0.8%
Total	1043	100%

there is a documented tendency for technologists to increase the exposure factors in DR exams. The exposure is increased by using higher technique factors than indicated on the technique guide for manual exams and by using plus density settings on AEC exams. This tendency is known as exposure factor creep.

The good news is that QC programs that track DR exposure indicators are effective in controlling exposure factor creep. Figure 10-12 shows exposure indicator values observed for a specific exam and view. The value of the DR exposure indicator is usually visible at the QC workstation. Some vendors have developed software that facilitates collecting exposure indicator data. If your DR device does not have this sort of software, an alternative method for collecting this data will need to be developed.

Automatic rescaling contributes to a common misconception that in DR exposure factor selection is irrelevant to the appearance of the image. This myth arises from misunderstanding about the differences between latitude, exposure latitude, and range-of-adjustment in DR. Latitude is used by imaging scientists and engineers to mean the ratio between the highest detectable radiation level and the lowest detectable radiation level for an image receptor. For DR receptors this may be a huge value, such as 10,000! Exposure latitude is used by technologists to mean the ratio of the highest exposure factor selection to the lowest exposure factor selection on the x-ray generator that will produce an acceptable radiographic image. Even in DR, exposure latitude is a much smaller value than image receptor latitude. Exposure latitude is reduced by the range of radiation levels that are produced by the range of tissue densities and thicknesses of the anatomy included in the radiographic projection. The ratio between the highest radiation levels in a projection, such as the areas near the skin or through the lung apices, to the lowest levels, such as the bones,

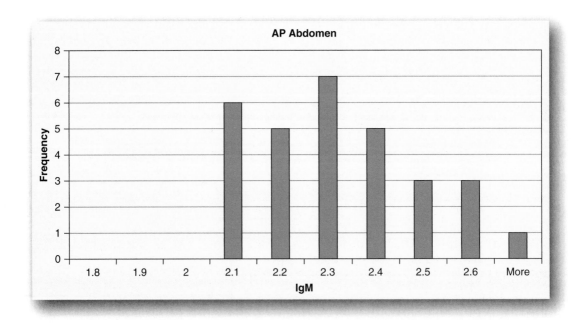

FIGURE 10-12. Distribution of DR exposure indicator values for specific radiographic views. The first and second histograms show the distribution of IgM values for AP abdomen exams. The target value was 2.2 ± 0.3. Even though the average value was similar after QC efforts, the distribution is clearly shifted toward lower exposures with none exceeding the maximum acceptable value of 2.5. The third histogram shows a much narrower distribution of values for AP chest exams.
Source: *Delmar, Cengage Learning (continues)*

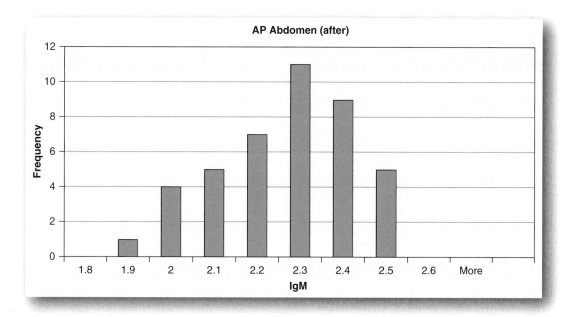

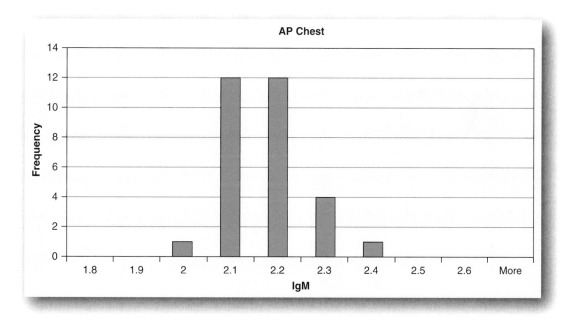

FIGURE 10-12. *(continued)*

is about 100. Even if the DR receptor had a latitude of 10,000, the exposure technique could only increase or decrease by a factor of 10 from the center of the receptor dynamic range and still acquire the entire range of radiation levels in the projection. That means that in this case the DR exposure latitude is only 100. This is still a large number compared to screen-film exposure latitude, which is about 2.

The exposure latitude is further limited by the range-of-adjustment of the DR system. Each DR system can only compensate for a limited amount of overexposure and underexposure for a single image. For example, one DR system can only display a range of 400 in radiation exposure once the settings for a specific acquisition have been determined by the operator, even though its receptor latitude is 10,000. This limits the exposure latitude to a factor of 4, which is still twice as good as screen-film.

The consequences of exceeding the limit-of-adjustment by underexposure and overexposure in DR have been traditionally neglected in the technical literature. Vendors who had been reluctant to acknowledge any limitations on their systems have begun to issue some cautions about gross overexposure. Underexposure in DR causes an increase in quantum mottle and a loss of contrast in dense features, as illustrated in Figure 10-13. It constitutes about 9% of all rejects. Overexposure can cause a similar loss of contrast in skin and dense features, as shown in Figure 10-14, and makes up about 5% of all rejects. Both underexposure and overexposure can confuse the exposure data recognition software, as shown in Figure 10-15. This image processing software decides which values in the image are of interest (VOI) and rescales the image accordingly.

If technologists are expected to make decisions about whether to repeat exams in Step 13 and Step 15, and whether to modify the appearance of the image before releasing to PACS, then the fidelity of the DR image that is displayed on a preview station, acquisition station, or QC workstation is a matter of concern. If the appearance of the image to the technologist differs from appearance to the physician, the technologist should not be allowed to modify the image. In order to ensure that the appearance of the image at the QC workstation matches the appearance at the physician's PACS workstation, both displays must be similarly

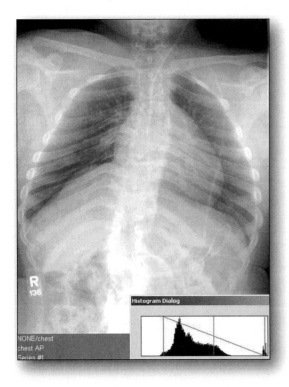
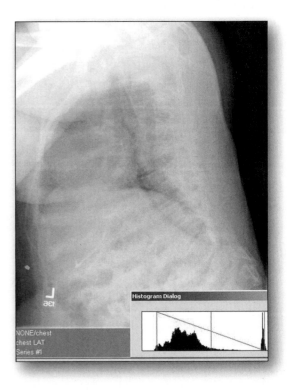

FIGURE 10-13. Underexposure in DR. Both views are underexposed. Note the grainy appearance and loss of contrast in dense features.
Source: *Delmar, Cengage Learning*

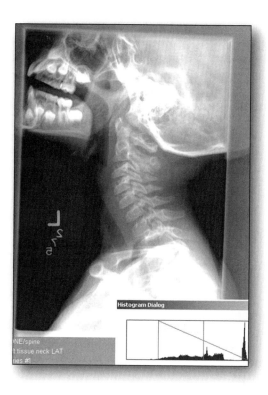 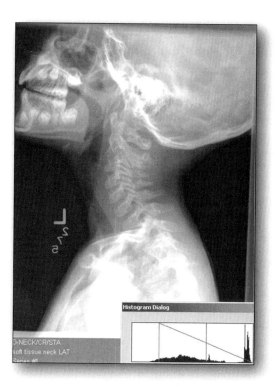

FIGURE 10-14. Overexposure in DR. The view on the left was overexposed. The exposure indicator was at the high end of the target range. The view on the right was repeated at one-half the mAs of the first image. Note the loss of contrast in the skin and dense areas in the overexposed image.
Source: *Delmar, Cengage Learning*

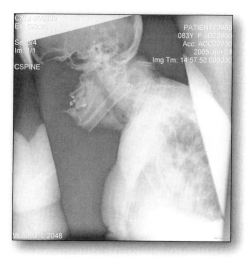

FIGURE 10-15. Exposure data recognition failure in DR. The image was grossly overexposed by a factor of almost 50. The detector was saturated. This is the result of exceeding the limit-of-adjustment.
Source: *Delmar, Cengage Learning*

calibrated. DICOM specifies a standard Gray Scale Display Function (GSDF), which helps in matching the appearance of the image on different electronic displays and helps to equalize the human observer's perception of contrast in light and dark areas of the image. The same function can be applied to laser film printers that can serve as the output device for DR in some imaging facilities. Some electronic displays automatically apply the GSDF and some automatically compensate for variations in ambient illumination and for changes in display performance. AAPM Task Group 18 has defined QC tests for electronic displays intended for primary interpretation. These QC tests should be repeated periodically to verify proper display performance. The frequency of testing depends on the specific display technology.

Because images appear at the QC workstation before they are available on PACS, physicians who have access to the QC workstation are likely to look at this display and to make decisions regarding the treatment of the patient. Imaging departments are wise to regard this as a display for diagnostic purposes and maintain it accordingly.

One of the frequent modifications of DR images before release to PACS is the annotation of the images to indicate laterality. This is needed when the lead marker is inadvertently excluded from the radiation field. Unfortunately, annotation post-exam is prone to human error and routine dependence on it should be discouraged. Just like conventional screen-film radiography, the lead marker should be included in the radiation field as a contemporaneous record in the DR image.

Errors in Delivery of the Images

When the acquisition station transfers the DR image to the PACS archive, there are several potential errors that can occur. For example, the transmission can be interrupted without any notification of the sender. The image can arrive safely only to be deleted from local cache. The image can arrive safely except that critical information present in the original image can be omitted from transmitted image, such as the exposure indicator, processing parameters, shutters, and annotations. This information may actually be present in the transmitted image but may not be displayable by the PACS viewer.

Unlike conventional screen-film radiography, in DR the technologist or supervisor must accept responsibility for appropriate delivery of all images to the physician. Processes must be in place to verify that all exams performed and all images acquired reach their intended destinations. In this regard, an image count of two does not necessarily mean that both the PA and LAT views arrived. Processes must be in place to correct delivery errors when detected.

Ultimately, the DR image is displayed for viewing by a physician. Regardless of whether the physician is viewing the image in soft copy, on an electronic display, or on a hard copy, a laser-printed film transilluminated on a light-box, there are a number of potential errors that affect image quality. The display device may have an incorrect GSDF calibration. The display may have an inadequate pixel matrix to display the full resolution of the DR image. This can either result in spatial resolution that is inadequate to visualize fine clinical details, or Moiré patterns (interference patterns) with periodic features in the DR image such as stationary grid lines. The value of the image can be compromised by incorrect or missing demographics or annotations, inadequate viewing conditions such as encountered environments with high ambient illumination and glare, and errors not detected and corrected by previous QC. It is important for the radiologist to feed back information about the ultimate quality of the images to the technologists who are producing the images.

Responsibilities for DR QC

In order to be effective, it is important to involve all local resources in a team approach to the QC effort. Active participation by the radiologist is an absolute requirement. The radiologist has the ultimate responsibility for quality of images. Within the imaging operation, resources and priorities are controlled by the radiologists. Radiologists set the standard: hospital staff can only produce the lowest level of quality that is acceptable to the radiologists. The radiologist must demand accountability for image quality and availability and must enthusiastically support the QC effort. Other members of the QC team will follow the example set by the radiologist.

The QC Team

The radiology administrator is also a key player in QC. The administrator is responsible for efficiency of imaging operations, and QC is a means of improving efficiency. The lead radiologic technologist is the first-line supervisor of QC operations. The clinical engineer is responsible for equipment life cycle management and is therefore intimately involved in calibrations and service. Clinical engineers are familiar with DR acquisition devices, x-ray generators, AEC devices, and electronic displays. Medical informatics is a relatively new discipline with an important role in modern imaging operations. A medical imaging specialist can assist with collection of QC data and troubleshooting of QC issues that arise from interactions between the RIS and the DR image acquisition stations, with networking, and with workstation configurations. The medical physicist is another key member of the QC team. No other person in the hospital has image quality as their first priority. The medical physicist is uniquely qualified to interpret the meaning of QC results in the context of clinical practice.

Radiologist Feedback

The pivotal role of the radiologist in providing feedback on QC merits some elaboration. Incidental comments and guidance regarding image quality is valuable. However, routine, systematic, documented assessment of image quality is much more valuable for the technical staff. In the film-based radiology department, periodically the radiologist would conduct a critique of a sample of films for interpretation. It is possible to institute a similar

process in the digital department. In order to minimize interference with the radiologist workflow, image critiques can be categorized into codes that are transcribed into a report for subsequent automated extraction. Critiques should include availability as well as quality items. A system such as this documents causes and frequency of substandard imaging and tracks improvement. This is a mechanism for establishing responsibility for the quality of service provided by the imaging operation. Figure 10-16 shows images that were released to the radiologist despite an active QC program.

Defining QC Responsibilities

Having considered specific QC activities that can help monitor and improve image quality, it is useful to construct a table that identifies each QC task and the party responsible for performing the task.

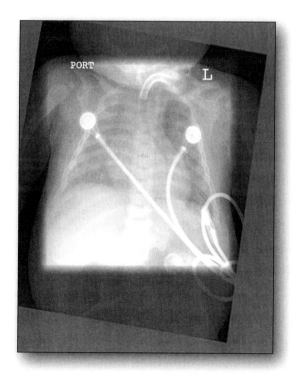
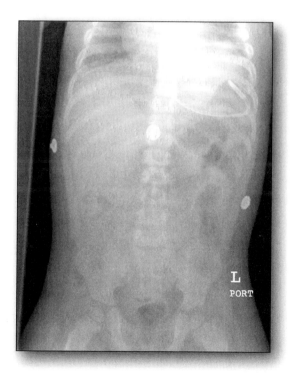

FIGURE 10-16. Substandard DR images released to the radiologist for interpretation. The radiologist reported a problem after receiving the image on the left. Note the periodic diagonal artifact going across the image from upper left to lower right. Later, the radiologist received the image on the right with a similar artifact, because no action was taken at the first report.
Source: *Delmar, Cengage Learning*

TABLE 10-3. QC Task Allocation Matrix

Task	Responsibility	Frequency
Verify patient ID and exam info	Technologist	Each exam
Verify patient positioning	Technologist	Each view
Verify image quality—release or repeat	Lead Technologist	Each image
Verify exam in PACS	Lead Technologist	Each exam
Reconcile patient data/image counts in PACS	Informatics	Incidental
Report substandard images	Radiologist	Incidental
Erase cassette-based image receptors	Technologist	Start-of-shift
Test image receptor uniformity	QC Technologist	Weekly
Clean cassette-based image receptors	Technologist	Monthly
Compile and review reject analysis data	QA Coordinator	Monthly
Verify display calibrations	Clinical Engineer	Quarterly
Review QC indicators	QA Committee	Quarterly
Verify receptor calibrations	Medical Physicist	Semi-Annual
Verify x-ray generator functions	Medical Physicist	Annual

This table is referred to as a **task allocation matrix**. Additional information can be added, such as the frequency that the task is performed and a reference for the procedure to be followed. An example is included as Table 10-3.

Digital Mammography QC

Although this chapter concentrated on DR for ordinary radiographic examinations, the QC concepts and principles are applicable in many respects to digital mammography. In the United States, the specifics of QC for digital mammography are mandated by the federal government under the Mammography Quality and Standards Act (MQSA). Section 900.12 states the following:

"(6) Quality control tests—other modalities. For systems with image receptor modalities other than screen-film, the quality assurance program shall be substantially the same as the quality assurance program recommended by the image receptor manufacturer, except that the maximum allowable dose shall not exceed the maximum allowable dose for screen-film systems in paragraph (e)(5)(vi) of this section."

The point is that the specific QC tests that are required for digital mammography are those specified by the imaging equipment manufacturer, with the exception of the limitation on maximum radiation dose, which is not more than that allowed for screen-film mammography.

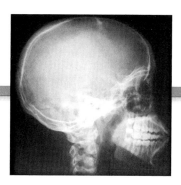
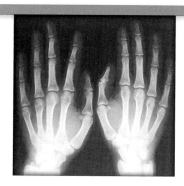
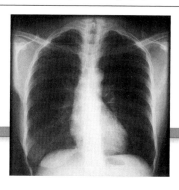

REVIEW QUESTIONS

1. Give three reasons why QC is still required when imaging operations are conducted using DR.

2. Name four components of QC.

3. Who can determine whether an image has sufficient diagnostic quality?

4. How would the process map for an integrated DR system differ from that of a cassette-based DR system, such as the one shown in Fig. 10-1?

5. The radiologist calls to report a PA chest image that is too dark and has too much contrast. The metadata of the image indicates that it was acquired as a LAT L-spine view. Referring to Fig. 10-1, identify each step in the process where QC failed.

6. The patient described in Question 5 had been scheduled for two exams, namely a two-view chest exam, and a lumbar spine exam. The DR acquisition system uses DICOM MWL for association of patient demographic and exam information with images. What was the first error that caused the problem?

7. A technologist notices that for similarly sized patients, the exposure indicator value for a PA chest view performed in Room 1 suggests that twice as much radiation was used compared to the value for the same view in Room 2. What are three possible explanations for the discrepancy?

8. In Question 7, does it matter whether the DR system is cassette-based or integrated? Justify your answer.

9. The chest exams in Question 7 were performed using AEC. If the kVp and mAs were the same in both cases, what is the most likely cause? Referring to the task allocation matrix (Table 10-3), which QC Team member could help correct the problem?

10. The radiologist calls to complain that images look good on the left display monitor of his workstation, but look bad on the right monitor. What is a likely cause of the discrepancy? Referring to the task allocation matrix (Table 10-3), which QC Team member could help correct the problem?

11. A technologist who is concerned about patient radiation exposure wants to decrease the radiographic technique for a PA chest view by 1/500. The DR manufacturer states that the receptor latitude is 10,000. Explain why the new lower technique is likely to make poor quality images.

12. Based on the results of reject analysis, shown in Table 10-2, a technologist has decided that by not "coning down," rejects from over-collimation can be eliminated, avoiding 40 repeated examinations each month. Give two reasons why under-collimation is likely to degrade the quality of many more images.

REFERENCES

Adams, H. G. & Arora, S. (1994). *Total Quality in Radiology. A Guide to Implementation* (p. 203). Delray Beach, FL: St. Lucie Press.

American College of Radiology Position Statement. *Quality Control and Improvement, Safety, Infection Control, and Patient Education Concerns*. Retrieved July 7, 2007 from http://www.acr.org.

American College of Radiology. *A Guide to Continuous Quality Improvement in Medical Imaging*. July 15, 2008 from http://www.acr.org.

Freedman, M., Pe, E., Mun, S. K., Lo, S. C. B., & Nelson, M. (1993). The potential for unnecessary patient exposure from the use of storage phosphor imaging systems. *Proceedings of SPIE, 1897,* 472–479.

Gur, D., Fuhman, C. R., Feist, J. H., Slifko, R., & Peace, B. (1993) Natural migration to a higher dose in CR imaging (p. 154). *Proceedings of the Eighth European Congress of Radiology.* Vienna, Austria.

National Council on Radiation Protection and Measurements. (1988). *Quality Assurance for Diagnostic Imaging,* NCRP Report No. 99 (p. 252). Bethesda, MD: National Council on Radiation Protection and Measurements.

Hendrick, R. E., & Berns, E. A. (2002). Quality Control in Digital Mammography (Chapter 4). In B. I. Reiner, E.L. Seigel, & J. A. Carrino (Eds.), *Quality Assurance: Meeting the Challenge in the Digital Medical Enterprise* (pp. 39–53). Great Falls: Society for Computer Applications in Radiology.

Kabir, M. Z., Yunus, M., & Kasap, S. O. (2004). Dependence of x-ray sensitivity of direct conversion x-ray detectors on x-ray exposure and exposure history, *Proceedings of SPIE, 5368,* 170–176.

Karellas, A., Vedanthum, S., Suryanarayanan, S., Belanger, P. L., & D'Orsi, C. J. (2001). Digital Mammography: Current State of the Art and Accreditation Issues. In R. L. Dixon, P. F. Butler, & W. T. Sobol (Eds.), *Accreditation Programs and the Medical Physicist* (pp. 295–325). Medical Physics Monograph No. 27, Madison: Medical Physics.

Overdick, M., Solf, T., & Wischmann, H. (2001). Temporal Artefacts in Flat Dynamic X-ray Detectors. *Proceedings of SPIE, 4320,* 47–58.

Papp, J. (2002). *Quality Management in the Imaging Sciences* (2nd ed., p. 287). St. Louis, MO: Mosby, Inc.

Samei, E., Badano, A., Chakraborty, D., Compton, K., Cornelius, C., Corrigan, K., Flynn, M., Hemminger, B., Hangiandreou, N., Johnson, J., Moxley-Stevens, D., Pavlicek, W., Roehrig, H., Rutz, L., Shepard, J., Uzenoff, R., Wang, J., & Willis, C. E. (2005). Assessment of display performance for medical imaging systems: Executive summary of AAPM TG18 report. *Medical Physics, 32(4),* 1205–1225.

Seibert, J. A., Shelton, D. K., & Moore, E. H. (1996). Computed Radiography X-ray Exposure Trends. *Academic Radiology, 4,* 313–318.

Seibert J. A., Bogucki T. M., Ciona T., Huda W., Karellas A., Mercier J. R., Samei E., Shepard S. J., Stewart B. K., Strauss K. J., Suleiman O. H., Tucker D., Uzenoff R. A., Weiser J. C., & Willis C. E. (2006) Acceptance Testing and Quality Control of Photostimulable Storage Phosphor Imaging Systems:Report of AAPM Task Group #10. American Association of Physicists in Medicine AAPM Report 93.

Shepard S. J., Wang J., Flynn M., Gingold E., Goldman L., Krugh K., Leong D. L., Mah E., Ogden K., Peck D., Samei E., & Willis C. E. (2009) An exposure indicator for digital radiography: AAPM Task Group 116 (Executive Summary). *Medical Physics, 36,* 2898–2914.

Siewerdsen, J. H., & Jaffray, D. A. (1999). A ghost story: Spatio-temporal response characteristics of an indirect-detection flat-panel imager. *Medical Physics, 26,* 1624–1641.

Williams M. B., Krupinski E. A., Strauss K. J., Breeden W. K. III, Rzeszotarski M. S., Applegate K., Wyatt M., Bjork S., & Seibert J. A. (2007) Digital radiography image quality: Acquisition. *Journal of the American College of Radiology 4,* 371–388.

Willis, C. E., Weiser, J. C., Leckie, R. G., Romlein, J., & Norton, G. (1994). Optimization and quality control of computed radiography. *SPIE Medical Imaging VI: PACS Design and Evaluation, 2164,* 178–185.

Willis, C. E. (1999). Computed Radiography, QA/QC. In *Practical Digital Imaging and PACS* (pp. 157–175), Medical Physics Monograph No. 28. Madison: Medical Physics.

Willis, C. E. (2002). Quality Assurance: An Overview of Quality Assurance and Quality Control in the Digital Imaging Department. In B. I. Reiner, E.L. Seigel, & J. A. Carrino (Eds.), *Quality Assurance, Meeting the Challenge in the Digital Medical Enterprise* (pp. 1–8). Great Falls: Society for Computer Applications in Radiology.

Willis, C. E., Thompson, S. K., & Shepard, S. J. (2004). Artifacts and Misadventures in Digital Radiography. *Applied Radiology, 33(1),* 11–20.

Zhao, W., DeCrescenzo, G., & Rowlands, J. A. (2002). Investigation of lag and ghosting in amorphous selenium flat-panel x-ray detectors. *Proceedings of SPIE, 4682,* 9–20.

Exposure Indicator
Standardization
Notes from the American Association
of Physicists in Medicine (AAPM)

Two authorities that have been actively engaged in standardization of the exposure indicator in digital projection radiography are the International Electrotechnical Commission (IEC) and the AAPM. Both groups have released their reports to the radiologic community, including the vendors of digital radiographic imaging systems.

The IEC report (2008) is entitled *"Medical Electrical Equipment-Exposure Index of Digital X-Ray Imaging Systems: Part 1 Definitions and Requirements for General Radiography.* The AAPM report (2009) on the other hand, is entitled *"An Exposure Indicator for Digital Radiography"*. Both reports address a host of topics including terminology, definitions, standard radiation exposure conditions (beam spectrum, beam geometry, measurement of the entrance exposure, calibration procedures) the indicated equivalent air kerma and the deviation index, for example, to mention only a few. A major section of the report includes several appendices which elaborate on a number of physical principles, such as standard beam conditions, and so on.

The AAPM however, point out that "users should be able to rely on manufacturer's claim of conformance to the IEC standard to identify equipment offering a standard exposure index as described. . . . ."

From a technologist point-of-view, this appendix will highlight the essential elements of the AAPM report in an attempt to identify the concepts needed for the clinical use of the standard. In doing so, a number of definitions and concepts will be quoted so as not to detract from the original meaning.

The AAPM has defined several terms, such as Digital Radiography (DR), Standard Radiation Exposure (K_{STD}), For-Processing Pixel Values (Q), Normalized For-Processing Pixel Values (Q_k), For-Presentation Image Values (Q_p), Indicated Equivalent Air Kerma (K_{IND}), Image Values of Interest (VOI), Target Equivalent Air Kerma Value (K_{TGT}) and the Deviation Index (DI). The interested reader should refer to the full report for complete definitions of all terms. Of these terms perhaps the most noteworthy ones of importance to the technologist are the following; DR, K_{STD}, K_{IND}, K_{TGT} and the DI (a central concept) and these are defined by the AAPM as follows:

1. Digital Radiography

"Radiographic imaging technology producing digital projection images such as those using photo-stimulable storage phosphor (computed radiography or CR), amorphous selenium, amorphous silicon, CCD, or MOSFET technology"

2. Standardized Radiation Exposure (K$_{STD}$)

"The air kerma at the detector of a DR system produced by a uniform field radiation exposure using a nominal radiographic kVp and specific added filtration resulting in a specific beam half value layer (HVL)"

3. Indicated Equivalent Air Kerma (K$_{IND}$)

"An indicator of the quantity of radiation that was incident on regions of the detector for each exposure made. The value reported may be computed from the median for-processing pixel values in defined regions of the image that correlate with an exposure to the detector. The median value is then converted to the air kerma K$_{STD}$ from a standard radiation exposure that would produce the same detector response. . . . . . The value should be reported in microgray units . . . ."

4. Target Equivalent Air Kerma (K$_{TGT}$)

"The optimum K$_{IND}$ value that should result from any image when the detector is properly exposed. K$_{TGT}$ values will typically be established by the user and/or DR system manufacturer and stored as a table within the DR system. The table is referred to . . . as K$_{TGT}^{(b,v)}$ where b and v are table indices for specific body parts and views"

5. Deviation Index (DI)

"An indicator as to whether the detector response for a specific image, K$_{IND}$ agrees with K$_{TGT}^{(b,v)}$"

In describing the method of standardization of the exposure indicator, the AAPM uses the following basic steps to emphasize where the K$_{IND}$ and the DI are determined:

1. The DR detector is first exposed to the radiation beam used for the examination and the exposure is converted into RAW data

2. The RAW data are corrected and the pixel values are now referred to as Q values

3. The Q values are "For-Processing" to include segmentation (extraction of useful information from the image histogram) and subsequent image processing

4. The result of number 3 above is "For-Presentation" values (Q$_p$)

It is from the Q values and the segmentation process that K$_{IND}$ and DI are determined, two concepts which are central to understanding standardization of the exposure indicator

Now, one can calculate the DI using the algebraic expression

$$DI = 10 \log_{10}\left[\frac{K_{IND}}{K_{TGT(b,v)}}\right]$$

where K$_{IND}$ (determined from the histogram) and K$_{TGT}$ defined above and has been deemed a "perfect exposure". The value of DI can now be used as an indicator by the technologist and the radiologist to determine whether the radiographic

TABLE 1. Exposure indicator DI control limits for clinical images.

DI	Range Action
> +3.0	Excessive patient radiation exposure Repeat only if relevant anatomy is clipped or "burned out" Require immediate management follow-up
+1 to +3.0	Overexposure: Repeat only if relevant anatomy is clipped or "burned out"
−0.5 to +0.5	Target range
Less than −1.0	Underexposed: Consult radiologist for repeat
Less than −3.0	Repeat

Source: From Shepard J; Wang, J; Flynn M; Gingold E; Goldman L; Krug K; et al. (2009): An Exposure Indicator for Digital radiography: AAPM Task Group 116 (Executive Summary) *Medical Physics* 36 (7) July 2009, pages 2898–2914 (Reproduced by permission of the AAPM)

exposure technique factors (mAs and kVp) used for the anatomical part and view under examination are correct.

It is clearly apparent from the algebraic expression above that when K_{IND} equals K_{TGT}, the DI is 0. The AAPM (2009) notes that "the index changes by ±1.0 for each +25%/−20% change in the reported K_{IND}". Furthermore the DI also provides the technologist/radiologist with information about the signal-to-noise (SNR) in the segmentation image. In assisting the technologist/radiologist in how to interpret the DI, the AAPM recommends that "a logarithmic scale in base 10 would provide approximate information in terms of both directions (overexposure or underexposure indicated by a positive or negative value, respectively) and magnitude (+1 is an approximate 125% of the intended exposure, −1 is 80% of the intended exposure) on needed corrections. An exposure resulting in a DI value of +1 would require an adjustment of −1 step on the density or mAs control of a properly calibrated modern radiographic system"

In addition and with respect to the clinical use of the DI, the AAPM (2009) suggests that "once $K_{TGT(b,v)}$ levels are set, it is useful to identify several types of 'control limits' on DI: a target range, a "management trigger" range, or a "repeat" range" as shown in Table 1.

The AAPM (2009) continues to explain that "the reason for this is that unlike film images, in which inadequate or excessive image optical density is a determinant of when a repeated film is needed, the reason for repeating a digital image is primarily noise related"

One of the other standardization activities centered around the EI, is DICOM integration. Both groups (IEC and AAPM) indicate that the DICOM standard incorporate the elements described in this appendix such as for example, the K_{IND}, DI, Q_p values and so forth.

Finally, the AAPM report makes several important recommendations relating to the EI for DR, however, only two would be quoted here"

1. "It is recommended that all DR systems regardless of the detector design provide an indicator of the x-ray beam air kerma expressed in

Gy that is incident on the digital detector and used to create the radiographic image"

2. "In addition to the indicated equivalent air kerma, it is recommended that the relative deviation from the value targeted by the system for a particular body part and view be reported. This index, the DI, should be prominently displayed to the operator of the digital radiography system after every exposure and immediately after any modification of the detected image values of interest"

Last, but not least, the AAPM emphasizes the following with respect to the "inappropriate clinical use of the DI":

"......: *even if images being produced clinically have corresponding DIs well with the target range, the clinical techniques used may still not be appropriate. One can just as readily achieve an acceptable DI for an AP L-Spine view with 65 kVp as with 85 kVp; evidence of underpenetration and concomitant excess patient exposure with the lower kVp may be clear from the contrast and underexposure of the spine regions, but may be windowed and leveled out in the digital image. Similarly, poor collimation, unusual patient body habitus, the presence of prosthetic devices, or the presence of gonadal shielding in the image may raise or lower DIs (depending on the exam and projection) and perhaps hide an inappropriate technique. It is essential that all aspects of good clinical technique be adhered to and an appropriate DI value should not be interpreted as proof of good work*"

References

Shepard J; Wang, J; Flynn M; Gingold E; Goldman L; Krug K; et al (2009): An Exposure Indicator for Digital radiography: AAPM Task Group 116 (Executive Summary) *Medical Physics* 36 (7) July 2009, pages 2898–2914 (Reproduced by permission of the AAPM)

IEC 62494-1(ed. 1.0) (2008): *Medical Electrical Equipment: Exposure Index of Digital X-Ray Imaging Systems-Part 1: Definitions and Requirements for General Radiography.* International Electrotechnical Commission. Pages 3–16.

Acceptance testing (AT) part of quality control, the first opportunity to determine whether imaging equipment meets certain baseline requirements before being used on a patient and is usually the responsibility of the medical physicist.

Algorithms in computers, specific step-by-step procedures for software functioning.

American Board of Imaging Informatics (ABII) founded by SIIM and ASRT in order to "enhance patient care, professionalism, and competence in imaging informatics."

Amorphous selenium (a-Se) photoconductor usually used in a direct flat-panel digital detector due to its X-ray detection properties and high spatial resolution capability.

Amorphous silicon (a-Si) photodiode flat-panel layer used in an indirect flat-panel digital detector.

Analog image radiology image obtained through continuous scanning by a light source transmitted through an image onto a photomultiplier tube that generates an analog output signal.

Analog-to-digital converter (ADC) device that converts an analog signal (electrical) into a digital signal (bits).

Analysis workstation in a PACS environment, computer hardware and software that facilitate the display of digital images for diagnosis and review.

Application service provider model system integrator that provides all PACS services to the client, including IT.

Bandwidth computer network data transfer rate.

Barium fluorohalides phosphor that can be used in computed radiology imaging.

Bit (binary digit) Discrete units used by computers for processing information.

Bit depth number of bits per pixel.

Bridge in computer networking, a device that links LANs (local area networks) to create an extended LAN.

Cassette-based system uses an external imaging plate that is exposed to possible damage within the scanning unit and from being physically transported between the scanning equipment and the reader unit.

Cassette-less systems use a single fixed image plate that is protected from the kind of damage found in cassette-based systems because it is encased in special housing that does not come into contact with the unit and it does not need to be physically transported at any time.

Certified Imaging Informatics Professional (CIIP) a designation awarded to qualified candidates who meet the criteria for ABII's mission to enhance patient care, professionalism, and competence in imaging informatics.

Cesium iodide (CsI) phosphor that can act as an X-ray scintillation layer in an indirect flat-panel digital detector.

Characteristic curve (H and D or Hurter-Driffield curve) in the imaging process, a plot of the optical density to the logarithm of the relative radiation exposure.

Charge-coupled device (CCD) digital detector based on an indirect conversion process and uses a CCD chip to convert light to an electrical charge.

Chemical processing in film-based radiography, use of chemicals to produce visible images.

Clinical trials used to compare the clinical usefulness of a new technique with existing techniques.

Closed-circuit television chain a video camera is coupled by coaxial cable to a television monitor to display the processed X-ray output image.

Communication protocol procedure for transferring information through a computer network in order for the parts of the network to communicate.

Communication standards systems such as DICOM and HL-7 that enable communication between digital imaging and information systems.

Communications media technologies for transmitting data, including phone lines, wire pairs (twisted pairs), coaxial cables, fiber optics, microwave, satellite and wireless transmission.

Communications technology the use of electromagnetic devices and systems for communicating over long distances.

Compression ratio ratio between the computer storage required to save an image and that of the compressed data of that image.

Computed radiography (CR) a cassette-based indirect digital image acquisition system that uses existing X-ray technology to produce data that is then processed by a computer into visible digital images.

Computer aided detection and diagnosis (CAD) in digital mammography, computer software used to provide additional information to the radiologist to form an accurate diagnosis.

Computer network system of interconnected computers that allows transfer of information through various forms of communication protocols.

Computer technology structure and function of a computer and how it can be used to solve problems.

Conduction band the higher energy band in the photostimulable storage phosphor that receives the electrons from the valence band at the ground state during ionizing radiation, creating a latent image.

Contrast enhancement post-processing technique also referred to as contrast scaling, gradation processing, tone scaling, and latitude reduction; third step in image processing in which adjusted or scaled raw data values are mapped to the for-presentation image for optimum contrast and brightness of an image.

Contrast ratio in an image intensifier tube, the ratio of the image brightness at the periphery to that at the center of the output screen.

Contrast-enhanced digital mammography technique that can be used in visualizing angiogenesis by using an iodinated contrast medium and image subtraction to obtain a clear image of iodine uptake around the lesion.

Control limits in acceptance testing, the maximum allowable deviation from normal before corrective action is initiated.

Conventional fluoroscopy use of an image intensifier coupled to a video camera that converts the image from the intensifier into an analog signal that can be viewed on a television monitor.

Convolution an example of filtering in the spatial location domain.

CR digital mammography system that uses computed radiography techniques in the detection of breast lesions.

CR reader scanner or processor used in computed radiography to render the image from an imaging plate visible. A laser is used to scan the imaging plate and return the electrons in the phosphor to ground state, releasing photoluminescence that is converted to an electrical signal and then digitized for subsequent processing and viewing.

CR workstation facilitates technologist interaction with the CR process, including access to patient data and image management.

Data acquisition collection of X-rays transmitted through a patient.

Data processing analog signals collected by X-ray are converted to digital signals by an analog-to-digital converter and the digital data is then processed by a computer.

Density resolution the effect of bit depth on the number of shades of gray in an image.

Desktop workstation in the PACS environment, the workstation used by technicians and physicians other than radiologists.

Detective quantum efficiency (DQE) measure of the efficiency and fidelity of image exposure measurement performed by a digital detector.

Diagnostic quality an image that is of an acceptable quality for accurate diagnosis.

DICOM *see digital imaging and communications in medicine*

DICOM conformance statements specifications for successful implementation of the DICOM data exchange standard.

DICOM objects types of data transferred between information systems, such as CR data, MRI, US, etc.

DICOM service class the type of function the DICOM is providing, such as transfer and storage of images, scheduling of data acquisition, image printing, transferring reports, etc.

Digital fluoroscopy application of digital image processing to fluoroscopy.

Digital fluoroscopy systems with flat-panel detectors fluoroscopy that uses flat-panel detectors instead of image intensifiers, video cameras, and TV monitors.

Digital image numerical representation of computer processing of digital data.

Digital image processing computer processing of digital data into a numerical representation of the patient that must then be converted to an analog image for human viewing.

Digital imaging and communications in medicine (DICOM) a data exchange standard that integrates information systems such as RIS and HIS.

Digital linear tape (DLT) magnetic tape used for long-term storage of images.

Digital mammography (DM) application of digital image processing to mammography.

Digital radiography radiography modalities that produce digital images that are displayed for interpretation and diagnosis, stored and archived for medical and legal purposes and retrospective analysis, and transmitted to remote locations for use by surgeons, emergency physicians, and others.

Digital subtraction angiography (DSA) process in which pre-contrast angiography images are subtracted from post-contrast images.

Digital tomosynthesis technique that used the principles of conventional tomography to produce images that are then digitally processed to enhance the appearance of lesions.

Direct conversion conversion of X-rays directly to electronic signals through the use of a photoconductor coupled to a matrix of electronic elements that produce electrical signals.

Direct detector flat-panel radiography detector that uses a photoconductor to convert X-ray energy directly into electrical charge.

Display workstation in the PACS environment, the system-to-user interface.

Dose creep the use of higher than necessary radiation dose to a patient due to technician overcompensation in avoiding the noise produced by underexposure.

Dual-sided reading the use of photodetectors on both sides of an imaging plate in order to increase the signal obtained and reduce the signal-to-noise ratio, thus improving image quality.

Dynamic FPD detector capable of producing fluoroscopy images that can be displayed and viewed in real time.

Dynamic range exposure latitude.

Edge enhancement post-processing operation also known as spatial frequency processing.

Electronic health record (EHR) comprehensive patient demographic and health records stored electronically and accessible to physicians.

Energy subtraction digital subtraction of angiography images taken at different kVs.

Enterprise-wide image distribution dissemination of diagnostic reports throughout the hospital system, eliminating the need for physicians to go to the radiology department to view films and read reports.

Erasure of IP removal of images from the imaging plate (IP) using a high intensity light to remove any residual energy remaining after scanning by laser beam. All IPs should be erased before subsequent use to avoid contamination of new images.

Exposure factor creep *see dose creep.*

Exposure field recognition important pre-processing method in CR, also referred to as exposure data recognition or segmentation, that identifies the appropriate raw data values to be used for grayscale rendition and to indicate the average radiation exposure to the IP CR detector.

Exposure index (EI) appears on the image and provides the technologist with visual feedback regarding radiation exposure to the patient, thus is a QC tool to facilitate optimization of radiation protection.

Exposure indicator *see exposure index.*

Exposure latitude in radiographic imaging, the response of the image receptor (screen-film or digital detector) to the radiation falling upon it, with CR detectors having a greater dynamic range than screen-film detectors and hence the detector can respond to both high and low levels of exposure and still provide a useful image.

Fading time taken for a latent image in an exposed IP to disappear.

Field-of-view (FOV) size of the matrix selected by the operator for examination depending upon the dimensions of the anatomy to be imaged.

Fill factor the ratio of the sensing area of a pixel to the area of the pixel itself; detectors with high fill factors (large sensing areas) provide better spatial and contrast resolution than detectors with low fill factors.

Film characteristic curve also known as the Hurter-Driffield (H and D) curve; indicates the degree of contrast or different densities that a film can display using a range of exposures.

Film speed sensitivity of radiographic film to radiation, inversely proportional to the exposure (E), expressed algebraically as film speed = 1/E.

Filmless imaging radiology that produces digital images without the use of film which improves diagnostic interpretation and image management and reduces radiation dose to patients.

Film-screen mammography mammography that uses film to produce images.

Film-screen radiography radiology that uses film to produce images.

Flat field a uniform field of radiation.

Flat fielding pre-processing technique properly referred to as system calibration that ensures detector performance integrity by removing artifacts.

Flat-panel a-Se detector detector that allows direct conversion of X-rays to electrical signals through the use of amorphous selenium (a-Se) as the photoconductor.

Flat-panel a-Si detector detector that uses amorphous silicon (a-Si) as a photodiode during the process of indirect conversion of X-rays to electrical signals.

Flat-panel digital radiography radiography that uses a flat-panel device to both detect X-rays and to digitize the signal.

For-presentation image digital image that has been pre and post processed into a DICOM image for presentation and transfer to the PACS for image display.

For-processing image raw digital data that has been pre-processed and is presented for post-processing.

Fourier transform (FT) converts a function in the time domain to a function in the frequency domain.

Frame rate from latent radiological images on the film created by X-ray photons.

Framework for MII system of medical imaging management including customized software, an informatics database, and the PACS database.

Geometric operation in image processing, allows the user to change the position or orientation of pixels in an image in order to enhance diagnosis.

Ghost image an image from a previous exposure that was not properly erased from an imaging receptor that is superimposed on a subsequent image.

Global processing operation all the pixels in the entire input image are used to change the value of a pixel in the output image.

Grayscale display function (GSDF) in QC, a DICOM standard that matches the appearance of an image on different electronic displays and helps to equalize the human observer's perception of contrast in light and dark areas of the image.

Grayscale image manipulation changes the contrast and brightness of an image displayed on the monitor in order to facilitate diagnostic interpretation.

Grayscale processing processing of an image that includes spatial filtering, image subtraction, and temporal averaging.

Hardcopy workstation in a PACS environment, the system-to-user interface that provides the means for image printing.

Hardware physical components of a computer.

Health care information systems clinical information systems, including administrative functions.

Health Insurance and Portability and Accountability Act (HIPAA) U.S. health care reform law passed in 1996 in order to protect patient's health information and patient privacy.

Health Level-7 (HL-7) data exchange standard that integrates hospital information systems such as the RIS and HIS.

High-resolution display workstation in the PACS environment, a workstation providing a high-resolution monitor for image viewing by radiologists for primary diagnosis.

High resolution IP imaging plate with a thinner phosphor layer than the standard resolution IP that provides a sharper image by reducing the lateral spread of the laser light during image retrieval.

Histogram a graph of the number of pixels in an image having the same density values plotted as a function of the gray levels.

Histogram analysis analysis of exposure data in an imaging system.

Histogram analysis errors errors introduced into the analysis of exposure data by such factors as incorrect exposure field location that generally result in rescaling errors and exposure indicator determination errors.

Hospital information system (HIS) information system used in hospitals that is now becoming integrated with PACS using data exchange standards such as DICOM and HL-7.

Host computer a minicomputer system capable of receiving dynamic digital data from the ADC and processing it for image display and storage.

Image acquisition refers to X-ray exposure of the phosphor plate storage, or imaging plate (IP). It also refers to the mechanism of X-ray interaction with the phosphor to produce a latent image and subsequent scanning of the IP by a laser beam to produce PSL.

Image acquisition modalities in the PACS environment are digital in nature, including film digitizers, CT, MRI, CR, DR, DF, DM, US, and NM.

Image analysis digital image processing in which measurements and statistics are performed, in addition to image segmentation, feature extraction, and classification of objects.

Image and Information management the use of PACS and information systems such as RIS and HIS to manage images and text produced in a digital radiology department.

Image artifacts a distortion or error in an image that is not related to the subject being studied and may mask or mimic a clinical feature, possibly leading to inaccurate diagnosis.

Image communications transmission of digital images using information technology such as the Internet or PACS.

Image compression reduction in the size of a digital image in order to decrease transmission time and reduce storage space.

Image data set all the information related to image acquisition, including matrix size, inherent spatial resolution, bit depth, number of slices, study sizes, and overall image quality.

Image display visible image of data collected from X-rays, usually on a computer monitor.

Image display optimization includes any factors that serve to enhance the radiographic image, such as image acquisition techniques, pre- and post-processing operations, and communication of the image from the technologic workstation to the PACS workstation.

Image enhancement improvement of image quality for the purposes of viewing needs, including contrast enhancement, edge enhancement, spatial and frequency filtering, image combining, and noise reduction.

Image intensification brightening of a fluoroscopic image through the use of an image intensifier.

Image intensifier artifacts unwanted interference in an image, including image lag, vignetting (loss of brightness at the periphery of an image), pincushion distortion, and S distortion.

Image intensifier tube replaces the conventional fluorescent screen of early fluoroscopes; includes input screen, photocathode, electrostatic lens, and output screen, all enclosed in an evacuated glass envelope.

Image intensifier-based digital fluoroscopy system of fluoroscopy that consists of an X-ray tube and generator, image intensifier, video camera, ADC, computer, DAC, and television monitor.

Image lag also known as memory effect; the persistence of an image in a flat-panel detector due to charge still being produced after the X-ray radiation beam has been turned off.

Image processing algorithm mathematical function used in computer processing of digital image data received from an ADC.

Image processing manipulation of displayed image using a variety of digital techniques to improve the image for the purpose of diagnostic interpretations.

Image restoration improvement in quality of image that has distortions or degradations; for example, sharpening of a blurred image.

Image storage archiving of radiographic images using various kinds of storage devices such as magnetic tapes, disks, and laser optical disks.

Image synthesis creation of a composite image from other images or nonimage data.

Imaging cycle X-ray exposure, readout, and erasure of an imaging plate during the imaging sequence.

Imaging modalities include computed radiography, flat-panel digital radiograpy, digital mammography, digital fluoroscopy.

Imaging plate (IP) the detector used in CR imaging, consisting of a photostimulable storage phosphor layered on a support base that can create and store a latent image when exposed to X-rays that is rendered visible by laser beam scanning and digital processing. The IP is reusable after erasure of the image by high intensity light beam.

Indicators in QC, factors that will be monitored as indicators in change of performance of any device.

Indirect conversion conversion of X-ray signals to electronic signals through use of an intermediary phosphor that produces light that is then converted into electrical signals by a charge-coupled device (CCD) array.

Indirect detectors flat-panel digital radiography detectors that use a phosphor to produce electrical charges.

Information systems computer-based systems that process raw data to produce information in a useable form that can be used for various purposes such as problem solving, patient diagnosis, etc.

Information technology uses computer technology and information technology to produce, manipulate, store, communicate, and disseminate information.

Information security system intended to protect data and information from unauthorized use.

Input computer data entry.

Integrating the Healthcare Enterprise (IHE) a standards-based initiative of the Radiological Society of North America and the Healthcare Information and Management System Society that provides a technical framework to facilitate communications between various computer-based health care information systems.

Integration in PACS environment, technology that enables various computer-based systems to communicate with each other to create a functional system that encompasses all radiology needs from patient scheduling to data imaging.

Internet a WAN (wide-area network) that uses TCP/IP to connect computers globally.

Intranet network that uses TCP/IP to connect computers within an organization.

Inverse Fourier Transform transforms an image in the frequency domain back to the spatial location domain for viewing.

Joint photographic experts group (JPEG) software for image compression.

Laser scanning releases the latent image in an imaging plate by scanning at a specific wavelength to produce the photostimulated luminescence in the storage phosphor that is proportional to the stored latent image.

Last-image hold (LIH) an image-processing technique that reduces radiation dose to the patient by allowing the X-ray beam to be turned on and off while retaining the previous image frame.

Latent image as X-ray photons pass through the patient to the imaging plate, electrons in the photostimulable storage phosphor are shifted from ground state to a higher state of energy (conduction band) and are stored in a pattern that reflects patient anatomical structures. The latent image is then rendered visible by laser scanning and digital processing.

Latitude in imaging, the ratio between the highest detectable radiation level and the lowest detectable radiation level for an image receptor.

Link in computer networks, a device that connects individual nodes.

Local area network (LAN) network that connects computers locally across short distances, for example, within a building or complex.

Local processing operation the output image pixel value is obtained from a small area of pixels around the corresponding input pixel; includes spatial filtering, edge enhancement, and smoothing.

Long-term storage methods of archiving radiology information and digital images; in the PACS environment these include magnetic disks and tapes and optical disks.

Lossless compression also known as reversible compression, in which no information is lost in the compression process.

Lossy compression also known as irreversible compression, in which information is lost in the compression process and is not generally used in primary diagnosis due to the possibility of incorrect diagnosis.

Low-intensity radiation sensitivity high sensitivity of digital detectors to low-intensity radiation that can cause scatter and off-focus radiation contribution to an image outside the collimation margins; causes some technologists not to collimate in order to reduce this visible distraction from the image of interest.

Low-pass filtering uses low-pass filter on the input image to reduce noise (smoothing), creating a blurred output image.

Magnification in conventional fluoroscopy, uses multifield image intensifiers to increase spatial resolution.

Mammography radiology of the breast.

Matrix a two-dimensional array of numbers the makes up a digital image.

Matrix size pixel matrices making up a digital image that vary according to the physical dimensions of the detector; as matrix size increases for the same field of view, the pixel size decreases and the image appears sharper.

Measured histogram also known as a scanned histogram, a measurement of the information on an IP.

Medical imaging informatics (MII) the application of information technology to medical imaging.

Medium resolution display workstation in the PACS environment, a workstation providing a medium-resolution monitor for image viewing by radiologists for review and secondary diagnosis of patient images.

Metadata demographic and exam data accompanying a DR image in an electronic file.

Modality worklist (MWL) a DICOM feature that takes advantage of existing RIS information to present a worklist of scheduled patients to the DR acquisition station from which the technologist can retrieve all relevant patient information.

Modem device used to send information between computers by converting a digital signal into an analog signal (modulate) to be transmitted over a communications link to a receiving computer and then converted back to a digital signal (demodulate) for processing.

Modulation transfer function (MTF) mathematical function that measures the ability of a detector to transfer its spatial resolution characteristics to the image.

Multiple exposure fields ability of CR systems to acquire multiple images on one imaging plate, necessitating strict alignment rules in order to ensure that each exposure field is recognized to prevent histogram analysis error.

Nearline storage archived patient information and images stored primarily for short-term usage and immediately accessible for review, such as in an automated library system.

Network protocol networking procedures that must be executed by hardware and software to transfer information between computers.

Network security procedures that safeguard confidential information that can be accessed by unauthorized users during data transfer, for example, a firewall.

Node computer connected via a single cable to a LAN or WAN.

Noise unwanted interference in X-ray signal detection of two main types: electronic noise (system or intrinsic noise) and quantum noise (quantum mottle) determined by the number of X-ray photons falling on the detector. Lower exposure produces fewer photons and a more noisy or grainy image and a higher signal produces a better image but at the expense of increased dose to the patient. Signal-to-noise quality can be improved by dual-sided imaging plates that produce more signal without increasing the radiation exposure to the patient and there are various software applications that can reduce noise during post-processing.

Offline storage long-term archiving of information and images on storage devices that must be retrieved by an individual and loaded into a drive to access the image.

Online storage short-term storage in which images are available for immediate viewing.

Optical density the log of the ratio of the intensity of the light falling upon radiology film to the intensity of the transmitted light through the film.

Output results of computer processing, usually displayed on a monitor.

PACS administrator individual trained in the use of computers and communication technologies; job position may involve the need for certification.

PACS certification provided by the PACS Administrators in Radiology Certification Administration (PARCA), any of the four levels of training and certification that qualify an individual to work as a PAC administrator.

PACS integration linking together of all the digital imaging modalities and hospital information systems.

Partnership model PACS model in which the manufacturer and the client work together to ensure optimal performance and integrity of the system through personnel training, system upgrading, and general system maintenance.

Photodetector a device, either a photomultiplier tube or a charge-coupled device, that converts PSL into an electrical signal.

Photostimulable luminescence (PSL) in CR imaging, the light emitted by the photostimulable phosphor on an imaging plate when scanned by a laser beam.

Photostimulable phosphor (PSP) a chemical layer on an imaging plate that is capable of creating and storing an image of patient anatomy as a result of X-ray photon stimulation that is subsequently released by laser scanning and digitally processed to create a visible image.

Picture archiving and communications systems (PACS) Systems used in the radiology department to transmit images to remote locations and to store images for long-term use.

Pixel (picture element) small square regions in an image matrix containing a discrete value that represents a brightness level reflecting the tissue characteristics being imaged.

Pixel pitch the physical distance between pixels, determined by the sampling frequency (pixels/mm) as the laser scans the imaging plate.

Pixel size calculated using the relationship pixel size = field of view/matrix size. In digital imaging, the larger the matrix, the smaller the pixel size, and hence better spatial resolution.

Post-processing manipulation of a CR image to enhance diagnostic ability, involving contrast enhancement (grayscale processing) and edge enhancement.

Pre-processing digital operation in CR involving shading corrections, pattern recognition, and exposure field recognition.

Process map a flowchart of the steps involved in performing a DR exam.

Processing function performed by computer hardware and software to process the raw input data into a useable form.

Provider in systems communications, PACS serves as a storage provider.

Pulsed fluoroscopy production of X-rays in short bursts or pulses by using a grid-controlled X-ray tube that reduces radiation dose to the patient as much as 90% compared to non-pulsed fluoroscopy.

QC tests *see quality control tools.*

Quality assurance (QA)/quality control (QC) strategies designed to ensure consistent and reliable quality of procedures and results as well as continuous improvement; in radiology, this includes ensuring optimal image quality, lowest possible radiation dosage to patients, and reduction of radiology operations costs.

Quality control tools include tests for computed radiology systems, dark noise, exposure index calibration, etc.

Quantization process by which brightness levels obtained from sampling are assigned an integer, known as the gray level.

Query/retrieve DICOM service class that retrieves stored images from the PACS.

Radiology information system (RIS) information system used in hospitals that is now becoming integrated with PACS using data exchange systems such as DICOM.

Random access memory (RAM) short-term computer memory.

Redundant array of independent disks (RAID) storage technology used primarily for short-term storage containing several magnetic or optical disk that can perform as a single large disk drive and functioning as an automated library system.

Reusable image media (RIM) in DR, receptors that are not consumed in the process of image

Right-handed X-Y coordinate system used to locate in the spatial domain any number that makes up an image; the X-axis describes rows or lines and the Y-axis describes the columns.

RIS/PACS broker device that links the primarily text-based data of the RIS with the image-based data of the PACS.

Router hardwire device that sends packets of data to remote computers.

Sampling measurement of pixel brightness level.

Sampling frequency expressed as pixels/mm, also referred to as pixel density. The higher the sampling frequency and the smaller the pixel pitch, the more pixels/mm and the higher the spatial resolution.

Saturation exposure level at which a large number of pixels will be at the maximum digital value (black) resulting in no signal differentiation and therefore no anatomical structure data.

Scaling the histogram based on the exposure to the detector, adjustment of the raw data histogram in order to optimize the for-processing image.

Scanning division of an image into an array of pixels.

Scanning technologies devices that acquire an image from an exposed imaging plate, including point-scan readers and line-scan CR readers.

Screen-film mammography (SFM) use of screen-film techniques in radiology of the breast.

Security threats attacks on computer data security of three major types: engineering attacks, hardware attacks, and software attacks.

Sensitivity number (S) the term used by Fuji Medical Systems (Japan) to describe the exposure indicator on their CR system.

Service class provider (SCP) any function in the DICOM system that serves the user, such as storage (PACS).

Service class user (SCU) any function in the DICOM system that uses the services of that system, for example, a CR unit is a service user since it uses the storage facility on the PACS (the provider).

Shading correction calibration to correct for the nonuniformity of DR receptors.

Short-term storage usually online storage of images for immediate access such as those held in computer RAM.

Software computer programs that use specific algorithms to process information.

Spatial frequency domain domain in which images are acquired and described according to the wavelength of the signal used to acquire the image.

Spatial frequency processing (edge enhancement) post-processing operation to control the sharpness of an image by adjusting the frequency components.

Spatial location domain domain in which an image is described using right-handed X-Y coordinates.

Spatial resolution sharpness of an image.

Speed class CR image acquisition operation that affects exposure index determination, rescaling, and image appearance analogous to film speed in screen/film acquisition but determined by the receptor exposure.

Standard resolution IP an imaging plate coated with a thick phosphor layer that absorbs more radiation than a high resolution imaging plate.

Storage in computer technology, information can be stored internally in the computer or externally, for example of disks or hard drives.

Storage technologies any device used for archiving radiology information and images.

Stored histogram also called known histogram; a copy of archived or stored anatomical images.

Task allocation matrix a table used in QC to identify each required task and the party responsible for performing the task.

Temporal frame averaging reduction of noise in an image by averaging frames collected over time.

Temporal subtraction digital subtraction of post-contrast angiography image from pre-contrast images over a time sequence.

Thin film transistor (TFT) array for readout of electrical charges generated by the photodiode flat-panel layer in an indirect flat-panel digital detector.

Turnkey model PACS model in which the manufacturer develops the system and sells it to a hospital, including implementation and training to ensure optimum functioning of the system.

Unsharp (blurred) masking subtracts the blurred image produced by the low-pass filtering process from the original image, resulting in a sharp image.

Valence band energy level of a photostimulable phosphor in which the electrons are at ground state.

Video camera in conventional fluoroscopy, a video camera, coupled to an image intensifier, which sends an analog signal to a television monitor for image display.

Voxel (volume element) the information contained in a volume of tissue that is converted into numerical values and expressed in pixels.

Wide-area network (WAN) computer networking system extending over large area, including global coverage, such as the Internet.

Window level (WL) the center of the range of numbers in a digital image.

Window width (WW) the range of numbers in a digital image.

Windowing digital image processing technique used to change the contrast (controlled by the window width) and brightness (controlled by the window level) of an image.

Workflow in radiology operations, the flow of patients and patient information and images through the hospital.

X-ray scintillator an X-ray detection medium that is part of an indirect flat-panel digital detector; usually the phosphors cesium iodide or gradolinium oxysulfide.

INDEX

A

AAPM. *See* American Association of Physicists in Medicine
ABII. *See* American Board of Imaging Informatics
Acceptance criteria, 71
Acceptance testing (AT), 71, 219
Active matrix array, 110
ADC. *See* Analog-to-digital converter
Administrative information system (AIS), 207
Advanced imaging technologists, role, 210
AEC. *See* Automatic exposure control
AIS. *See* Administrative information system
ALARA. *See* As low as reasonably achievable
Alignment precautions, 91
American Association of Physicists in Medicine (AAPM)
    EI standardization, 116–117
    implementation issues, 47
    Task Group 10, vendor interaction, 232
American Board of Imaging Informatics (ABII), 211
American Registry of Radiologic Technologist (ARRT), 211
Amorphous selenium (a-Se) digital detectors, thickness
        requirement, 113
Amorphous selenium (a-Se) photoconductor, 110
Amorphous selenium (a-Se) TFT direct digital detector, 140
Amorphous silicon (a-Si) DM system, 158–159
Amorphous silicon (a-Si) photodiode flat-panel
    array, 108–109
    layer, 108
Amorphous silicon (a-Si) photodiode TFT indirect flat-panel
        digital detector, system components, 108f
Amorphous silicon (a-Si) TFT direct flat-panel digital detector,
        system components, 109f
Analog images, 24
Analog-to-digital converter (ADC), 7, 54, 137. *See also* Digital
        mammography
    addition, 138f
    digitization, 14
    electronic/analog signal, input, 110
    electrostatic image, input, 104
    processing role, 30
    signal
        change, 24
        digitization, 49
        input, 24
    usage, 138
Analysis workstations, 179–181
ANRAD dynamic FPD, 141
Application Service Provider (ASP) model, 172
Archive medium, film problems, 7
Archive server, 172
ARRT. *See* American Registry of Radiologic Technologist
Artifacts. *See* Computed radiography readers; Image artifacts;
        Image intensifier; Imaging plate
    operator error, 69f, 70f
        relationship. *See* Object artifacts
As low as reasonably achievable (ALARA) philosophy, 17
    requirements, 120
    violation, 83, 90

ASP. *See* Application Service Provider
AT. *See* Acceptance testing
Atomic number (Z), 113
Automated QC testing, results. *See* Digital radiography
Automatic black border feature, activation, 95f
Automatic exposure control (AEC), 85
    periodic checks, 232
Automatic rescaling, 80

B

Backscatter, transmission (impact), 68f
Bandwidth, 175
Barium Fluoro Halide, phosphor type, 49–50
Barium fluorohalide (BaFX-X), 103
Barium-fluoro-halide coating, usage, 10
Barium fluorohalides, PSP, 160
Bar test pattern, impact, 122f
Beam alignment, 90–94
BG. *See* Brightness gain
Billing preparation, 207
Binary digits (bits), 8
Bit depth, 29
    impact, 31f
Blur, level, 97
Blurred masking, 39
Body part, overexposure, 96
Breast tomosynthesis
    imaging technique, 164
    technologic principles, 165f
Brightness gain (BG), 133–134
Brightness transformations, 32–33

C

CAD. *See* Computer-aided diagnosis
Cassette-based CR system, 54
    exposure field, location, 90–91
Cassette-based DR system
    demographic system, 226f
    ghost image, example, 231f
    nonuniformity, correction, 230f
Cassette-less CR system, 54
    spatial resolution, 97–98
Cathode-ray tube (CRT) display
    requirements, 179
    technology, 157, 206
Centering problems, results, 95f
Central processing unit (CPU), 201
Certified Imaging Informatics Professional (CIIP), 211
Certified PACS Associate (CPAS), 211
Certified PACS Interface Analyst (CPIA), 211
Certified PACS Systems Analyst (CPSA), 211
Certified PACS Systems Manager (CPSM), 211
Cesium iodide (CsI) a-Si TFT indirect digital detector, 140
Cesium iodide (CsI) phosphor, 108
Characteristic curve. *See* Film characteristic curve